COMMUNICATION FOR NURSING AND HEALTH CARE PROFESSIONALS

COMMUNICATION FOR NURSING AND HEALTH CARE PROFESSIONALS

A Canadian Perspective

Robert J. Meadus

CANADIAN SCHOLARS

Toronto | Vancouver

Communication for Nursing and Health Care Professionals: A Canadian Perspective
Robert J. Meadus

First published in 2023 by
Canadian Scholars, an imprint of CSP Books Inc.
425 Adelaide Street West, Suite 200
Toronto, Ontario
M5V 3C1

www.canadianscholars.ca

Library and Archives Canada Cataloguing in Publication

Title: Communication for nursing and health care professionals : a Canadian perspective / Robert J. Meadus.
Names: Meadus, Robert J., author.
Description: Includes bibliographical references and index.
Identifiers: Canadiana (print) 20230213413 | Canadiana (ebook) 20230213464 | ISBN 9781773383651 (softcover) | ISBN 9781773383675 (EPUB) | ISBN 9781773383668 (PDF)
Subjects: LCSH: Communication in nursing.
Classification: LCC RT23 .M43 2023 | DDC 610.7301/4—dc23

Cover design by Rafael Chimicatti
Cover image by Shutterstock/Den Dubinko
Page layout by S4Carlisle Publishing Services

23   24   25   26   27   5   4   3   2   1

Printed and bound in Ontario, Canada

Canada

Table of Contents

CHAPTER 1

Introduction to Communication

LEARNING OBJECTIVES

After reading this chapter, you will be able to

1. Define *communication*
2. Discuss the importance of learning about effective communication
3. Recognize the purpose of communication for all health care professionals
4. List the basic components of communication
5. Discuss the models of communication
6. Describe the levels of communication
7. Identify conditions that influence the outcome of the communication process
8. Identify both verbal and nonverbal behaviours of communication

KEY TERMS

Decoder

International model

Kinesics

Linear model

Paralanguage

Proxemics

Transactional model

Transformational model

INTRODUCTION

Working in a health care setting requires an understanding of others and ourselves to meet the needs of clients through the process of communication. The focus of this chapter is to introduce the concept of communication and its basic components. Strategies for learning and developing effective communication skills are introduced, including a review of communication models. The chapter concludes by highlighting modes of verbal and nonverbal communication and factors that facilitate or hinder communication.

You may be thinking, *Everyone can communicate, so why do I, as a health professional student, need to learn about communication?* In a health care setting, effective communication skills are considered a critical competency for all health care professionals. Therapeutic communication can be challenging. However, in most client care situations, the health care provider can enhance the encounter if highly developed communication skills are used. These skills, if learned and used effectively, lead to a greater knowledge and understanding of ourselves and others through interpersonal interactions in provision of client care. In this chapter, as in other chapters throughout this book, information is presented on how aspects of communication can be applied in the practice area. This information will help you develop professional skills so that you can become competent in any area of clinical practice.

COMMUNICATION

Communication can be defined as more than a one-way process that involves the sending and receiving of information between a sender and a receiver. The message depending upon the method for communication may be verbal and nonverbal (e.g., gestures, facial expressions, and body movements) behaviours (Ratna, 2019). Regardless of the communication method, the key is mutual understanding of the message by the sender and receiver. Effective communication occurs when the message intended is the message received. However, due to the many facets of complex information exchange within health care, many underlying factors may facilitate or hinder communication (Guttman et al., 2021). These factors are discussed in further detail later in this chapter. Clear communication is critical to information exchange, the establishment of relationships among health care professionals, and the people seeking services. Communication is central to building rapport and trust, and is considered the first step in the engagement of clients and families who seek health services. Therefore, you must learn about communication and develop skills in this area to be effective in clinical practice settings facilitating best client outcomes (Kwame & Petrucka, 2021).

In nursing, the focus is on client care and the activities of providing care. A knowledge of effective communication concepts and skills is essential for delivery of quality services in all aspects of the health care system (Jang et al., 2022). These skills are not innate but can be learned through discussions and practice in classroom and clinical environments. In the health care setting, nurses and other health care providers obtain and exchange information through assessments, interactions, and collaboration with clients, families, colleagues, and other team members. Communication is a significant factor in client satisfaction, safety, and complaints of care with health care delivery (Derman, 2020; Ratna, 2019). Today's health care system presents challenges in professional communication, especially related to interprofessional collaboration and safe person-centred care. As part of its safety competency framework, the Canadian Patient Safety Institute (CPSI, 2020) recommends guidelines for health care organizations. This includes training and education designed to promote effective communication skills for all health professionals. This organization reports miscommunication as the leading cause of poor-quality care and major harmful events, such as injury or death, for persons receiving health care.

MODELS OF COMMUNICATION

This section provides an overview of communication models that illustrate theories of communication. These early models were influenced by the telecommunications industry, and the basic terms introduced, such as *sender, receiver, message, decoder,* and *channel,* are reflected in the evolution of future models (McHugh Schuster & Nykolyn, 2010). The simplest, the linear model, which was introduced in the 1940s, focused only on the sender and receiver of messages. In the 1950s, an international model included the concept of feedback, relevant to the understanding and interpretation of messages. Through further research, in 1970, a transactional model of communication was produced with an enhanced process that details how various factors impact the sending and receiving of messages. In the 2000s, a more complex model with a direct focus on the health care environment and health care professionals was developed: the patient-safe transformational model of communication. This model focuses on outcomes and higher-level competency and is recommended for use in all interpersonal communication and professional client-safe communication (McHugh Schuster & Nykolyn, 2010).

The Linear Model

This early model of communication developed by pioneer Claude Shannon, a mathematician and engineer, in the late 1940s identified communication as a linear one-way process. This model, based upon his work in telecommunications with Bell Telephone Laboratories, is known as the sender-and-receiver model. It emphasizes the basic unit of communication as consisting of a sender, receiver (or decoder), and message set within the context of the situation. However, it does not consider the setting or circumstances of the sender and receiver (Shannon & Weaver, 1949).

Figure 1.1 illustrates communication as a simple one-way process in which a message is sent to the receiver. In this model, the focus is on the sending and receipt of messages. The sender is the originator of the message, which may be conveyed

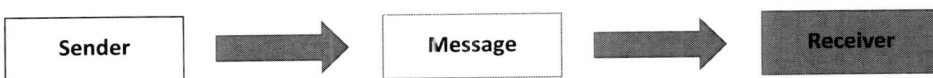

| Sender | ➡ | Message | ➡ | Receiver |

Figure 1.1: The Linear Model Developed by Shannon

Source: Adapted from Shannon & Weaver Model of Communication, https://www.communicationtheory.org/shannon-and-weaver-model-of-communication/

using verbal and nonverbal behaviours through a particular channel (e.g., video, telephone, or writing). The channel used in message transmission may experience noise (interference), such as background noise (environment), which may interrupt or distort the message. The receiver interprets (decodes) the message to determine its meaning, which is influenced by the receiver's values, beliefs, and attitudes.

Case Example

[Sender] Client, Mr. Stone, rings his call bell.

[Message] "I am having pain."

[Receiver] Personal care attendant: "I'll check and see when you had something for pain."

[Context] Hospital environment—answering the client's call bell

This form of communication is a common approach used by health care professionals within the context of work performance with a focus on task completion and not engagement of assigned clients (interpersonal communication). This model may be used in emergency situations when seeking client information quickly in the provision of care. It is not useful in creating an understanding of the interpersonal communication between the health care provider and client in building therapeutic relationships (Arnold & Boggs, 2020).

The International Model

This model, developed by Wilbur Schramm in the early 1950s, depicted human communication as more than a one-way process. This model introduced the element of feedback to reflect communication as a reciprocal two-way flow of information between people. This model also introduced the element of fields of experience, which highlights the fact that messages are created and interpreted by individuals. All of these messages are shaped by the person's—the sender's and receiver's—unique perspectives, values, culture, and personal history, which are not evident in the linear model (Foulger, 2004).

The model illustrated in figure 1.2 begins with the transmitter (sender) encoding the information in some form of behaviour (the message) based upon their thoughts, feelings, and intent. This is then communicated to another person (receiver). The message sent though the medium or channel is influenced by the senses (hearing, sight, touch, smell, taste) of the receiver. The message may experience interference from the environment (e.g., noise) that influences the decoding and interpretation

Interference

Sender

Receiver

Feedback Loop

Message Encoded

Medium

Message Decoded

Communication
Zone

Field of Experience

Field of Experience

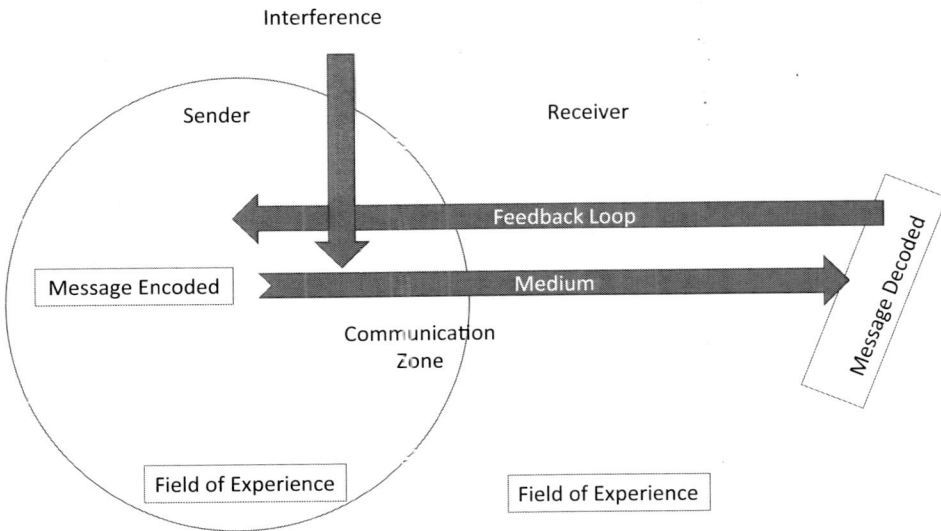

Figure 1.2: The International Model Developed by Schramm

Source: Adapted from Carey, J. W. (2018). *A cultural approach to communication.*
https://brewminate.com/a-cultural-approach-to-communication/

by the receiver. Through the process of feedback (verbal and nonverbal responses), the sender can determine if the message has been interpreted correctly (McHugh Schuster & Nykolyn, 2010).

The Transactional Model

Developed by Dean Barnlund in the early 1970s, this model enhanced the work of other scholars and described the communication process as a simultaneous flow of messages and feedback between individuals. During this exchange, the person speaking (communicator) interprets the information while considering their partner's verbal and nonverbal behaviours to create common meaning of the message in the exchange. In this model, the terms *sender* and *receiver* are illustrated as communicators reflecting the continuous flow of messages and feedback during the interactions. Compared with the previous two models, Barnlund's model (see figure 1.3) outlines more detail within the communication process and considers other factors that influence the flow and exchange of messages and feedback (Barnlund, 1970).

This model built on aspects of the interactional model, introduced the term *context* (environment), and expanded the concept of noise to mean any interference or distortion that impacts the message being transmitted. Figure 1.3 illustrates that the sending of messages along with feedback is influenced by the moods, timing, and judgments of the communicators as well as the physical, cultural, and social settings that affect the communication situation (contextual factors). As demonstrated in the following

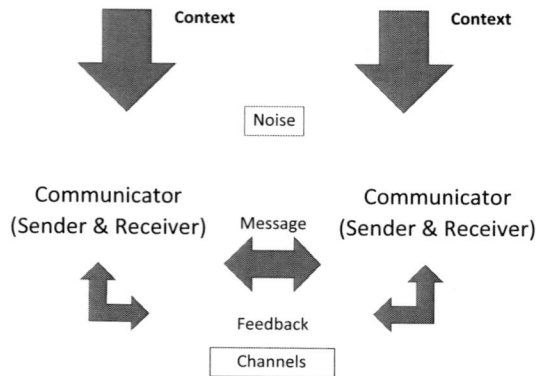

Figure 1.3: The Transactional Model Developed by Barnlund

Source: Adapted from Crawley, D. (2019). *Communication style: 3 ways to choose the right one.* https://doncrawley.com/how-to-choose-communication-style/

case example, the licensed practical nurse (LPN) considers the emotions of the client (e.g., fear) in encoding the message. The client decodes the message and is influenced by the contextual factors of the nurse. The LPN in this interpersonal communication can determine that the communication was successful based on the client's response.

Case Example

LPN: (*enters the room*) "Good morning, Mrs. Bellows." (*looks out of window*)

Client: "Hello ..." (*head is down, looks like she was crying; tears run down face*)

LPN: "I see that you were crying." (*sits down, moves chair closer to Mrs. Bellows, establishes eye contact with client, and leans in*) "Could you please tell me what is going on?"

Client: "Well, this is all new for me, having foot surgery. I'm not sure what to expect, and having so much pain after surgery ... I will become dependent on painkillers."

LPN: (*nodding head as client talks*) "Once you have your surgery, you will have pain, but the doctor will prescribe a medication to reduce the pain. The nurses will assess your pain during your recovery and provide the medication on a regular basis depending upon your pain level. If you take more medication than you are supposed to, it is possible to become addicted. However, it is also important to relieve your body of the pain so it can focus on healing itself."

Client: (*smiles*) "Thanks very much. It helps to know I will not become dependent on the medication and the nurses will assess my pain level as I recover from the surgery. I want to get better and be able to move around on that foot. A quick recovery will help me to go home sooner, I hope."

Transformational Model

A more detailed and complicated model that reflects the client–health care communication interaction with a focus on positive outcomes and links to client safety was introduced by Pamela McHugh Schuster and Linda Nykolyn (2010). This model outlines the process of communication highlighted by concentric circles that portray factors contributing to the process of communication within health care settings.

The centre (core) of the model reflects two persons communicating (e.g., nursing student and client) who come together to share information to meet a physical, identity, social, or practical need influencing person-centred care. The interaction is influenced by each person's biopsychosocial history, the context of the situation (second circle), and the flow and interpretation of information. The outer circles identify the other factors (third circle) that lead to miscommunication (e.g., stereotypes, medical jargon, illegible handwriting) and client-safe communication strategies, such as trust, rapport, touch, and empathy (fourth circle), leading to transformation for positive client outcomes. In comparison to other communication models, this one serves to guide identification of workplace and personal factors of care providers that impact outcomes in the communication process. The fourth circle, illustrating the client-safe communication strategies, can be used as a tool in clinical practice to guide change leading to transformation (outer circle) to support and promote communication for competent, safe client care.

LEVELS OF COMMUNICATION

In your professional development as a health care provider, you will be exposed to different levels of communication depending upon the audience for the intended message: intrapersonal, referred to as self-talk; interpersonal communication; public communication; transpersonal communication; and small group communication (Beebe et al., 2020).

Intrapersonal communication (*intra-* is a prefix meaning "within") involves messages that individuals engage in daily with themselves when they are unsure or have doubts about something. For example, as a nursing student you are giving an intramuscular injection to your client. You may doubt your ability to carry out the procedure and think, *I have only practised this technique in the learning lab*, but as you enter the client's room, you say to yourself, *I can do this; it will be fine*. In this instance you think about a message, send it, and are influenced by the message that follows (self-talk). This communication with yourself helps you to become more self-aware and reflective, aiding the therapeutic use of self in the delivery of client-centred care.

Interpersonal communication (*inter-* is a prefix meaning "between") occurs between people, as demonstrated by nurses in their day-to-day clinical practice. The communication includes all aspects of sending and receiving a message along with feedback. For example, a nurse who enters a client's room observes that the client grimaces when he turns over in bed. The nurse interprets this nonverbal behaviour as indicating that the client is experiencing pain. The nurse uses verbal communication: "Mr. Sheripo, please describe your pain. On a scale of 1 to 10, how would you rate your pain?" He describes it as a 9. The nurse asks the client if he would like something for pain, and he states, "That would help. Thanks." The nurse leaves and returns with an oral pain medication for Mr. Sheripo. In this scenario, the nurse validated the client's nonverbal behaviour. Thus, the understanding of the message was achieved through feedback in the communication exchange.

Public communication involves the nurse in the role of presenter of information. For example, a nurse may be invited as a speaker to a particular group on a health-related issue affecting the community or may present on an area of completed research on the coping strategies for high-school students that present with major depressive disorder.

Small group communication consisting of two or more persons may be what nurses are involved in as part of their clinical role. In the health care setting, nurses may be members of a particular group or lead a group that provides a service to clients and their families. In the clinical setting, nurses may lead a variety of groups (e.g., medication teaching or group therapy), depending upon their level of education and expertise. Nurses are also able to refer clients to a particular inpatient or outpatient therapeutic group or self-help group depending upon the clients' plan of care and community resources.

Transpersonal communication is related to the concept of spirituality and is considered part of a holistic approach to person-centred care (Cooper et al., 2022; Pinto & Pinto, 2020). Although it is recognized by health care professionals as important, many lack the confidence to utilize its approach in practice (O'Brien et al., 2019). Zumstein-Shaha et al. (2020) contend that a nursing-focused spirituality begins with the nurse's own sense of spirituality. In person-centred care, listening to clients' expressions of spiritual or religious issues enhances health care providers' personal reflections on spirituality. Within the therapeutic process of relationship building, nurses become aware of the interdependent elements of mind, body, and spirit to connect with clients (Rogers & Wattis, 2020).

COMMUNICATION: VERBAL AND NONVERBAL BEHAVIOUR

Communication is a bidirectional process that entails the conveying of information through both verbal (e.g., spoken, written, digitally transmitted) and nonverbal behaviours. However, sometimes our personal perceptions influence what is said and how the message sent or received is interpreted by others. The challenge in communication is achieving common meaning of the content of the message for the sender and receiver (Ogbogu et al., 2022). Clear communication is critical in all health care interactions for promotion of quality care and client safety (Horváth & Molnár, 2021). Communication breakdown can lead to harmful events, such as injury or death, in any health care setting (Guttman et al., 2021). According to Shea (2017), roughly 90 percent of communication is nonverbal and 10 percent is verbal. As the term implies, verbal communication involves information that is spoken but also includes the written word. In face-to-face communication, talking is the common mode of engaging with others. Verbal and nonverbal communication is influenced by language, culture, beliefs, values, emotions, age, gender, social status, education, and environment. Individuals may express their emotions nonverbally. Thus, it is important for nurses to assess and validate within the nurse-client relationship.

Nonverbal communication, often referred to as cues, involves information that is sent without words, meaning behaviours displayed through gestures, facial expressions, or other means. The components of this form of communication are body language (kinesics), including facial expressions, eye contact, touch, and gestures; personal space (proxemics), posture, position, physical appearance and dress; and paralanguage, or voice tone, inflection, and rate of speech (Ogbogu et al., 2022; Resat, 2019). In a health care environment, the health care provider needs to assess not only what is said verbally but also what is communicated nonverbally. Clients may have trouble expressing or may mask their feelings, such as sadness or fear, and not disclose. Clients are also aware of the nurse's nonverbal behaviour when engaged in an exchange. To aid development of therapeutic communication, health care professionals need to have awareness of their own verbal and nonverbal behaviours as well as those of their clients and other team members. All verbal and nonverbal behaviour in the information exchange should be congruent, meaning that the spoken word corresponds to the nonverbal message. If the verbal message is contradicted by the nonverbal message, miscommunication occurs (Wanko Keutchafo et al., 2020). Such an event is called a double or mixed message. Verbal and nonverbal communication skills are key to positive communication, leading to enhanced client outcomes (Afriyie, 2020).

Case Example

The nurse (not looking at the client) enters his room and states, "Good morning, Mr. Smith, I'll help you set up your breakfast tray." The client is talking, but the nurse is constantly looking at the wall clock. What message is the nurse sending to the client? The nurse's spoken words say one thing but their body language and behaviour say another. The client may be thinking the nurse is in a hurry and not interested in helping.

Body Language

Body language is a form of nonverbal behaviour that is displayed by gestures, facial expressions, eye contact, sitting position, and physical contact and is used by persons to convey messages either together with or completely without words (Ogbogu et al., 2022). As a health care professional, it is critical that you have awareness of your own nonverbal behaviour and also have the ability to read body language, as the majority of persons use nonverbal communication as their main means of expression (Resat, 2019). Body language may vary across different cultures, age groups, and genders (Ali, 2018). This knowledge aids nurses' development and understanding of nurse-client encounters in meeting health needs.

Facial expression is the primary source of communication next to the spoken word. The face is most powerful and can give multiple messages, such as sadness, happiness, fear, disgust, anger, surprise, pain, and doubt, without the use of words (Holland et al., 2019). According to Ali (2018), basic human emotions revealed by facial expressions are universal regardless of culture or age. When meeting a client, it is imperative that the health care provider is aware of their own facial expressions and nonverbal behaviours to ensure a warm, friendly demeanour. Societal and

Exercise 1.1: Body Language

Purpose: To gain awareness of body language and its influence on nonverbal communication

Procedure
1. Pair up with another student and search websites to assess a variety of facial expressions.
2. Taking turns, each of you will role-play and demonstrate the facial expressions while the other tries to determine the emotion being expressed. Notice how much eye contact you make.

Discussion
1. List other examples of facial expressions that may influence communication.
2. Discuss feelings you experienced during this exercise.
3. Describe any frustrations you experienced in completing this exercise.
4. Describe how miscommunication occurs in determining the meaning of facial expressions.
5. Share what your learned about yourself from this exercise and how you would apply this knowledge to your clinical practice.

cultural factors impact eye behaviour: where to look, at whom, and for how long. Eye contact is important in engaging clients as it demonstrates interest in the other person. In some cultures, direct eye contact is not appropriate and is considered rude and threatening, while in other cultures, fleeting eye contact or keeping the eyes down is a show of respect (Henderson & Barker, 2017). Health care professionals need to know how to make appropriate eye contact in all health care interactions. Through self-awareness, the nurse becomes aware of their verbal and nonverbal cues and corrects misunderstandings within the nurse-client interaction. It is also important for the health care provider to recognize and evaluate the client's body movements, facial expressions, and eye contact during interactions. These behaviours may indicate that the client is anxious, sad, happy, or experiencing pain or some other health concern. For example, upon entering a client's room, the client's body language suggests they are having pain. The client is holding their right side and has a facial grimace but states they are fine. The health care provider can question the client further to check for congruency between what is said and what is observed (Ali, 2018).

Proxemics

Proxemics relates to personal space or how close one person is to another. Personal space, also referred to as your protective bubble, helps you gauge how comfortable others feel when someone invades their space. According to Hecht et al. (2019), an individual's personal space remains stable over time and thus persons tend to avoid inappropriately close interpersonal spaces. Health care professionals need awareness and understanding of the social meaning of space in interpersonal communication. In the health care setting, physical closeness is necessary as personnel from a variety of disciplines need to enter clients' personal spaces to deliver care.

As a health care professional, depending upon your role in client interactions or provision of care, completing or assisting with a procedure or doing an assessment may entail invading a client's personal space. As nurses, we should not assume that we have the right to do so, as clients do not have to submit to invasion of their personal space. In these situations, the health care professional should ask the person what distance they are comfortable with in regard to their personal space. Respecting clients' personal space and considering their preferences supports a person-centred approach. This strategy promotes better communication and will offset any misunderstandings.

Sitting Position

Another important aspect of body language that is relevant in the communication process is how health care professionals sit when engaging with clients. The recommended approach is to sit at a slight angle to the client and to avoid poor posture (e.g., slouching) or crossed legs and arms. Poor posture and crossed legs and arms indicate lack of interest, defensiveness, and being closed to communication (Stickley, 2011). As personal space is influenced by culture and individual preference, the health care provider should be tuned in to any cues of discomfort from the client. In the health care environment, health care professionals need to avoid negative body language in all client encounters. During interactions, the health care provider needs to consider the position of the client in order to facilitate effective communication. For example, if the client is confined to a bed or seated in a chair, attempts should be made to sit beside the person at eye level. This may require elevation of the head of the client's bed. These strategies support effective communication and a person-centred approach in the health care interaction (Knollman-Porter & Burshnic, 2020).

Self-Reflective Exercise

Can you think of other examples of negative body language that health care professionals should avoid?

Touch

Touch is integral to health professionals who are working in clinical practice areas such as nursing, medicine, physiotherapy, or osteopathy. In these areas, touch is expressed in the provision of care in different ways, for example, physical care (giving a bed bath), treatments (irrigating a wound), procedures (obtaining blood), and information gathering (taking temperature or blood pressure). Touch is a powerful tool in communication and can be interpreted as an expression of caring, compassion, empathy, comfort, or support (Kelly et al., 2018). See the following vignette from a client named Meg, who recalls being in hospital 30 years ago and how touch was demonstrated by the nurse providing care (Durkin et al., 2021).

> The thing that stands out in my mind, it's a very small thing, but the fact that I still remember it obviously means that it was very significant for me. I'd had surgery and it didn't go well and I was bed bound for over a week ... anyway, I just wasn't allowed out of bed. The thing that really struck me and touched me was the care and yes, the compassion, of a nurse who gave me a bed bath. It was just that sense of her carefulness and her tenderness, really, real care, so it was—I don't know how to explain it really. It was just the feeling of being really cared for and cared about and treated with enormous respect. (Meg) (Durkin et al., 2021, p. 1985)

Touch is a basic element of connecting with clients through the establishment of the therapeutic nurse-client relationship. However, some clients may not be comfortable with touch for a variety of reasons, including individuals experiencing psychosis (impairment of reality) or some other form of cognitive impairment. In other instances, touch may be misinterpreted and should be used cautiously for a person who has been sexually or physically abused. For health professionals, best practice is to always seek client permission before its use. This provides clients a choice and "empowers them to have control over their body and physical space" (Fleishman et al., 2019, p. 4). To be competent in clinical practice, health care providers require knowledge and awareness on the topic of touch as a communication tool, its cultural implications, and its use in person-centred care. The use of touch for health care professionals will be further discussed in the chapters on therapeutic communication (chapter 2) and the nurse-client relationship (chapter 3).

MASKS AND COMMUNICATION

As health care professionals, wearing face masks is a component of care, and masks are used throughout a variety of clinical and nonclinical situations. While face masks are considered an important piece of personal protective equipment, they present a challenge in interpersonal communication (Kilgore et al., 2021; Mheidly et al., 2020). Face masks hamper communication, both verbal and nonverbal, affecting interactions with clients and health care colleagues. Facial expressions and gestures play a large role in communication. The wearing of a face mask involves covering the mouth and the nose, impacting speech and the ability to understand facial expressions and lip movements (Homans & Vroegop, 2022; Kilgore et al., 2021).

For clients with a neurocognitive disorder or communication, hearing, or sight difficulty, the wearing of masks by health care providers leads to frustration and miscommunication (Marler & Ditton, 2021). These clients are hindered in their understanding of speech and comprehension of nonverbal behaviours such as lip movements, vocal tones, and facial expressions. To improve communication, a variety of strategies to support clients and health care interactions are suggested. One method of communication support is the use of gestures, defined as "the movements people make with their hands and arms in isolation or combined with a spoken message to relay meaning" (Knollman-Porter & Burshnic, 2020, p. 8). Other recommended strategies are using written information (e.g., on whiteboards, flashcards, notepads) and pictures (e.g., a board containing images of care-related topics such as thirst, pain, bathroom), and modifying speech (e.g., monitoring rate, tone). Also, best practice is to communicate one-on-one with the client directly in a well-lit, quiet environment (Knollman-Porter & Burshnic, 2020; Marler & Ditton, 2021; Mheidly et al., 2020). Furthermore, transparent face masks are suggested in place of surgical face masks as they allow others to see the nurse's facial expressions and emotions while providing the nurse with personal protection (Chu et al., 2021; Mheidly et al., 2020).

FACTORS CONTRIBUTING TO EFFECTIVE COMMUNICATION

According to Ratna (2019), effective communication occurs only if the sender and the receiver mutually understand the intended meaning of the message. This process occurs through the use of verbal and nonverbal communication in the health care professional–client interaction. However, within the health care setting, factors related to the health care provider and to the client, as well as within the environment, may facilitate or hinder communication. Health care professionals interact with a variety of people, clients, and family members in their clinical practice activities. Several factors influence the understanding of the message received, such as the client's age, gender, education, background, history, and particular disorder or health condition. For example, clients who experience a cardiovascular accident (stroke) have impaired cognitive ability and difficulty with speech, while other clients may have sensory impairments of hearing or vision. In these situations, the health care provider caring for these clients will need to adjust their communication style during interactions. Also, the sender and the receiver of messages are influenced by their own thoughts, needs, and emotions. A client who is experiencing pain because of a broken hip will have little interest in learning about deep breathing and coughing if the pain issue is not addressed. A health care professional who is having personal family issues may not be fully present while at work. These situations demonstrate factors that affect the development of client-centred communication and the establishment of therapeutic relationships.

Another factor that contributes to ineffective communication is the use of language. All health professionals require knowledge and awareness of when and where to use professional jargon. When communicating with other health care providers it is appropriate, but when working with clients it requires adjustment to promote understanding of the information. Language also needs to be considered with respect to cultural implications. The use of dialect or foreign accents or language may lead to misunderstandings during care delivery and within therapeutic relationships. In these cases, an interpreter (see chapter 4) should be available to promote mutual understanding of the interaction (Gerchow et al., 2021). These situations also require the health professional to listen, take time, and not rush the client. This approach demonstrates respect for the client and helps to lessen any anxiety. It prevents confusion, enhancing development of the therapeutic relationship and promoting client safety (Conroy et al., 2017).

The health care environment is complex, busy, and noisy, which impacts communication for health care professionals and clients. Nurses who provide client care experience many distractions and interruptions and an increased workload due to the introduction of information technology as well as less staff. These barriers place limitations on their ability to engage in client-focused interactions and only allow them to complete task-focused care (Kwame & Petrucka, 2021). These factors demonstrate that work life conditions of health care professionals are demanding and support the notion that the communicative competence of staff who work in these settings is critical.

Self-Reflective Exercise

Think about a time when someone invaded your personal space. Think about your feelings in that situation. How did you handle the experience? How does this situation relate to your role as a student in a health professional program?

CHAPTER SUMMARY

This chapter introduced information on the evolution of communication models and basic aspects that impact effective communication for health care providers. Effective and client-centred communication is critical for health care professionals in all clinical settings. Today health care environments are chaotic, leading to poor client outcomes and dissatisfaction with care. To be effective in their roles, health care professionals need knowledge and awareness of factors that facilitate or hinder communication processes. Communication competency comprises both verbal and nonverbal behaviours evident in all components of interpersonal communication. With support and education, health care professionals can become more effective in communicating with clients, families, colleagues, and other members of the health care team. This knowledge and these skills lead to positive client outcomes, respectful communication, and a culture of safety.

REVIEW QUESTIONS

1. Review the common elements of the communication process.
2. Compare and contrast the similarities and differences among the communication models.
3. Define the terms *kinesics, paralanguage*, and *proxemics*.
4. Describe the different levels of communication and provide examples of how they can be used in practice.
5. How do our emotions affect our ability to send, receive, and comprehend messages?
6. List four factors that facilitate effective communication.
7. List four barriers that impede communication.

REFERENCES

Afriyie, D. (2020). Effective communication between nurses and patients: An evolutionary concept analysis. *British Journal of Community Nursing, 25*(9). https://doi.org/10.12968/bjcn.2020.25.9.438

Ali, M. (2018). Communication skills 3: Non-verbal communication. *Nursing Times, 114*(2), 41–42. https://www.nursingtimes.net/clinical-archive/assessment-skills/communication-skills-3-non-verbal-communication-15-01-2018/

Arnold, E. C. & Boggs, K. U. (2020). *Interpersonal relationships: Professional communication skills for nurses* (3rd ed.). Elsevier.

Barnlund, D. C. (1970). A transactional model of communication. In K. K. Sereno & C. D. Mortensen (Eds.), *Foundations of communication theory* (pp. 82–102). Harper and Row.

Beebe, S. A., Beebe, S. J., & Redmond, M. V. (2020). *Interpersonal communication: Relating to others* (9th ed.). Pearson.

Canadian Patient Safety Institute. (2020). *The safety competencies: Enhancing patient safety across the health professions* (2nd ed.). https://www.patientsafetyinstitute.ca/en/toolsResources/safetyCompetencies/Documents/CPSI-SafetyCompetencies_EN_Digital.pdf

Carey, J. W. (2018). *A cultural approach to communication.* https://brewminate.com/a-cultural-approach-to-communication/

Chu, J. N., Collins, J. E., Chen, T. T., Chai P. R., Dadabhoy, F., Byrne J. D., Wentworth, A., DeAndrea-Lazarus, I. A., Moreland, C. J., Wilson, J. A. B., Booth, A., Ghenand, O., Hur, C., & Traverso, G. (2021). Patient and health care worker perceptions of communication and ability to identify emotion when wearing standard and transparent masks. *JAMA Open Network, 4*(11), 1–13. https://doi.org/10.1001/jamanetworkopen.2021.35386

Conroy, T., Feo, R., Boucaut, R., Alderman, J., & Kitson, A. (2017). Role of effective nurse-patient relationships in enhancing patient safety. *Nursing Standard, 31*(49), 53–61. https://doi.org/10.7748/ns.2007.e10801

Cooper, K. L., Chang, E., Luck, L., & Dixon, K. (2022). Spirituality and standards for practice: A critical discourse analysis. *Journal of Holistic Nursing, 40*(1), 16–24. https://doi.org/10.1177/08980101211009049

Crawley, D. (2019). *Communication style: 3 ways to choose the right one.* https://doncrawley.com/how-to-choose-communication-style/

Derman, G. S. (2020). How does interpersonal communication affect health and patient safety? *International Journal of Social and Economic Services, 10*(1), 49–53. https://ijses.org/index.php/ijses/article/view/267/255

Durkin, J., Jackson, D., & Usher, A. (2021). The expression and receipt of compassion through touch in a health setting: A qualitative study. *Journal of Advanced Nursing, 77*(4), 1980–1991. https://doi.org/10.1111/jan.14766

Fleishman, J., Kamsky, H., & Sundborg, S. (2019). Trauma-informed nursing practice. *OJIN: The Online Journal of Issues in Nursing, 24*(2), 1–8. https://doi.org/10.3912/OJN.Vol24No2Man03

Foulger, D. (2004). *Models of the communication process*. http://foulger.info/davis/research/unifiedModelOfCommunication.htm

Gerchow, L., Burka, L. R., Miner, S., & Squires, A. (2021). Language barriers between nurses and patients: A scoping review. *Patient Education and Counseling*, *104*(3), 534–553. https://doi.org/10.1016/j.pec.2020.09.017

Guttman, O. T., Lazzara, E. H., Keebler, J. R., Webster, K. L. W., Gisick, L. M., & Baker, A. L. (2021). Dissecting communication barriers in healthcare: A path to enhancing communication resiliency, reliability, and patient safety. *Journal of Patient Safety*, *17*(8), e1465–e1471. https://doi.org/10.1097/pts.0000000000000541

Hecht, H., Welsch, R., Viehoff, J., & Longo, M. R. (2019). The shape of personal space. *Acta Psychologica*, *193*, 113–122. https://doi.org/10.1016/j.actpsy.2018.12.009

Henderson, S., & Barker, M. (2017). Developing nurses' intercultural/intraprofessional communication skills using the excellence in cultural experiential learning and leadership social interaction maps. *Journal of Clinical Nursing*, *27*(17–18), 3276–3286. https://doi.org/10.1111/jocn.14089

Holland, C. A. C., Ebner, N. C., Lin, T., & Samanez-Larkin, G. R. (2019). Emotion identification across adulthood using the dynamic face database of emotional expressions in younger, middle aged, and older adults. *Cognition and Emotion*, *33*(2), 245–257. https://doi.org/10.1080/02699931.2018.1445981

Homans, N. C., & Vroegop, J. L. (2022). The impact of face masks on the communication of adults with hearing loss during COVID-19 in a clinical setting. *International Journal of Audiology*, *61*(5), 365–370. https://doi.org/10.1080/14992027.2021.1952490

Horváth, A., & Molnár, P. (2021). A review of patient safety communication in multicultural and multilingual healthcare settings with special attention to the U.S. and Canada. *Developments in Health Sciences*, *4*(3), 49–57. https://doi.org/10.1556/2066.2021.00041

Jang, H., Lee, M., & Lee, N.-J. (2022). Communication education regarding patient safety for registered nurses in acute hospital settings: A scoping review protocol. *BMJ Open*, *12*(2), 1–6. https://doi.org/10.1136/bmjopen-2021-053217

Kelly, M. A., Nixon, L., McClurg, C., Scherpbier, A., King, N., & Dornan, T. (2018). Experience of touch in health care: A meta-ethnography across the health care professions. *Qualitative Health Research*, *28*(2), 200–212. https://doi.org/10.1177/1049732317707726

Kilgore, B., Harriger, C., Gaeta, L., & Sharpp, T. J. (2021). Unmasking misunderstandings: Strategies for better communication with patients. *Nursing*, *51*(1), 56–59. https://doi.org/10.1097/01.NURSE.0000724368.90257.74

Knollman-Porter, K., & Burshnic, V. L. (2020). Optimizing effective communication while wearing a mask during the COVID-19 pandemic. *Journal of Gerontological Nursing*, *46*(11), 7–11. https://doi.org/10.3928/00989134-20201012-02

Kwame, A., & Petrucka, P. M. (2021). A literature-based study of patient-centered care and communication in nurse-patient interactions: Barriers, facilitators, and the way forward. *BMC Nursing*, *20*(158). https://doi.org/10.1186/s12912-021-00684-2

Marler, H., & Ditton, A. (2021). "I'm smiling back at you": Exploring the impact of mask wearing on communication in healthcare. *International Journal of Language & Communication Disorders*, *56*(1), 205–214. https://doi.org/10.1111/1460-6984.12578

McHugh Schuster, P., & Nykolyn, L. (2010). *Communication for nurses: How to prevent harmful events and promote patient safety.* F. A. Davis Company.

Mheidly, N., Fares, M. Y., Zalzale, H., & Fares, J. (2020). Effect of face masks on interpersonal communication during the COVID-19 pandemic. *Frontiers in Public Health*, *8*, 1–6. https://doi.org/10.3389/fpubh.2020.582191

O'Brien, M. R., Kinloch, K., Groves, K. E., & Jack, B. A. (2019). Meeting patients' spiritual needs during end-of-life care: A qualitative study of nurses' and healthcare professionals' perceptions of spiritual care training. *Journal of Clinical Nursing*, 28, 182–189. https://doi.org/10.1111/jocn.146.48

Ogbogu, P. U., Noroski, L. M., Arcoleo, K., Reese, B. D. Jr., & Apter, A. J. (2022). Methods for cross-cultural communication in clinic encounters. *The Journal of Allergy and Clinical Immunology in Practice*, *10*(4), 893–900. https://doi.org/10.1016/j.jaip.2022.01.010

Pinto, C. T., & Pinto, S. (2020). From spiritual intelligence to spiritual care: A transformative approach to holistic practice. *Nurse Education in Practice*, *47*, 1–2. https://doi.org/10.1016/j.nepr.2020.102823

Ratna, H. (2019). The importance of effective communication in healthcare practice. *Harvard Public Health Review*, *23*, 1–6. https://doi.org/10.54111/0001/w4

Resat, F. A. (2019). The body language of culture. *International Journal for Innovation Education and Research*, *7*(8), 32–39. https://doi.org/10.31686/ijier.Vol7.Iss8.1639

Rogers, M., & Wattis, J. (2020). Understanding the role of spirituality in providing person-centred care. *Nursing Standard.* https://doi.org/10.7748/ns.2020.e11342

Shannon, C. E., & Weaver, W. (1949). *The mathematical theory of communication.* University of Illinois Press.

Shea, S. C. (2017). *Psychiatric interviewing. The art of understanding* (3rd ed.). Elsevier.

Stickley, T. (2011). From SOLER to SURETY for effective non-verbal communication. *Nurse Education in Practice*, *11*(6), 395–398. https://doi.org/10.1016/j.nepr.2011.03.021

Wanko Keutchafo, E. L., Kerr, J., & Jarvis, M. A. (2020). Evidence of nonverbal communication between nurses and older adults: A scoping review. *BMC Nursing*, *19*(53), 1–13. https://doi.org/10.1186/s12912-020-00443-9

Zumstein-Shaha, M., Ferrell, B., & Economou, D. (2020). Nurses' response to spiritual needs of cancer patients. *European Journal of Oncology Nursing*, *48*, 1–7. https://doi.org/10.1016/j.ejon.2020.101792

CHAPTER 2

Therapeutic Communication

LEARNING OBJECTIVES

After reading this chapter, you wil be able to

1. Define *therapeutic communication*
2. Describe therapeutic and nontherapeutic communication techniques
3. Differentiate between verbal and nonverbal communication
4. Discuss self-awareness
5. Describe the process of reflection
6. Differentiate between positive and negative listening responses
7. Define *active listening*
8. Describe effective listening skills to use with clients
9. Identify the aspects of SOLER and SURETY models

KEY TERMS

Active listening

Client-centred care

Closed-ended questions

Focused questions

Negative listening responses

Nontherapeutic communication
  techniques

Open-ended questions

Reflection

Self-awareness

Therapeutic communication
  techniques

Validation

Why questions

INTRODUCTION

This chapter provides an introduction to the aspects of therapeutic communication and its components necessary for the establishment of a nurse-client relationship. It discusses a variety of communication techniques, both verbal and nonverbal, that are used by health care professionals, including nurses, to therapeutically engage clients. The therapeutic use of self (self-awareness), reflection, and attentive listening skills are presented.

An important competency for the professional nurse is having the knowledge, self-awareness, and skill to use effective communication in practice. Today, the emphasis for health care personnel is to focus on a "client-centred" approach to ensure the best possible health outcomes. Client- or person-centred care is a recommended standard in placing people as professional partners in health care. This entails respecting and responding to individual client care needs, values, and preferences in their health care journey (Moore et al., 2021). A core component of client-centred care is the use of therapeutic communication to facilitate the delivery of holistic, effective nurse-client relationships in all health care environments (Kwame & Petrucka, 2021). Therapeutic communication is considered a primary professional competency and is highlighted in standards of nursing practice for nurses and nurse practitioners (College of Registered Nurses of Newfoundland & Labrador, 2019). The use of therapeutic communication enables nurses to build a therapeutic alliance with clients through all aspects of their care journey. In using therapeutic communication, the nurse is providing a safe place for the client to explore the meaning of their illness experience, building trust, and promoting coping and recovery (Xue & Heffernan, 2021).

Exercise 2.1: Therapeutic Communication

Purpose: To identify nurse behaviours that are considered components of therapeutic communication

Procedure
In groups of two to three students, brainstorm about behaviours that are essential for the development of therapeutic communication. The following questions can guide the discussion:

1. What is therapeutic communication?
2. What behaviours displayed by the nurse are considered therapeutic for the client?
3. What factors impact the ability to use therapeutic communication in a health care setting?
4. What words best describe therapeutic communication?
5. Generate a word cloud to illustrate those words identified among group members.

Discussion
How difficult was it for your group to arrive at a consensus on the words used to describe therapeutic communication? Discuss findings with the class. How does the information in this exercise reflect on your role as a nursing student in clinical practice?

SELF-AWARENESS

In nursing, understanding of self is an interpersonal process that facilitates the use of therapeutic communication in nurse-client interactions. Self-awareness is learning about the components of self (self-concept, self-esteem, self-identity) and how, as a health professional, coming to know "self" through reflection on thoughts, beliefs, emotions, biases, attitudes, and behaviours increases self-understanding, enhancing competency of one's professional role as a nurse (Younas et al., 2020). Getting to know the "true self" is a lifelong process that starts with conscious awareness of who they are as a person (Rasheed et al., 2019).

For example, using the concept of communication, reflect on what you think of yourself as a communicator. Think about the ways you currently communicate with others. Nurses' self-awareness and understanding of their own communication behaviours and those of their clients promotes personal and professional growth, leading nurses to be more effective in clinical practice. Also, enhancing awareness of self provides a bridge to understanding others better, which is critical in the health professions (Rasheed et al., 2021). Becoming self-aware additionally heightens nurses' critical thinking and clinical decision-making skills (Han & Kim, 2016). A nurse scholar, Rungapadiachy (2007), identified three layers of self-awareness. The first is superficial, awareness of one's age and gender, and the second is selective, perception of things we feel we may need to be aware of, like our physical appearance or attitude toward something. The third is deep awareness, which reflects our deepest thoughts and secrets—things that we do not share with others.

Similarly, the Johari window (Luft 1970) is a psychological tool that can be used by nurses and other health professionals for understanding and improving self-awareness. The model divides personal awareness into four quadrants (open, blind, hidden, and unknown), and each quadrant reflects different information about oneself. The tool can be used as a self-examination by nurses to foster their development of a person-centred approach or enable them to evaluate their behaviour in interpersonal relationships. The open quadrant reflects things that they, as well as everyone, know about themselves. For example, Betty works on a surgical unit. Her co-workers know she values answering client call lights quickly, is knowledgeable about principles of burn care, and likes the Toronto Maple Leafs. The blind quadrant refers to attributes that are unknown to oneself but are known by others. For example, when nervous, you tend to rub your arm, and your classmates may become aware of this behaviour while working with you on a group project. The hidden quadrant includes things that you are aware of but keep from others: a family member's death by suicide or the fact that you were caught smoking on school property in high school. The unknown quadrant symbolizes information about behaviours, feelings, and beliefs that remain undiscovered by oneself and others. For example, how will you, as a first-year nursing student, function in your first clinical rotation,

Table 2.1: The Johari Window

1 **Open:** Known to self and to others	2 **Blind:** Not known to self, but known to others
3 **Hidden:** Known to self but not to others	4 **Unknown:** Not known to self or others

Source: Oliver, S., & Duncan, S. (2019). Editorial: Looking through the Johari window. *Research for All, 3*(1), 1–6. https://doi.org/10.18546/RFA.03.1.01

giving an enema or intramuscular injection to a client for the first time? Depending upon your communication style, what you learn about yourself through feedback from others, and telling others more about yourself, quadrants one, two, and three become larger, while the fourth becomes smaller (Oliver & Duncan, 2019).

Exercise 2.2: Johari Window Framework

Purpose: To develop awareness of self

Procedure
Using the Johari window framework, reflect on each area and identify aspects of yourself, fitting information within each quadrant.

Discussion
Describe your experience in trying to complete the framework. What did you learn about yourself in attempting this exercise? Do you feel the assignment was useful in helping you to become more aware of your personal beliefs, attitudes, values, and motivations?

REFLECTION

Another useful strategy for the professional nurse is the use of reflection in gaining knowledge of self, which leads to professional development and improved competency in clinical practice (Barbagallo, 2019). According to Bagheri et al. (2019), reflection is valuable for nursing students as it allows them to reflect on their experiences in practice from a critical perspective. It helps them examine not only their role, behaviours, actions, communication skills, and beliefs, but also those of others in the clinical context of the nursing situation. Through reflection, students are also able to explore potential biases or stereotypes they hold and gain understanding of how these beliefs may influence practice and therapeutic engagement with clients (Blake & Blake, 2019; Reljic et al., 2019). Using reflection, nurses learn to examine their practice, challenge assumptions, build on their knowledge, and promote practice change (Nagle & Foli, 2020). In the nursing literature, the concept of reflective practice has been described, and several models have been identified to aid nurses' reflective process. One of the most famous reflection models commonly used by nurses and nursing students is the one developed by Gibbs (1988).

Case Example

Ann Carson, a 26-year-old woman, comes to the emergency department complaining of abdominal pain, nausea, vomiting, and restlessness. Ann's partner, who accompanied her to the hospital, states, "Ann has ulcerative colitis and experiences a lot of pain." Her partner demands that Nurse Mary give her pain medication. As Mary leaves Ann's room, she comments to Ben, another nurse, "I can't believe this one is back again. She was here three weeks ago with the same complaint. She needs to do something about her drug-seeking behaviour."

Gibbs's Step-by-Step Process

- Description: Describe what happened.
- Feelings: What were you thinking and feeling?
- Evaluation: What was positive and negative about the experience?
- Analysis: Do an analysis of the situation.
- Conclusion: What else could you have done?
- Action plan: For the same circumstances, what could you do in the future?

Source: Gibbs, G. (1988). *Learning by doing: A guide to teaching and learning methods.* Oxford Brookes University.

Gibbs's model is a structured, step-by-step process that prompts the user to reflect on an experience or situation using self-awareness and critical thinking to explore the main issues associated with an event in order to build on clinical insight, enhance clinical judgment, and promote practice change.

Self-Reflective Exercise

Choose a situation that you were involved in recently with a family member or friend. Using Gibbs's reflective mode, write your description of the situation and then apply the rest of Gibbs's steps to reflect on the situation.

ACTIVE LISTENING

Active listening ("tuning in") is an essential communication tool used by nurses and other health professionals to create an environment that promotes therapeutic engagement with clients. According to McCann et al. (2019), being listened to and feeling heard helps to reduce conflict, alleviate pain, and foster emotional well-being. It has been suggested that nursing students incorporating active listening and self-awareness into their practice leads to an improvement in client-centred care (Haley et al., 2017). McKenna et al. (2020) contends that nurses must "consistently implement active listening techniques with patients and their families" (p. 614). However, listening as a primary communication technique is underused and can be a challenge in health care environments (Ellison & Meyer, 2020). To listen actively is to be attentive to what the client is saying, both verbally and nonverbally, understand the message, and validate through feedback the intended message. In today's health care system, it is paramount that clients feel they are heard, and nurses can facilitate the listening process by demonstrating interest, respect, compassion, and acceptance during client engagement (Loos, 2021). Ellison and Meyer (2020) contend that therapeutic listening is an essential component of effective communication and requires a conscious commitment from the health care provider to be present and attentive within the interaction. This requires that the nurse be both physically and emotionally present in the clinical situation. Some attributes of listening identified are empathy, silence, attention to both verbal and nonverbal behaviours, and the ability to be nonjudgmental (Ellison & Meyer, 2020; McCann et al., 2019).

Read the poem entitled "Listen, Nurse," written by registered nurse Ruth Johnston and published in the *American Journal of Nursing* in 1971 (p. 303). Although the poem was written and published many years ago, the words reflect the true essence and importance of listening to clients that is so relevant in the current health care system. The link for the poem is https://journals.lww.com/ajnonline/Citation/1971/02000/Listen,_Nurse.27.aspx.

Nurses and other health care providers need to understand the reasons for not listening and further develop skills for active, therapeutic listening. It has been proposed that nurses spend, on average, 80 percent of their day in some form of communication and that about 45 percent of that time is spent listening (Younis et al., 2015). Some barriers reported that impact listening are lack of interest, feeling tired, being too busy, prejudices, lack of time, lack of privacy, nurse-client language barriers, and noisy environments (Ellison & Meyer, 2020). The essence of active listening is taking the time to listen and placing the client at the heart of the interaction. Two facilitative skills for attentive listening identified in the literature are known by the acronyms SOLER (Egan, 2007) and SURETY (Stickley, 2011).

Table 2.2: SOLER

SOLER
Squarely: "Sit squarely" to the client. This indicates you are interested in the client and are there to listen.
Open posture: Keep an open posture, meaning that your legs and arms are uncrossed. This behaviour suggests you are open to what the client has to say. A closed position can convey a lack of interest to the client.
Lean forward: Leaning slightly forward conveys that you are interested in what is being said and are trying to be attentive.
Eye contact: Establish eye contact and do not use a stare gaze. Eye contact should be fleeting, and you should take occasional breaks in eye contact with the client. Keep in mind the cultural implications of eye contact.
Relax: Be aware of your own body language. Demonstrate a sense of being relaxed, and do not fidget.

Source: Egan, G. (2007). *The skilled helper: A problem-management approach to helping* (8th ed.). Brooks/Cole.

Table 2.3: SURETY

SURETY
S: Sit at an angle to the client. Keep in mind our "bubble" personal space as comfort for client and nurse. Assess for any discomfort from client.
U: Uncross arms and legs. Crossed arms and legs communicate defensiveness, lack of interest, or superiority.
R: Relax. Maintain an appropriate position that shows active listening. Have an awareness of your own body language while engaged with the client.
E: Retain appropriate eye contact, with breaks on occasion. Have awareness of cultural implications with respect to eye contact.
T: Touch is an important communication tool. Nurses use touch to demonstrate caring, compassion, empathy, and comfort. Nurses need awareness of when touch is appropriate and inappropriate in nonverbal communication. Touch is personal and perhaps cultural, so it is important to assess the client's response to touch.
Y: Your intuition—trust your instincts and use intuition (knowledge and expertise) in clinical situations.

Source: Stickley, T. (2011). From SOLER to SURETY for effective non-verbal communication. *Nurse Education in Practice,* *11*(6), 395–398. https://doi.org/10.1016/j.nepr.2011.03.021

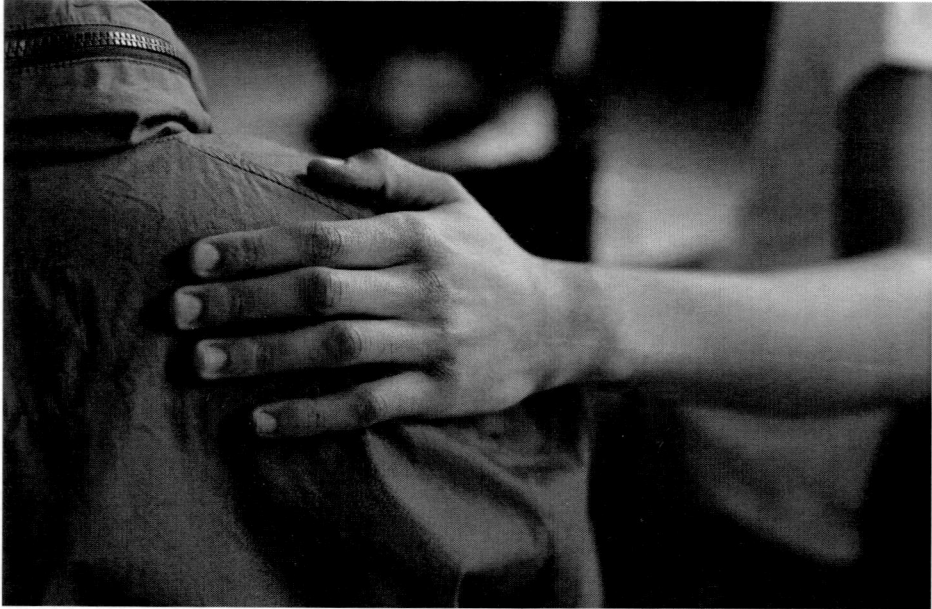

Figure 2.1: Appropriate touch as a communication tool
Source: Adobe Stock/pressmaster

The SOLER and SURETY models for nonverbal behaviour are obviously similar, and both provide guidance for nurses as well as other health care professionals on ways to create a safe space for therapeutic engagement. The slight amendments to the SURETY model include touch and intuition, which are vital components of clinical practice for nurses. For beginning nursing students, these acronyms can serve as a useful reminder of the elements necessary for active listening as they develop knowledge of and skill in therapeutic communication.

Research Highlight: Improving Therapeutic Communication in Nursing through Simulation Exercise

Background

Effective communication is critical within the nursing discipline as it fosters positive client outcomes, safety, and trust in clinical encounters. Nurses' skills in communication help to build relationships with other health care providers as well as students in the health professions. Nursing students may find communication skills a challenge and experience anxiety in clinical rotations regarding their ability to communicate appropriately in client situations. Laboratory simulation is considered a useful strategy to improve students' confidence and their self-efficacy in utilizing effective therapeutic communication.

Purpose of the Study

- To assess student use of previously learned communication skills
- To explore student communication skills and areas for improvement in a post-simulation environment

Method

Using a quasi-experiment one-group, pre-test/post-test design, a convenience sample (n = 32) of nursing students completed a simulation exercise during a weekly laboratory simulation on communication skills. Students completed a pre-test questionnaire consisting of five questions focused on their self-efficacy of therapeutic communication skills. Students were randomly divided into groups and were assigned roles (e.g., client, nurse, rater). Students who played the client role were provided a script, while the raters were responsible for completing a rubric that outlined therapeutic and nontherapeutic responses. A nursing faculty member was also assigned to each simulation and completed the evaluation rubric. At the conclusion of the simulation, a faculty member and students discussed the simulation as part of a debriefing exercise.

Findings

Wilcoxon tests indicated that student responses for the pre-test and post-test survey were all significant, with $p < .01$, meaning there was improvement in student self-efficacy in therapeutic communication skills. Students reported feeling better prepared to assess their therapeutic and nontherapeutic skills. They also described the ability to refine personal objectives for improving their communication skills.

Implications for Nursing Practice

Communication simulations could be used as a teaching strategy in nursing courses (e.g., therapeutic communication, mental health, medical-surgical, fundamentals). The simulation exercise can be developed to be more or less complex depending upon the particular course and level of student. Proficiency in therapeutic communication reflects a need for adequate educational preparation for students in the speciality of nursing.

Source: Blake, T., & Blake, T. (2019). Improving therapeutic communication in nursing through simulation exercise. *Teaching and Learning in Nursing, 14*(4), 260–264. https://doi .org/10.1016/j.teln.2019.06.003

ACTIVE LISTENING RESPONSES

According to Beebe et al. (2020), listening is a complex process that involves more than hearing. These authors suggest that listening consists of five elements:

- **Selecting**: Having competing sounds to listen to requires you to be sensitive to the sound or nonverbal behaviour that symbolizes meaning.
- **Attending**: After selecting a sound, attend to it. Focus on the message.
- **Understanding**: Relate the message to what you hear and assign meaning.
- **Remembering**: Be in the moment through being self-aware—physically and emotionally present with the client.
- **Responding**: Respond to others to inform them that you've received the message and understand. Lack of response may indicate lack of understanding or not listening. (Beebe et al., 2020)

Many competing obstacles within the nursing environment impact the listening process. Self-awareness by the nurse provides the opportunity to focus on the client and use appropriate body language, eye contact, nodding, leaning forward, and verbal indicators (e.g., "Go on") to show attention, understanding, and acceptance (Loos, 2021). These behaviours facilitate communication and indicate that the health care provider is fully engaged with the client.

The nurse, if effectively listening in interpersonal interactions, is not only using their ears but also their eyes (eye contact), mind (cognition), heart (compassion), and a person-centred, focused approach to therapeutically communicate in clinical situations. This is evident in the Chinese character for listen, "ting," (figure 2.2), which symbolizes complete engagement in therapeutic listening.

TING

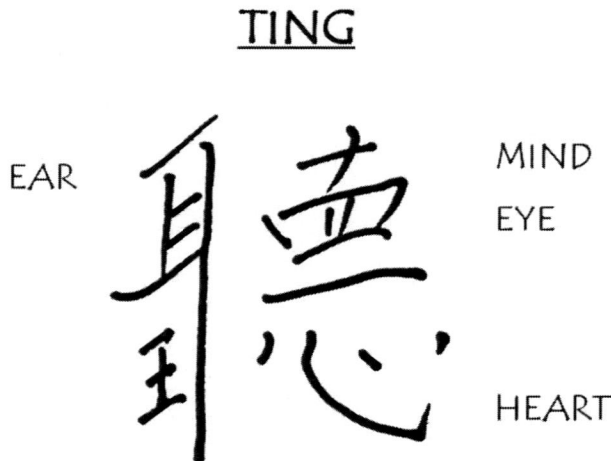

EAR   听   MIND
EYE
HEART

Figure 2.2: The Traditional Chinese Character for Listening

Meeting the Client

Individuals usually make judgments, either positive or negative, based on how a person appears on first encounter. Nurses' attire and behaviours (verbal and nonverbal) determine how professional and competent they are seen by clients, which influences the establishment of a therapeutic nurse-client relationship (Willis et al., 2018). The phases of the therapeutic nurse-client relationship are pre-interaction, orientation, working, and termination (Arnold & Boggs, 2020; Peplau, 1997). The pre-interaction phase allows the health care provider time to prepare prior to meeting the client. The orientation phase involves the client and nurse meeting for the first time, also known as the introductory phase. Here the focus is developing rapport and laying the groundwork for the establishment of trust. From there, the continuum of relationship building moves into the working phase, where the client, as partner, works to identify their health concerns as the health care provider goes through the process of assessment and data collection. With ongoing collaboration and shared decision-making, a personal health care plan is designed to meet the client's continuing needs. The final phase, termination, occurs when the client is discharged or transferred to another level of care (Peplau, 1997). The phases of the nurse-client relationship are discussed in greater detail in chapter 3. Health care professionals, in getting to know clients, demonstrate a professional presence and model professional behaviour by applying a person-centred approach. This action requires that they have an awareness of ways to promote effective communication when meeting the client and other family members who may be present. Several recommended strategies include the following (Guest, 2016):

- Ensure nonverbal communication is open and positive (see the SOLER and SURETY acronyms).
- Begin the interaction by introducing yourself, using first and last names, and explaining your role and the purpose of the encounter or interaction (Canadian Nurses Association, 2017).
- When greeting a client, use their proper name. Ask them how they would like to be addressed, and if their name is difficult to pronounce or unfamiliar, have them repeat the name. Adjust verbal communication depending upon client status, diagnoses, or unfamiliar language. Seek the assistance of an interpreter if necessary.
- Provide privacy and have an awareness of the environment to eliminate or minimize distractions and interruptions.
- When talking, it is important to sit at eye level with the client and consider proxemics during the interaction.
- Use active listening skills and appropriate communication techniques, such as open-ended, closed-ended, and focused questions; reflection; and paraphrasing.

- Ask the client if they have any questions. Keep in mind that you should use language they understand and avoid medical jargon.
- Thank the client for their participation, explain what will happen, and provide educational material (e.g., brochures, pamphlets), depending upon the interaction.

THERAPEUTIC COMMUNICATION TECHNIQUES

Therapeutic communication includes the use of several skills: active listening, positive body language, appropriate verbal responses, and the nurse's ability to interpret and effectively analyze the client's verbal and nonverbal behaviours. These skills allow the health care provider to interact therapeutically with clients in all clinical situations. An important part of clinical nursing is assessment, where the nurse, through observation, questioning, and responding, collects the client information necessary to provide care interventions. In using observation, the nurse can assess the client's nonverbal behaviours and invite the client to validate, clarify, correct, or elaborate on those observations. During an interview or interaction, the nurse is meeting face-to-face, so they can recognize behaviours and verbalize their perceptions with the client. Several nurse responses are highlighted in the following examples:

- "I notice you got teary-eyed when you mentioned that your wife is unable to visit."
- "You said you feel fine, but I notice that you grimace when you sit up in bed."
- "I noticed you were pacing around the unit this morning."

Questioning

Questioning is a valuable therapeutic tool that health care professionals, including nurses, use daily in their engagement with clients. Through questioning, the nurse gains information about the client's reason for hospitalization, expressions of their feelings, and clarification or validation of the client's message. Also, depending upon the agency's client assessment forms for data collection, nurses may use a combination of open-ended, closed-ended, and focused questions to interact therapeutically with clients. This section presents information on the verbal and nonverbal communication techniques used by health care professionals during the client-centred encounter.

Open-Ended Questions

This technique is an excellent approach to establish rapport with the client in building a therapeutic alliance. These questions do not require a yes or no answer but encourage a whole lot of possible responses and information. Open-ended questions are useful in obtaining information about feelings, thoughts, perceptions, and symptoms. Open-ended questions usually begin with words such as *how* and *what*. Examples of open-ended questions include the following:

- "Tell me something about your family."
- "What is it like for you to be in hospital?"
- "How are you feeling?"
- "What brings you to the clinic today?"

Closed-Ended Questions

Closed-ended questions are useful in gaining specific information or when there is a yes or no answer. They are particularly useful in obtaining information in emergency situations and in some instances where the client is unable to provide a lengthy response. The health care provider should not use exclusively closed-ended questions during completion of a full nursing assessment or interview; it is best to use a combination of open-ended, closed-ended, and focused questions. This type of approach allows the collection of data from the client's perspective, which is important in the development of a person-centred health care plan. Examples of closed-ended questions include the following:

- "Are you having pain?"
- "Do you have any allergies?'
- "Do you want a slice of toast?"
- "Is your sling too loose?"

Focused Questions

Focused questions require more than a yes or no response but focus on specific areas of concern. They are useful in emergency situations and when inquiring about the client's health concerns or experienced symptoms during data collection and assessment. Examples of focused questions include the following:

- "Tell me more about the ringing in your left ear."
- "How would you describe the pain in your foot?"
- "How would you describe your bowel movements?"
- "When did your chest pain begin?"

The following sections detail additional therapeutic communication techniques.

Silence

You may have heard the proverb "Silence is golden," which implies the importance of using silence (brief pauses) in conversation. However, nursing is a profession that abounds with verbal interactions in the provision of client care. As a nursing student, you may find a period of silence uncomfortable when interacting with a client. Sometimes we don't know what to say or how to deal with the emotions or thoughts expressed by the client. Keep in mind that silence if used effectively is a productive communication technique. Silence (5 to 10 seconds) gives the client, as well as the nurse, time to organize their thoughts and reflect on what has been said or where they are in the conversation. Silence also provides the nurse the opportunity to assess the client's nonverbal behaviours and validate, clarify, or explore further topics that arose during the interaction. Silence also gives the health care provider an occasion to be present with the client in the moment without verbal communication (Carroll, 2020). Depending upon the client's condition, the nurse just sitting can demonstrate compassion and respect for the client (Kemerer, 2016). Health care professionals must keep in mind that if they are sitting, the focus is the client; the nurse must not be texting or using some other electronic device (Fogger, 2019).

Exploring

Exploring is a technique that enables the nurse to inquire about an experience, idea, subject, or relationship in more detail. For example, if a client tells you they work as a supervisor at the paint factory, you can further explore this area, asking, "Tell me more about your job." Or, if a client tells you about their fears of upcoming electroconvulsive therapy (ECT), you can open with "Tell me about those fears you are having about the treatment."

Clarification/Validation Techniques

An important factor in communication is that the message being sent is understood, so feedback regarding validation/clarification may be necessary. The key to the interaction is that both the client and the nurse have mutual understanding so there are no misperceptions. The use of validation/clarification technique provides the opportunity for increased understanding and accuracy of both verbal and nonverbal behaviours. The client may be somewhat vague in their message, so the nurse can seek clarification or validation. The following are several examples of this:

- "I hear you saying that you have been having trouble with sleep the past few months. Is that correct?"
- "I'm not sure that I understand. Please give me more information."
- "Do I understand you correctly that you said ...?"

- "I hear you saying that you are having difficulty trusting your wife after what happened. Is that correct?"
- "Do you mean …?"

Paraphrasing

A nurse can use this technique to confirm their interpretation of the client's previous message before moving on in the interaction. The nurse restates the content of the client's message using their own words or phrases. Paraphrasing is a responding skill as it indicates to the client that the nurse is focused on what has been said and is actively listening. It also confirms understanding and clarity of the intent of the message:

> Client: "I am so tired of all of this; the treatments are making me feel worse. I don't know if I can go on."
> Nurse: "Am I correct in saying you feel exhausted and you wish to discontinue your treatments?"

Reflection

This technique is used to reflect on the client's feelings communicated in the verbal or nonverbal message. It enables the nurse to further explore those feelings and label them for the client. This technique helps the client to understand their own thoughts and feelings once they are brought into awareness. For example, the nurse might ask the following:

- "You seem sad this morning. What are you thinking about?"

The nurse could also link the client's feelings with context:

- "It sounds like you feel unsure of what to do because you have not had an opportunity to discuss the treatment with your wife."

Restatement

Using this technique, the nurse simply restates a few of the key words from the client's statement. Be careful not to use this technique excessively as it may inhibit or block further communication. It could be seen as "parroting," which may feel disparaging for the client.

> Client: "I can't sleep. I am up all night."
> Nurse: "You can't sleep at night."

Summarization

Summarizing the content following a lengthy interaction or teaching session with a client or family member is useful. Summarization provides an opportunity to clarify concerns or ask additional questions before the teaching session or conversation ends. Also, this technique is suitable when providing discharge information to the client and family members when leaving the hospital, clinic, or other health facility. For example, a nurse may educate the client and family members about the care of a chest incision, asepsis, hand hygiene, or signs of infection.

- "During this teaching session, we have covered information about care of the chest incision ..."
- "In our conversation, we talked about your readiness to return to work, and medication management for your blood pressure.... Is there anything else?"

NONTHERAPEUTIC COMMUNICATION TECHNIQUES

These are techniques that the nurse and other health care providers may use, either intently or not, because they lack awareness of their impact on the therapeutic communication process and establishment of a therapeutic relationship. These negative approaches impair all aspects of client engagement as they reflect a lack of respect and interfere with the establishment of trust, building of rapport, and understanding of the illness experience. With knowledge and recognition of these barriers, the novice nurse can take steps to avoid such ineffective techniques. As stated earlier in this chapter, the use and development of self-awareness and reflection will enhance clinical judgment, foster understanding, and promote behaviour change in the skill of therapeutic communication for the health care professional.

Asking Excessive Questions

Bombarding the client with excessive questions (especially closed-ended) and using the interview or assessment process as an interrogation is an ineffective approach. It demonstrates to the client that the nurse is in control and is not treating them as an equal partner in the nurse-client relationship. In the interview, the client is the focus and the nurse needs to provide a welcoming and supportive environment that encourages the telling of their illness experience. The nurse's best approach is to use a combination of open-ended, close-ended, and focused questions, all of which clarify issues and demonstrate a client-centred focus for engagement.

Avoid asking excessive questions: "What lead you to cut yourself? Do you do it very often? Did someone tell you to do this?"

It's better to say, "Tell me about the situation that caused you to harm yourself."

Requesting an Explanation (Asking Why Questions)

This type of question can be intimidating to the client as they feel the need to explain or defend their actions and feelings. These questions are negative and can be interpreted by the client as being treated like a child by the health care provider, closing communication.

For example, avoid the following:

- "Why are you late for the group session?"
- "Why did you do that?"
- "Why didn't you keep your appointment?"

It's better to say:

- "I noted you were late for today's group session. How are things going with you?"
- "What is going on? You usually do not react like that."
- "I notice you did not make your appointment this morning. What happened?"

Giving Advice

The client may look to the nurse for advice, believing they know best. This notion implies that clients are incapable of making decisions and fosters dependence. In giving advice, the health care provider hinders client problem-solving. The nurse's role is to avoid giving advice and, in collaboration with clients, help them to explore options and arrive at solutions themselves. Giving advice is very different from providing information. In therapeutic engagement, the nurse is helping the client through interactions and providing appropriate information to ensure informed decision-making.

For example, avoid saying the following:

- "I think you should ..."
- "If I were you, I would ..."

It's best to say, "What do you think you should do?" or "What do you think are some possible solutions?"

There are other nontherapeutic communication responses that are also considered "roadblocks" to the communication process. The key for the health care professional is to recognize them and avoid their use in all client interactions. As stated earlier in this chapter, gaining therapeutic communication skills is a lifelong process.

Through reflection and self-awareness, nurses gain insight into their communication practices, recognize the need for change, and note improvement. Table 2.4 provides explanations and examples of other negative listening responses that can shut down the communication process.

Table 2.4: Negative Listening Responses

Response	Explanation	Response Example
Changing the subject (topic)	The health care provider changes the subject/topic and cuts off the client. This may be because of a lack of time or because the health care provider does not want to discuss the topic.	Client: "I did not sleep well last night." LPN: "Is your wife coming in today?"
Belittling feelings	The health care provider does not fully explore the client's experience, demonstrating a lack of empathy.	Client: "I am very concerned about my surgery." Nurse: "It is only a minor procedure."
Giving false reassurance	The health care provider makes stereotypical/trite comments, demonstrating a lack of understanding and interest.	Client: "This is the first time I have had this type of procedure." Nurse: "I wouldn't worry about that if I were you. Everything will be fine. Dr. Smith has done the procedure numerous times."
Giving approval	The health care provider uses social comments to pass judgment on the behaviour/opinion/ideas of client as "good" or "bad." These comments can be misinterpreted by client.	"That's good; you took the sleeping pill." "I am glad that ..." "I am happy you decided to go ahead with chemotherapy."
Making false inferences	The health care professional jumps to conclusions. Information is not validated; there is incongruence between verbal and nonverbal behaviours.	"What you are really saying is that you drink because your wife left you."
Interrupting	The health care professional uses constant interruptions while the client is speaking, demonstrating a lack of respect and that they are not listening to client.	Client: "I have been having the pain, but I'm—" Nurse: "How can you describe the pain?"

Exercise 2.3: Who Am I?—Getting to Know Aspects of Self

Purpose: To gain awareness of aspects of self and how these components shape your development as a health care professional

Procedure

Break into groups of two and work individually on each question. After completing each question, discuss your answers with your partner and reflect on the similarities or differences noted in your responses. How does this exercise relate to your role as a health care professional student?

1. Who am I? Identify and record three words that describe you as a person.
2. What is important to me, and what do I value?
3. What do I know about myself and am willing to share with others?
4. What do I know about myself and am not willing to share with others?
5. Am I open to my feelings, and can I express them?
6. Write a sentence or two on why you chose to become a nurse.
7. What did you learn about yourself from doing this exercise?
8. Did you have difficulty in finding only three words to describe yourself?
9. Identify differences or similarities among your classmates' responses.

Exercise 2.4: Requesting an Explanation—Asking Why Questions

Purpose: To gain an understanding of why questions and the need to avoid their use in therapeutic communication

Procedure

Review the why questions and change them into a better format that makes them less judgmental and defensive.

1. "Why didn't you take your medications?"
2. "Why do you think that?"
3. "Why are you crying?"
4. "Why do you continue to ring your call bell?"
5. "Why are you such a difficult patient?"
6. "Why do you keep pulling off your dressing?"

Exercise 2.5: Active Listening—Use of SOLER and SURETY

Purpose: To understand the components of the SOLER and SURETY facilitative skills for listening

Procedure

This exercise will help you gain some awareness of your verbal and nonverbal behaviours. Pair off with another student and role-play the following case. Each of you will have the opportunity to play the role of the client and the nurse.

Scenario

Mrs. Alma Wang is a 65-year-old woman who is being admitted from the emergency department to your unit for assessment of abdominal obstruction. Upon admission, Mrs. Wang is sitting in a wheelchair accompanied by the hospital porter and Mrs. Wang's daughter, Amy. As a first-year nursing student, you are assigned to care for Mrs. Wang, who has been assigned to Room 245 at the end of the nursing unit.

For the role play, set up two chairs. Position chairs so that you are face-to-face and able to make eye contact. One student will play the role of the client and the other will be the nurse. Later, you will switch roles and complete the exercise again. Follow and use the aspects of the SOLER and SURETY models to set up the environment and assess your attentive listening skills. Answer the following questions:

1. How will you introduce yourself to Mrs. Wang and her daughter?
2. Identify some open- and closed-ended questions and focused questions that could be used in this scenario.
3. What characteristics would be displayed by the nurse that would indicate to Mrs. Wang that the focus is on her as the client?

In your role play, Mrs. Wang informs the nurse that "I have been having this sharp pain in my stomach for the past two weeks. I have a lot of gas when I go to the bathroom. Do you think I should change my diet?"

4. Identity some clarification, validation, and focused questions that could be used in response to Mrs. Wang.
5. How should the nurse respond to Mrs. Wang when she asks, "Do you think I should change my diet?"

Exercise 2.6: Communication Techniques

This exercise consists of activities related to communication techniques used by health care professionals.

A. This exercise involves reading the responses and identifying the type of technique and whether it is therapeutic or nontherapeutic.

Example: Client: "I have nothing to live for … I wish I was dead."
Nurse: "I feel that way sometimes as well."
Nontherapeutic: Belittling of client feelings.

Client: "I wish I did not have to stay here for another two weeks."
Nurse: "Did you want to go to the lounge and play some pool?"

Client: "I am really concerned about having my surgery tomorrow."
Nurse: "No need to worry; you are in good hands with Dr. Smith."

Client: "I am not sure that chemotherapy is appropriate at this time."
Nurse: "I think you should take the treatment that is offered to you."

B. Review the following nurse-client interaction and answer the questions.

Nurse: (*knocks and enters the room*) "Good afternoon, Mrs. Brown." (*smiles*)
Client: "Hello …" (*Mrs. Brown looks sad and has red eyes. She has been crying. She turns away and looks out the window.*)
Nurse: "I see that you have been crying." (*Nurse pulls up a chair and sits close to the bed, leaning in and looking at Mrs. Brown lying on the bed. Passes her a box of tissues.*) "Please tell me what is going on."
Client: "I just feel so overwhelmed, too much on my mind."
Nurse: (*looking at Mrs. Brown*) "You're concerned about your lung biopsy tomorrow?"

Answer the following questions:
1. List the behaviours that indicate the nurse is an effective listener.
2. Identify the types of verbal and nonverbal communication responses the nurse uses.
3. Is the nurse using behaviours that facilitate the establishment of a therapeutic relationship?

CHAPTER SUMMARY

This chapter presented an overview of the components of therapeutic communication required for the development of therapeutic relationships with clients. If health care professionals have knowledge and skill in therapeutic communication, a person-centred approach is facilitated, which leads to positive health outcomes. In their work, nurses use observation, questioning, and responding to obtain client information. Through self-awareness and reflection, nurses and other health care professionals can build skill in therapeutic communication and enhance their clinical practice. The use of the Johari window or Gibbs's reflective cycle can assist health care providers to strengthen their clinical insight and judgment, leading to personal growth and practice change. The key for therapeutic communication is being an active listener, using effective communication techniques (open- and closed-ended questions and focused questions), and avoiding nontherapeutic listening responses. The use of the acronyms of SOLER and SURETY by health care professionals is essential in therapeutic engagement. Effective communication is a skill, so as beginning practitioners, listening to your clients and using reflection and self-awareness will assist you in becoming competent in therapeutic communication.

REVIEW QUESTIONS

1. Define *therapeutic communication*.
2. Describe how nurses use touch as a form of communication.
3. List the five elements necessary for effective listening.
4. Identify four strategies nurses use to promote effective communication when meeting a client.
5. Describe why nurses' use of self-awareness is critical in their development as health care professionals.

REFERENCES

Arnold, E. C., & Boggs, K. U. (2020). *Interpersonal relationships: Professional communication skills for nurses* (8th ed., pp. 176–205). Elsevier.

Bagheri, M., Taleghani, F., Abazari, P., & Yousefy, A. (2019). Triggers for reflection in undergraduate clinical nursing education: A qualitative descriptive study. *Nurse Education Today, 75*, 35–40. https://doi.org/10.1016/j.nedt.2018.12.013

Barbagallo, M. S. (2019). Completing reflective practice post undergraduate nursing clinical placements: A literature review. *Teaching and Learning in Nursing, 14*(3), 160–165. https://doi.org/10.1016/j.teln.2019.02.001

Beebe, S. A., Beebe, S. J., & Redmond, M. V. (2020). *Interpersonal communication: Relating to others* (8th ed.). Pearson.

Blake, T., & Blake, T. (2019). Improving therapeutic communication in nursing through simulation exercise. *Teaching and Learning in Nursing, 14*(4), 260–264. https://doi.org/10.1016/j.teln.2019.06.003

Canadian Nurses Association. (2017). *Code of ethics for registered nurses* (2017 ed.). https://www.cna-aiic.ca/en/nursing/regulated-nursing-in-canada/nursing-ethics

Carroll, K. (2020). Insights of silence. *Nursing Science Quarterly, 33*(3), 222–224. https://doi.org/10.1177/0894318420920615

College of Registered Nurses of Newfoundland & Labrador. (2019). *Standards of practice for registered nurses and nurse practitioners.* https://www.crnnl.ca/site/uploads/2021/09/standards-of-practice-for-rns-and-nps.pdf

Egan, G. (2007). *The skilled helper: A problem-management approach to helping* (8th ed.). Brooks/Cole.

Ellison, D. L., & Meyer, C. K. (2020). Presence and therapeutic listening. *Nursing Clinics of North America, 55,* 457–465. https://doi.org/10.1016/j.cnur.2020.06.012

Fogger, S. A. (2019). Learning to communicate professionally. In N. L. Keltner & D. Steele (Eds.), *Psychiatric nursing* (8th ed.. pp. 75–82). Elsevier.

Gibbs, G. (1988). *Learning by doing: A guide to teaching and learning methods.* Oxford Brookes University.

Guest, M. (2016). How to introduce yourself to patients. *Nursing Standard, 30*(41), 36–38. https://doi.org/10.7748/ns.30.41/.36.s43

Haley, B., Heo, S., Wright, P., Barone, C., Rettiganti, M. R., & Anders, M. (2017). Relationships among active listening, self-awareness, empathy, and patient-centered care in associate and baccalaureate degree nursing students. *NursingPlus Open, 3,* 11–16. https://doi.org/10.1016/j.npls.2017.05.001

Han, S., & Kim, S. (2016). An integrative literature review on self-awareness education/training programs in the nursing area. *Perspectives in Nursing Science, 13*(2), 59–69. https://doi.org/10.16952/pns.2016.13.2.59

Johnston, R. (1971). Listen, nurse. *American Journal of Nursing, 71*(2), 303.

Kemerer, D. (2016). How to use intentional silence. *Nursing Standard, 31*(2), 42–44. https://doi.org/10.7748/ns.2016.e10538

Kwame, A., & Petrucka, P. M. (2021). A literature-based study of patient-centered care and communication in nurse-patient interactions: Barriers, facilitators, and the way forward. *BMC Nursing, 20*(158). https://doi.org/10.1186/s12912-021-00684-2

Loos, N. M. (2021). Nurse listening as perceived by patients. *The Journal of Nursing Administration, 51*(6), 324–328. https://doi.org/10.1097/NNA.0000000000001021

Luft, J. (1970). The Johari window: A graphical model of awareness in interpersonal relations. In *Group processes: An introduction to group dynamics* (pp. 11–20). National Press Books.

McCann, S., Barto, J., & Goldman, N. (2019). Learning through story listening. *American Journal of Health Promotion, 33*(3), 477–481. https://doi.org/10.1177/0890117119825525e

McKenna, L., Brown, T., Williams, B., & Lau, R. (2020). Empathic and listening styles of first year undergraduate nursing students: A cross-sectional study. *Journal of Professional Nursing, 36*(6), 611–615. https://doi.org/10.1016/j.profnurs.2020.08.013

Moore, H. L., Farnworth, A., Watson, R., Giles, K., Tomson, D., & Thomson, R. G. (2021). Inclusion of person-centred care in medical and nursing undergraduate curricula in the UK: Interviews and documentary analysis. *Patient Education and Counseling, 104*(4), 877–886. https://doi.org/10.1016/j.pec.2020.09.030

Nagle, A., & Foli, K. J. (2020). Student-centred reflection in debriefing: A concept analysis. *Clinical Simulation in Nursing, 39*, 33–40. https://doi.org/10.1016/j.ecns.2019.10.007

Oliver, S., & Duncan, S. (2019). Editorial: Looking through the Johari window. *Research for All, 3*(1), 1–6. https://doi.org/10.18546/RFA.03.1.01

Peplau, H. E. (1997). Peplau's theory of interpersonal relations. *Nursing Science Quarterly, 10*(4), 162–167. https://doi.org/10.1177/089431849701000407

Rasheed, S. P., Sundus, A., Younas, A., Fakhar, J., & Inayat, S. (2021). Development and testing of a measure of self-awareness among nurses. *Western Journal of Nursing Research, 43*(1), 36–44. https://doi.org/10.1177/0193945920923079

Rasheed, S. P., Younas, A., & Sundus, A. (2019). Self-awareness in nursing: A scoping review. *Journal of Clinical Nursing, 28*(5–6), 762–774. https://doi.org/10.1111/jocn.14708

Reljic, N., Pajnkihar, M., & Fekonja, Z. (2019). Self-reflection during first clinical practice: The experiences of nursing students. *Nurse Education Today, 72*, 61–66. https://doi.org/10.1016/j.nedt.2018.10.019

Rungapadiachy, D. M. (2007). *Self-awareness in health care: Engaging in helping relationships.* Palgrave Macmillan.

Stickley, T. (2011). From SOLER to SURETY for effective non-verbal communication. *Nurse Education in Practice, 11*(6), 395–398. https://doi.org/10.1016/j.nepr.2011.03.021

Willis, N. L., Wilson, B., Woodcock, E. B., Abraham, S. P., & Gillum, D. R. (2018). Appearance of nurses and perceived professionalism. *International Journal of Nursing Studies, 3*(3), 30–40. https://doi.org/10.20849/ijsn.v3i3.466

Xue, W., & Heffernan, C. (2021). Therapeutic communication within the nurse-patient relationship: A concept analysis. *International Journal of Nursing Practice, 27*(6), e12938. https://doi.org/10.1111/ijn.12938

Younas, A., Rasheed, S. P., Sundas, A., & Inayat, S. (2020). Nurses' perspectives of self-awareness in nursing practice: A descriptive qualitative study. *Nursing & Health Sciences, 22*(2), 398–405. https://doi.org/10.1111/nhs.12671

Younis, J. R., Mabrouk, S. M., & Kamal, F. F. (2015). Effect of the planned therapeutic communication program on therapeutic communication skills of pediatric nurses. *Journal of Nursing Education and Practice, 5*(8), 109–120. https://doi.org/10.5430/jnep.v5n8p109

CHAPTER 3

The Nurse-Client Relationship

INTRODUCTION

This chapter examines aspects of the therapeutic nurse-client relationship, which is considered foundational to nursing practice (Steuber & Pollard, 2018). A critical component in the development of a therapeutic nurse-client relationship is the use of effective communication by health care professionals in the provision of client care (Granados-Gámez et al., 2022). Caring is an important factor in nursing practice and is significant in the development of a helping relationship. Caring-within-practice is demonstrated in nurse-client encounters through the partnership of getting to know each other in the professional relationship (Hines, 2017). These caring interactions between the client and the care provider facilitate the formation of nurse-client relationships (Cussó et al., 2021). The chapter highlights the key traits (e.g., respect, genuineness, rapport, trust, empathy, confidentiality) that nurses must exemplify in order to establish a therapeutic alliance. Obstacles to effective nurse-client relationships are also explored. The phases of the therapeutic nurse-client relationship and aspects of the interpersonal relations theory, created by Peplau (1997), are described, and the concepts of self-disclosure and boundaries, which affect therapeutic nurse-client relationships, are examined.

CARING

Caring is a universal phenomenon that is shared among all health care professions. However, how the members of a particular profession demonstrate caring through their practice is what makes them distinct from one another (Martinez, 2019). Caring, a concept based on a human science perspective, is recognized as central within the discipline of nursing (Jaastad et al., 2022). Although there are multiple definitions of *caring* within the nursing literature, caring behaviours are identified as an essential aspect of nurse-client relationships (Persaud & Thornton, 2018). According to Lowry (2009), caring involves "the will to care, the intent to care, and caring actions" by the nurse (p. 32). Caring is demonstrated through continual interactions established through the nurse-client relationship, which may evolve in minutes or over extended periods of time, depending upon the client's reason for seeking health care.

In a meta-synthesis of the literature on caring, Finfgeld-Connett (2007) identified caring as an interpersonal process characterized by expert nursing practice, interpersonal sensitivity, and intimate relationships. The two types of caring behaviours identified are instrumental and expressive (Romero-Martin et al., 2019). Clients value these behaviours in bedside nurses. Instrumental caring behaviours reflect physical and technical skills, and expressive caring behaviours encompass nurses' ability to engage therapeutically with clients through the nurse-client relationship (De los Santos & Labrague, 2021).

Several nurse scholars identified caring as a central concept in their theories on caring, with aspects of unique interconnectedness between the nurse and client supporting a person-centred practice. Scholars such as Benner and Wrubel (1989), Leininger (1995), and Watson (2018a) classified caring as the core of nursing and relationships as central within professional nursing practice. Watson (2018b) stated that "caring can be effectively demonstrated and practiced only interpersonally" (p. 5) and such caring promotes health and growth for both the client and nurse. Jean Watson began to write about caring in the late 1970s and has continued to refine her caring theory. In 2013, she founded the Watson Caring Science Institute. The goal of this international nonprofit organization is to advance the unitary philosophies, theories, and practices of unitary caring science. Her theory of human caring involves 10 primary "caritas processes" that guide nurses to understand care as a phenomenon in an interpersonal relational process. She suggests that transpersonal relationships and the human-to-human caring moments in practice can create a caring-healing environment that serves to benefit the caregiver and the care recipient (Wei & Watson, 2019).

Care in nursing is experienced, established, and delivered through therapeutic nurse-client relationships. This relationship does not exist in isolation but includes clients, their families, nurses, and other health care team members (Feo et al., 2017). Within this caring relationship, the nurse "presence"—described as a *way of being* and a *way of relating, a way of being-with and being-there*—characterizes the therapeutic process occurring within the relationship. This nurse-client connection provides a safe space for clients to share and find meaning in the health-illness experience (Covington, 2005). Caring involves the therapeutic use of self by the nurse as a fundamental factor in establishing a therapeutic relationship. "It is through the use of nurse-self" (Wagner, 2002, p. 121) that caring and relational practices are of benefit to the client in establishing and developing a therapeutic encounter. Travelbee (1971) was the first to describe the nurse as an "instrument in therapeutic use of self." This attribute is defined as "the ability to use one's personality consciously and in full awareness in an attempt to establish relatedness and to structure nursing interventions" (p. 19). Such interventions through nurse-client collaboration promote safe, quality care outcomes for those accessing health care services (Pratt et al., 2021).

As a nursing student, you may observe a situation in the clinical area in which a nurse demonstrates a lack of caring. Some nurses may develop a level of detachment or feel emotionally fatigued due to job dissatisfaction or work demands, impairing their ability to care for clients (Powell, 2020). As highlighted in chapter 2, self-awareness and reflection are important personal strategies for nurses to use in building competency, self-understanding, and healthy self-care practices.

Self-Reflective Exercise

Think about the concept of caring and how it relates to the discipline of nursing. How do you define *caring*? Identify behaviours that reflect how nurses demonstrate caring within their clinical practice.

THE THERAPEUTIC RELATIONSHIP

What is a therapeutic relationship? Is this type of relationship the same as a social relationship? As a student entering a health professional program, you are very familiar with social relationships. A nursing pioneer, Hildegard E. Peplau, the founder of psychiatric–mental health nursing, first described the nurse-client relationship in the book *Interpersonal Relations in Nursing*, in 1952. Peplau's (1997) interpersonal relations theory is used by nurses as a vehicle to foster connections between the client and nurse in a professional therapeutic relationship and to assist clients to regain health and well-being. The theory described the nurse-client relationship as occurring through three interlocking, overlapping phases: orientation, working, and termination. The phases have changed over time to include a pre-interaction phase, which does not involve the client but provides the health care provider preparation time prior to the initial client encounter (Arnold & Boggs, 2020). These phases are discussed in more detail later in this chapter.

The therapeutic nurse-client relationship is defined as "one that is grounded in an interpersonal process that occurs between the nurse and the client. Therapeutic relationship is a purposeful, goal directed relationship that is intended at advancing the best interest and outcome of the client" (Registered Nurses' Association of Ontario, 2006, p. 13). In the health care system, clients enter an unfamiliar and sometimes unfriendly environment and need nurses who are welcoming, friendly, genuine, caring, and approachable. These behaviours are critical in building a therapeutic alliance with clients, enhancing the establishment of the professional nurse-client relationship.

Although effective health care communication is recognized as a core component of the health care system, it is a challenge as it is often considered the norm rather than the exception (Younis et al., 2015). Nurse-client interaction is valuable as it has been shown to promote client health and well-being, satisfaction, healing, recovery, and safety (Conroy et al., 2017; Nisa et al., 2019). Nursing students often find such interaction challenging and lack the confidence to engage in professional health care relationships (Cannity et al., 2021; Stevens et al., 2020). However, that is why it is essential to learn about nurse-client relationships and therapeutic communication: to facilitate effective interactions with clients, family members, and other health care professionals. Nurse educators have a responsibility to emphasize the relational aspects of care when working with students in both the classroom and the clinical practice area. The nurse-client relationship provides the foundation for all other nursing interventions. Having knowledge of nurse-client relationships and therapeutic communication will help students develop skill in this area, enhancing their competency as practitioners in everyday practice.

Table 3.1: Comparison of a Nurse-Client Relationship and Social Relationship

Nurse-Client Relationship	Social Relationship
Purpose: Professional helping	Purpose: Friendship, socialization, and enjoyment
Client-focused	Shared focus
Purposeful and time-limited	Open with respect to content and time
Mutually determined goals, short and long term	No specific goals
Intimate personal information restricted	Exchange of information not restricted
Nurse responsible for guiding interaction and meeting client needs	Shared responsibility for the interaction
Client issues/concerns explored/discussed with potential solutions	Mutually met needs
Solutions implemented by the client; nurse and client evaluate the degree of change in client	Giving advice, meeting dependency needs for all participants
Nurse uses communication skills in interaction, knowledge of human behaviour, and personal strengths to enhance client growth	Superficial communication; little evaluation of the interaction occurs
Nurse is objective, free from bias, and nonjudgmental	Subjective emphasis on one's own feelings and opinions
Self-disclosure used sparingly, and nurse needs to reflect on its benefit for client growth	Self-disclosure used by participants
Relationship is established when nurse meets client; relationship is terminated when client's health-related goal(s) is met or they are discharged or transferred to another health care facility	The relationship may be long term or short term, depending upon the participants

COMPONENTS OF A THERAPEUTIC RELATIONSHIP

The following elements are considered inherent to the professional therapeutic nurse–client relationship (College of Nurses of Ontario, 2019).

Respect

Showing respect for clients regardless of their diagnosis, culture, behaviour, values, and personal beliefs is critical in building interpersonal relationships. The nurse is accepting and nonjudgmental and through engagement comes to understand the client's health-illness perspective. Psychologist Carl Rogers called this *unconditional positive regard* (Frankel et al., 2012). Actions and attitudes displayed by the nurse show a willingness, in partnership with the client, to help the client use their strengths and resources to meet their health-related goals.

Case Study 3.1

Mrs. Elizabeth Wang, a 63-year-old woman, had abdominal surgery three days ago. She is lying in her bed after having a restless night's sleep. She is thinking, *I hope the doctor makes his rounds to check on my progress since surgery.* The day nurse enters the room and asks, "Good morning, honey. How are we doing today? Can you turn over on your back because I need to check your abdomen dressing before the doctor arrives? If you can turn quickly, that would be great."

1. What communication behaviours in this interaction show respect? How many can you identify?
2. In the above scenario, the nurse demonstrates a lack of respect through their actions. Reflect on the information about therapeutic communication presented in chapter 2. As the nurse in this situation, identify the behaviours (verbal and nonverbal) that would display unconditional positive regard for the client.

Nurses can communicate respect by doing the following (Clucas et al., 2019):

-   Asking clients how they prefer to be addressed (calling them by full name and title, first name, formal/informal)
-   Knocking and announcing themselves before entering the client's room or space
-   Spending time with the client (not just to complete a task)
-   Being honest in all communications
-   Asking before touching
-   Providing privacy
-   Maintaining confidentiality

- Taking time to answer the client's questions and concerns
- Involving the client in all care-treatment decisions
- Respecting the client's opinions, values, ideas, and preferences
- Providing appropriate information
- Valuing the client as a person
- Displaying an atmosphere of cultural safety in all communications

Genuineness

Genuineness or authenticity in nurses is important in the development of the nurse-client relationship. Genuineness is the nurse's ability to be real when engaging with the client (Schnellbacher & Leijssen, 2009). In this relational process, the nurse has awareness of feelings that may arise in the relationship. It implies congruence between what the nurse is feeling and the expression of that feeling. The nurse has knowledge and awareness of if and when to use self-disclosure and uses actions such as listening and therapeutic communication techniques appropriately and effectively in getting to know and understand the client's experience (Schnellbacher & Leijssen, 2009). The nurse, working in partnership with the client, enhances the client's ability to identify issues and work on strategies to cope with factors impacting their health. When the nurse is genuine within the relationship, the base for trust can be established, which is crucial for the therapeutic alliance (Greene & Ramos, 2021).

Case Study 3.2

The client is a 70-year-old divorced man with a history of prolonged substance use. He has been admitted to the medical unit for assessment of enlarged spleen, jaundice, and persistent cough. Since being admitted to the unit, he has been mildly confused and anxious but reports no abdominal pain. The day nurses noted that he tends to use his call light frequently but is in no extreme distress. The night nurse, who has been on the unit for an hour, notices that he has rung his call light. After waiting 10 minutes, the nurse stands at the doorway to his room and asks (in a loud tone, rolling their eyes with hands on hips), "You rang your call light. How can I help you?"

1. What does the behaviour displayed by the nurse indicate to the client?
2. How could the nurse's bias about substance use impact client care?
3. As a nursing student providing care, how would you respond in this situation?

Rapport

Rapport building starts as soon as the nurse meets the client. Think about the first time you meet someone; what is the first thing you do? When meeting the client and their family members for the first time, it is important to introduce yourself and explain your role, the reason for the interaction, and the information to be collected. Nurses show care and interest by knowing the client's name. At this time, if unsure, ask the client to pronounce their name, and also ask how they would prefer to be addressed. Rapport building leads to the development of trust within the nurse-client relationship. According to English et al. (2021), a "simple welcome" that includes greeting with a smile, small talk, eye contact, use of verbal and nonverbal communication, and taking the time to connect as human beings enhances rapport building with clients. Rapport building is considered essential if nurses use a person-centred approach in their clinical practice. Despite the heavy workloads and demands on nurses' time, taking time to incorporate simple gestures, such as greeting clients in a friendly and welcoming manner, are essential for communication competency and establishment of professional relationships (Bladh & Van Leeuwen, 2017).

Trust

Trust is considered one of the most critical components of the therapeutic nurse-client relationship (College of Registered Nurses of Newfoundland and Labrador [CRNNL], 2014). Nurses' interpersonal caring attributes and professional competency over the course of an interaction support the development of trust (Ozaras & Abaan, 2018). Trust cannot be presumed; it must be earned, and once broken it is difficult to re-establish. Some examples of nursing interventions that promote trust include the following (Greene & Ramos, 2021; Ozaras & Abaan, 2018):

- Keeping promises
- Showing warmth and kindness
- Smiling
- Being honest (e.g., saying "I don't know the answer to your question, but I will try to find out" and then following through)
- Ensuring confidentiality
- Being consistent in adhering to unit guidelines
- Providing clear and concise reasons for certain policies, procedures, and rules
- Providing privacy
- Using active listening
- Using attending behaviours—SOLER/SURETY
- Providing a safe environment

- Using the client's proper name—avoiding the use of labels/bed number of client, or medical diagnosis or treatment (e.g., the difficult client in Room 245 or the colostomy in Room 225)
- Being accessible
- Setting limits
- Being sensitive to client needs (e.g., providing a blanket if cold)
- Being flexible
- Considering the client's preferences, requests, and opinions in care decisions
- Maintaining professional boundaries
- Providing support and reassurance during procedures/treatments
- Spending time with the client
- Demonstrating caring

Empathy

Empathy is a critical component in the development of therapeutic nurse-client relationships (Patterson, 2018). Moudatsou et al. (2020) suggest that empathy is a communication skill consisting of three dimensions—emotional, cognitive, and behavioural—that is used by many health professionals to develop relationships. When a health care provider utilizes empathy, they demonstrate to the client that they have some awareness and interpersonal understanding of the client's feelings and communicate those feelings to the client without losing objectivity (Deligianni et al., 2017). This is like "walking in the client's shoes," even though the nurse has not had the same experience as the client. The nurse communicates understanding and meaning of the client's feelings through the use of empathy, an essential aspect of therapeutic communication techniques. Empathy is an interpersonal process that provides the nurse an opportunity to get to know the client in the context of human interaction (McKinnon, 2018). Through knowing the client, they come to understand the client's feelings, and they convey such perception to the client through validation. This acknowledgement helps the client to create a stronger bond with the nurse because they feel understood, thus building trust (Mikkelsen et al., 2019). It is important to note that empathy sometimes gets confused with sympathy. *Sympathy* is a word that is derived from the ancient Greek word *sympatheia*, which literally means "to suffer with." Today, sympathy is considered a nontherapeutic response by health care providers as it is regarded as a "pity-based" response and more subjective than objective (Guerrero, 2019).

It is important for nursing students to build knowledge and skill in therapeutic communication techniques. Many of the techniques (behaviours) discussed in chapter 2 are applicable for use when communicating empathically with clients. Students communicate *empathy* by demonstrating to clients, verbally and nonverbally, an understanding of how they are feeling. Several strategies—such as listening, showing courtesy/respect, observing, using attending behaviours, using verbal and nonverbal behaviours and validation techniques—indicate that understanding to clients. An empathic approach helps promote client recovery and achievement of their health care goals (Burkhartzmeyer et al., 2021). See the following case example, which demonstrates how the communication technique of empathy is used by the nurse.

Case Example

Mrs. Tina Bellows is a 40-year-old female who was admitted to the medical surgical unit with a diagnosis of infection in her right toe. The client has a history of cardiovascular disease controlled by medication and diabetes mellitus type 2 treated with insulin. Her hemoglobin A1C (blood glucose) levels have been unstable for about two weeks. It has been noted that her right toe is warm to the touch and slightly red, with a 2 cm broken area that is not healing. She has an intravenous of normal saline (NS 0.9%) running at 100 cc/hour in her left arm and is receiving 1 g of cefazolin intravenously every eight hours.

Nurse: (*knocks and enters client's room*) "Good morning, Mrs. Bellows. I am here to change your toe dressing. How are you feeling right now?"

Client: (*lying in bed and looking up at nurse*) "Not very well. My toe is painful all the time. My A1C levels are out of whack, and I don't know how long before things get better."

Nurse: (*pulls up a chair next to bed, looks at client, and speaks in a soft tone*) "I understand it has been quite a difficult time for you with everything going on. It is hard to stay positive with your ongoing health concerns. I just want to let you know that you are in the right place because Dr. Smith and I and the rest of the health care team will do our best to care for you."

Student Tip

As you enter clinical practice settings, you may experience some anxiety as you work to build helping relationships with clients. With support from your clinical faculty and your use of reflection and self-awareness, you will learn to become comfortable with therapeutic communication throughout your development as you become a professional nurse. The key is to always remember to centre yourself when you enter the client's space and be present in the moment when interacting (Turner et al., 2019).

Confidentiality

Professional nursing organizations have articulated the importance of protecting clients' privacy and confidentiality for information obtained in the context of a therapeutic nurse-client relationship (Canadian Nurses Association [CNA], 2017; CRNNL, 2019). The CRNNL (2019) Standards of Practice, Standard 3: Client Centred Practice (3.5) states that a nurse "Upholds and protects clients' privacy and confidentiality in all forms of communication including, but not limited to, e-records, verbal, written, and social media" (p. 7). Although this document is directed at practising nurses, the duty to maintain privacy and confidentiality also extends to nursing students. Nurses, regardless of the clinical area, have an ethical and legal responsibility to keep client information private, secure, and confidential. Privacy laws in Canada at the federal and provincial level mandate an individual's right to privacy of their personal health information. In Canada, all provinces and territories have passed their own health privacy laws, and hospitals are usually covered by these provincial laws. Nurses and nursing students should be familiar with these laws as well as employer policies that outline practices for privacy and confidentiality of client information. For example, in Newfoundland and Labrador, the provincial government passed the Personal Health Information Act (Government of Newfoundland and Labrador, 2008), which outlines the procedures for collecting, using, disclosing, and storing personal health information. Within this act, reference is made to the "circle of care," which "means the persons participating in and activities related to the provision of health care to the individual" (p. 19). This includes any health care provider who is directly involved in the treatment plan and provides care to the individual.

When nurses meet clients for the first time (orientation phase), confidentiality is discussed, and this is also repeated throughout the other phases of the nurse-client relationship. It is considered one of the parameters in establishing the nurse-client relationship. The client is informed of why information is collected, how it is stored, and the possibility of sharing information for those involved in the "circle of care" for development of a health care plan. During nursing assessment, family members may be interviewed to provide collateral information to support assessment. In some instances, family members may ask the nurse about private information that the client shared with those in the "circle of care." Nurses are legally and ethically responsible to keep the information private unless the client has given consent to share with family members. All client information is privileged material and should be treated confidentially. Nurses in all clinical areas can access client health information records for those under their care and should not access the records of other clients. All clients should be informed that there are limitations to confidentiality: nurses have a duty to report information about a client at risk for suicide or causing harm to others. In these situations, information must be shared with others.

Student Tip

These ethical principles and documents will guide you in the development of relationships with clients, families, and colleagues around the use and sharing of client information.

POWER

Health care institutions and hospitals have traditionally been associated with hierarchical patriarchal structures that impact health care communication. Although there is no agreed upon definition of *power* within the health professions, it has been conceptualized as a multifaceted concept that may positively or adversely affect client care (Fawcett & Zhang, 2021; Griscti et al., 2017). According to Fawcett and Zhang (2021), "the perspective of power each of us hold determines how we act with each other and with those who seek our care" (p. 94). Health care professionals, including nurses, need an awareness of how a hierarchical health care system influences their work environment, their relationships with clients and families, and other health care workers. Nurses can use power to advocate for clients as well as to influence change within the health care system (Fackler et al., 2015). In a nurse-client relationship, there is a power imbalance because of the nurse's authority in the health care system and the client's vulnerability. The health care provider has knowledge of and access to the client's personal health information, which, from a negative perspective of power, can be seen as control or power-over. However, within the nurse-client relationship, power may be evident as cooperation that involves the client and health care provider in a partnership, meaning power is shared (Fawcett & Zhang, 2021; Flagg, 2015). From this perspective of shared decision-making, meaningful client engagement within the relationship supports a person-centred approach in the health care system. It is important that the nurse is vigilant and maintains the therapeutic relationship to prevent abuse of such power (CNA, 2017; College and Association of Registered Nurses of Alberta [CARNA], 2020; College of Registered Nurses of Manitoba [CRNM], 2019).

In the current health care system, the focus is on working to achieve active client participation in care decision-making related to their values and preferences. This requires honest, effective communication by health care professionals in the provision of client care, appropriate use of language, and a collaborative relationship in clinical practice. When health care providers interact with clients, their power is evident, but being aware of this will help them recognize and understand its influence, leading to an improvement in care. In nurse-client scenarios, determine if the power dynamics reflect a positive approach.

Case Example

Lynn Tanner is a 49-year-old unmarried female who was diagnosed five years ago with breast cancer and underwent a mastectomy of her left breast and follow-up chemotherapy. Two years ago, Ms. Tanner experienced a recurrence of cancer in her other breast and underwent another mastectomy and round of chemotherapy. Last month, she experienced a recurrence of cancer in her left lung. She has been admitted to hospital for a removal of her affected lung and to begin a regime of chemotherapy. As the nurse, you enter her room to check her vital signs and begin some preop teaching.

Nurse: "Hi, Lynn. I know you are scheduled for surgery tomorrow, so I am here to check your blood pressure, temperature, and pulse. I will also provide you with some preop information. How are you feeling this morning?"

Client: "I am not sure, really. I just feel so tired of all of this and having to face another surgery and chemotherapy. It will make no difference; the cancer just keeps coming back."

Nurse: "Well, I think it is important for you to follow through with the surgery and treatment. You are still a very young woman and have a lot to live for."

SHARED DECISION-MAKING

Shared decision-making (SDM) is a collaborative approach between health care professionals and clients that is considered an essential element of effective health care (Baca-Dietz et al., 2021). SDM emphasizes a person-centred approach in the provider-client relationship, fostering self-determination, autonomy, and choice through partnership in the decision-making process (Muscat et al., 2020; Pavlo et al., 2019). According to Truglio-Lordrigan and Slyer (2018), communication and relationship building are foundational for the shared decision-making process. The individuals within the relationship work on building trust and respect in a relational way through collaboration and sharing of power. Through open communication, information is obtained from an assessment of the client's issues, feelings, preferences, and reason for seeking health care. This assessment helps health care professionals get to know the client, the client's family, and their understanding of the health care issue. Using this knowledge in collaboration with the client, possible options for action are discussed, goals are set, and progress is evaluated on an ongoing basis (Lenzen et al., 2018). An important role for health care providers in integrating SDM into practice is to provide clients—taking into account their health literacy skills—with the appropriate information in order to facilitate an interactive decision-making process

(Muscat et al., 2020). Although shared decision-making is the focus within health care relationships, it is an individual choice. Some clients may decide not to be involved and let health care professionals included in their "circle of care" make their care decisions. Other clients, because of their health status and diagnosis, may not be able to be fully involved in the shared decision-making process.

PHASES OF A THERAPEUTIC NURSE-CLIENT RELATIONSHIP

The foundation of nursing practice is the nurse's ability to engage in interpersonal relationships with clients. In today's chaotic health care system, the nurse may have an opportunity to meet the client only briefly or have more prolonged encounters, depending on the client's health-related needs. Hildegard Peplau (1997) was a nurse theorist and a pioneer in the development of the theory and practice of psychiatric mental health nursing. Peplau was the first nurse who emphasized the importance of the nurse-client relationship as the foundation of nursing practice. Although she developed her interpersonal relations theory from her work in psychiatric nursing, her theoretical model has been adopted and recognized as a critical tool for all areas of nursing practice. The structure of nurse-client relationships is described through four distinct overlapping phases (Arnold & Boggs, 2020; Peplau, 1997): pre-interaction, orientation (introductory), working, and termination. It is important for health professionals to keep in mind that the phases are not a sequence of processes but are used to guide nursing approaches according to the client's status and health care needs (Steele, 2019).

Pre-Interaction Phase

This phase provides an opportunity for the health care provider to obtain client information from the clinical chart or from discussions with other health care team members. This is the only phase of the nurse-client relationship in which the client does not directly participate. During this time, the nurse can reflect on feelings, fears, assumptions, or concerns prior to the first interaction. For example, the nurse takes a call from a nurse in the emergency room (ER) about a client transfer to the medical floor. The floor nurse receives a brief report from the ER nurse on a 35-year-old woman who has been involved in a motor vehicle accident. The client received some facial lacerations, a fracture of her left femur, and some chest contusions. Her husband, who was driving the car, sustained only minor abrasions on his upper and lower extremities. The client will be transferred to the unit in the next hour. Being aware of this information allows the floor nurse to prepare the client's assigned room and think about an approach to use with the client.

Orientation Phase

Initially in this phase, the nurse and client get to know each other. During this process, clients learn about the role of the health care provider in helping them with their health-illness needs. The nurse works to create an environment for establishing trust and rapport. The nurse also addresses the parameters of the relationship (e.g., purpose, roles, and framework for assessment), identifies the client's strengths and weaknesses, and explores both the client's feelings and their own. Confidentiality is discussed and termination is introduced and discussed throughout the relationship. The nurse should use appropriate therapeutic communication techniques as outlined in chapter 2, for instance, during the initial building of trust and rapport, which includes making introductions; learning the client's name, professional status, and title; and sharing essential information about the purpose and nature of the relationship. From the client assessment, the nurse determines what health issue is of most concern from the client's perspective.

Case Example

Nurse: (*knocks on client's room door, smiles, and enters to begin assessment*) "Good Morning, Mrs. White. My name is John Rideout. I am the registered nurse, and I will be taking care of you today. How are you feeling since coming to the floor? The goal right now is to get you ready for your upcoming surgery scheduled for 1100 hours. The anesthesiologist will be here in about a half hour to complete your preop assessment."

Client: "Thank you, John. I'm feeling a little groggy from the pain medication they gave me in emergency last night. My husband, Paul, should be here shortly. He went home to talk to my parents, who are looking after the kids. I would like to see the clergy before going for surgery. Is that possible?"

Nurse: (*looking at the client*) "Not a problem. I will see who is on call and notify them that you would like to see them before surgery. I will have to prepare you for the procedure by assisting you with a preop bed bath and helping you put on a special operating room gown. Do you have any questions about the upcoming procedure?"

Client: "No, John, but will I be coming back to this floor after surgery?"

In this scenario, as evidenced by the nurse-client dialogue, the immediate concern for the client is the surgical preparation for treatment of her fractured femur. The nurse is focused on that issue and is attending to building trust and rapport by introducing themselves, assessing the client's immediate concerns, and providing information in preparation for the upcoming surgical procedure.

Working Phase

In this phase, the nurse works to build the relationship with the use of appropriate therapeutic communication (e.g., listening, asking open-ended questions, validating), maintaining trust and rapport. The nurse is collecting further data as part of the ongoing assessment process and promoting client insight and problem-solving around health-related goals. In collaboration with the client, the nurse determines the client's main issues and how they may impact recovery. The nurse uses a shared decision-making approach with the client to promote guidance on overcoming resistance behaviours, while evaluating issues and goals, and refining them as necessary for goal attainment. Clients may disclose more personal concerns or issues that they are experiencing. For example, you may work with a client who is experiencing major depressive disorder and has low self-esteem. They may disclose their use of substances as a way to deal with their ongoing depression. In this instance, the focus is on respecting the client's perspective and not giving advice but promoting self-care, helping the client initiate change to effectively cope with their illness.

Termination Phase

Termination is discussed in the orientation and the working phase of the relationship to help prepare the client for discharge. The termination phase may occur for a variety of reasons: clients may have accomplished their goals, been transferred to another facility, or been discharged to home.

Termination is a critical part of the therapeutic nurse-client relationship and provides an opportunity for the client and nurse to recognize and explore feelings about termination. A review, evaluation, and summary of strategies for post-discharge occurs. This may involve providing the client with information about contact agencies in case issues arise or a referral for community follow-up with a nurse or other health care providers. However, in many inpatient and outpatient health care settings, the client's goals may not be completed before discharge or transfer to another level of care.

It is important that the client is prepared for termination well in advance of the date and time of the final nurse-client interaction. This provides the health care provider and the client time to explore feelings about termination. Some clients may not feel they are ready for discharge and have fears about how they will cope when at home. The nurse and the client may feel a sense of loss or sadness due to the termination of the relationship. These feelings are normal and should be acknowledged and discussed with the client prior to relationship termination.

Student Tip

Keep in mind that you may not have time to develop all phases of the nurse-client relationship due to client status and the length of your clinical practice experience. During your clinical rotations, you may also have to terminate relationships with assigned clients early due to the completion of your clinical rotations. You may feel a sense of loss or sadness, which is a normal response to the ending of a professional relationship. It is okay for nursing students to express care and concern and convey best wishes for the client's future (Ashton, 2016). You may benefit from discussing your feelings with your clinical faculty and also through reflection on the practice experience.

ROLES OF THE NURSE

In Peplau's (1991) interpersonal relations theory, several defined sub-roles that the nurse may undertake throughout the interpersonal process in building the nurse-client therapeutic relationship are highlighted. As a professional health care team member, nurses' roles may vary depending upon their particular clinical practice area. These six roles, when engaging with clients, are stranger, resource person, teacher, leader, surrogate, or counsellor. In the role of stranger, the nurse and the client come together in their initial meeting as strangers but come to know each other through trust formation and the development of the therapeutic nurse-client relationship. As the relationship develops, the nurse may take on other roles, depending on the health care needs of the client. Within this relationship, the nurse serves as an important resource person for the client and family members. Through a collaborative approach, the nurse uses appropriate language that the client understands, supplies information, interprets clinical data, and answers questions related to their particular health care needs. In the sub-role of teacher, the nurse, following an assessment of the client and family's learning needs, provides instruction, education, and evaluation to support self-care. For example, a client who is prescribed a medication to manage their diabetes receives instruction on its use, common adverse effects, and contraindications. In the counsellor role, the nurse uses effective therapeutic communication techniques to explore the client's understanding of their illness experience. This helps the nurse and the client have a greater understanding of the client's present health-illness concerns. This knowledge aids the nurse's guidance and support, which contributes to the best client outcomes and self-care initiatives. In the role of surrogate, the nurse works to promote client autonomy through advocacy and shared decision-making within the therapeutic relationship. This process promotes client independence rather than dependence on health care providers. In the active leader role, the nurse assists the client to be an active participant through collaboration in the development of treatment goals and a personal health care plan. Think about the different roles that you may undertake as a professional nursing student while completing your clinical practice experiences.

Professional Boundaries

Professional boundaries are a critical aspect of the nurse-client relationship, and the nurse has the responsibility for maintaining the boundaries that establish the parameters of the relationship. The nurse-client relationship is client-focused, and boundaries represent invisible structures imposed by legal, ethical, and professional nursing standards that help to keep the relationship therapeutic, safe, and respectful (CARNA, 2020). In maintaining professional boundaries, the nurse helps to build the foundation for the relationship and nurtures the sense of trust in the client (Smythe et al., 2018). The nurse is obligated to inform clients, family, and other health care providers when a potential conflict exists (see case example).

Case Example

You are a nurse working on an acute psychiatric admission unit with several registered nurses (RNs) and licensed practical nurses (LPNs) on each shift. During the day shift, you noticed that one of the LPNs was selling chocolates as a fundraiser for the community church choir and was approaching staff. Later during the shift, you observe the LPN approaching unit clients with the order form. Although you observe no clients being pressured to purchase, the LPN informs them that it is a fundraiser for the community church. Does this behaviour influence the therapeutic relationship? Is this a boundary violation? As a colleague of the LPN, what would you do?

Boundaries of the therapeutic relationship are classified as boundary crossings and boundary violations (CARNA, 2020; CRNM, 2019).

Boundary Crossings

Boundary crossings are identified as brief, intentional excursions across boundaries that are done to meet a client's therapeutic need. An example is self-disclosure, where brief personal information from the nurse is shared with the client. The reason for the disclosure is of therapeutic benefit to the overall care of the client and is not done to meet the personal needs of the nurse. Nurse self-awareness and reflection, and dialogue with other nurses or health care providers, is essential in these situations. Continual crossing of the boundary line should be avoided, as it may lead to boundary violations that are harmful or exploitive (Hall, 2011; Peternelj-Taylor & Yonge, 2003). An example of appropriate and healthy self-disclosure would be a nurse showing empathy for a client who is grieving from the loss of a child by briefly relating their own personal experience with loss.

Boundary Violations

Boundary violations occur when an act or behaviour is unacceptable and the client's needs are no longer the focus of the therapeutic relationship. Boundary violations occur when the nurse confuses their own needs with those of the client. The nurse loses sight of their own boundaries or has not understood the client's boundaries, which leads to harm and damage to the therapeutic relationship. Several common professional boundary violations have been identified and will be discussed here: dual relationships, gifts and money, excessive self-disclosure, secretive behaviour, overinvolvement, sexual behaviour, and social media (CARNA, 2020; Manfrin-Ledet et al., 2015).

Dual Relationships

This happens within the therapeutic nurse-client relationship when the nurse has other demands or stresses in addition to the nurse-client relationship. For example, the nurse becomes a business partner with or romantic partner to the client. As a result of these dual relationships, possible conflicts of interest arise, which impact clinical objectivity and impair professional judgment. In these violations, the nurse's needs are being met by the client (Baca, 2011).

Gifts and Money

Nurses must evaluate the implications of gifts from clients. There should be no exchange of money. Gifts considered "token gifts," such as chocolates, flowers, cards, or notes of thanks, usually given as a show of appreciation for care, are acceptable as they can be shared with all staff. Expensive gifts are not acceptable; in these instances, agency policy regarding gifts can be explained to the client and family members. However, if the client insists on giving a gift, the nurse can refer them to a supervisor to discuss acceptable ways to provide a gift (e.g., to the hospital foundation).

Excessive Self-Disclosure

Nurses in a professional therapeutic nurse-client relationship can use self-disclosure, but it is best to use it sparingly and with purpose (Knapp, 2015). It is considered useful if it helps to build rapport and provides therapeutic value for the client. The self-disclosure is not acceptable if it is done to meet the needs of the nurse as it creates confusion and impacts the parameters of the nurse-client relationship. Nurses should not discuss personal problems or aspects of their intimate life with clients.

Secretive Behaviour

This type of violation involves the nurse keeping certain behaviours or knowledge from the client and/or others with selective sharing of information. This can occur if the nurse withholds information about illegal or unhealthy activities the client is involved in; client abuse or neglect; or personal, social, or business financial arrangements between the nurse and the client or family member (Manfrin-Ledet et al., 2015)—for example, if the nurse is in the process of moving to a new house and hires the client's moving company because they will be given a reduced rate.

Sexual Behaviour

Romantic or sexual relationships are never appropriate between nurses and clients. Clients are vulnerable, and the responsibility is on the nurse to maintain professional boundaries even if the client initiates the sexual behaviour (Manfrin-Ledet et al., 2015). In their professional role, nurses should not initiate sexual interactions, use sexually suggestive comments or off-colour jokes, or engage in inappropriate touching. Nurses need to be cognizant of the importance of maintaining healthy boundaries in the nurse-client relationship; often they are unaware they have crossed a boundary. In some instances, nurses may be on the receiving end of sexual behaviour exhibited by clients. This behaviour may involve sexual comments, inappropriate touching, indecent exposure, or off-colour jokes.

If you experience inappropriate sexual comments from clients, you can follow these recommendations (Smith et al., 1997):

- Clarify your role as nurse and care provider.
- Set appropriate verbal boundaries. State, for example, "I'm uncomfortable when you speak (or touch me) that way. Please don't."

- Set physical boundaries. Ask a colleague to assist with care if necessary.
- Consult with the unit manager—does the situation warrant reassignment?
- Document interactions with the client as directed by your manager and hospital policy.
- Seek support from colleagues and/or a counsellor from the employee assistance program.
- Treat the client respectfully when redirecting inappropriate behaviour.

Overinvolvement

In some circumstances within the professional-client relationship, the nurse may become overinvolved, which is considered a boundary violation. In such cases, the nurse may display a variety of behaviours:

- Giving extra time and attention to certain clients
- Visiting the client in off-duty hours
- Doing things for the client that they can do for themselves
- Keeping secrets with the client
- Believing that they are the only one who understands the client's needs
- Dressing differently when assigned to certain clients
- Switching assignments or shifts to work with certain clients
- Showing jealousy when other nurses are assigned to the client
- Wanting to spend their break times with clients
- Thinking or daydreaming about client when away from work (CARNA, 2020).

The opposite of overinvolvement is disengagement. This occurs when nurses find themselves withdrawing from a client due to the client's behaviour, diagnosis, or intensity of suffering. These feelings may lead nurses to reject the client, label them, and use judgmental communication (Arnold & Boggs, 2020). Nurses' use of self-awareness and reflection should help to maintain appropriate boundaries in all aspects of the professional-client relationship.

Social Media

Today social networking is a popular and common method of communication. According to Catlin (2013), the most significant area of boundary violation involves nurses' use and misuse of social media. Nurses need to be keenly aware that postings on social media sites can impact their personal and professional lives. Even though clients may ask, nurses should not disclose their personal email address or phone number. The following principles provide guidance related to nurses' use of social media (Canadian Nurses Protective Society, 2021; CARNA, 2020; Catlin, 2013; CRNNL, 2013):

- Nurses must protect client privacy and confidentiality.
- Nurses must not post any client information or pictures on social media sites.
- Nurses should not "friend" or "follow" past or present clients.
- Nurses should separate the use of social media for professional and social purposes. Any posting on any social media platform may come to be viewed by clients, colleagues, and employers.
- Nurses should not post disparaging remarks about employers or co-workers. These actions can result in employment and/or personal liability consequences.

Student Tip

These principles and professional practice documents on the use of social media will guide your practice during client encounters.

Other relationship boundaries that may occur in all helping relationships are transference and countertransference. *Transference* occurs in relationships when the client unconsciously or inappropriately transfers onto the nurse feelings, desires, and behaviours related to significant others in their past. This transference can be positive or negative and may involve feelings of hostility, jealousy, or love. The nurse is in a position of authority in the relationship, so the client could displace feelings of hostility toward the nurse if the nurse reminds them of a former boss who was autocratic. As another example, the client could displace feelings of love toward the nurse because the nurse reminds them of their grandfather, who was kind and caring (O'Brien, 2013).

Countertransference is the nurse's unconscious personal response or feelings toward the client, which can be related to either positive or negative associations. These responses can impact the development and maintenance of the nurse-client relationship (O'Brien, 2013). For example, the client may remind the nurse of their grandmother, who cared for them during illness. This could result in the nurse doing everything for the client, promoting dependence. A nurse might show strong feelings toward a client who reminds them of their father, who abused alcohol. This could cause the nurse to disengage from the client, impacting the nurse-client relationship. To work through and identify transference and countertransference issues, nurses need to be self-aware and have knowledge of issues occurring in the nurse-client relationship. Such insight will help them to seek guidance from colleagues, unit managers, or other health team members, leading to professional growth and improved client care.

Case Study 3.3

Mr. Austin Miller is a 65-year-old retired teacher who lives with his partner, William. He is admitted to your hospital on the surgical unit with a diagnosis of acute cholecystitis. He is scheduled to undergo a cholecystectomy the next day. This is the first time that he had to be scheduled for a surgical procedure. You are a first-year nursing student who is assigned to this client and will help to prepare him for the surgical procedure.

1. Describe how you will initiate your first encounter with Mr. Miller.
2. After you complete the introduction, identify several open-ended questions you can use to engage the client.
3. Mr. Miller states, "This is the first time that I have ever had to have surgery. I am very nervous. I am not a young man, you know. When can William visit after I have the surgery?" How would you respond to the client?
4. Identify the type of therapeutic communication techniques that you used in responding to Mr. Miller.
5. Identify some caring behaviours that you would use in development of the nurse-client relationship.
6. How do you show respect to Mr. Miller in your nursing behaviours?
7. What did you learn from doing this exercise that could be used in your clinical practice?

Case Study 3.4

Ms. Penny Smith is a 25-year-old female admitted to the emergency department (ED) following an accident with a city bus. She was riding her bicycle to dance class but was hit on the side when the bus was making a turn. She was thrown from her bike and landed on the ground, hitting her head. On arrival to the ED, she is awake and alert but having a lot of pain in her left hip and right foot. While being assessed, she is worried about her future and thinking about whether she will ever dance again.

1. You are the nurse working in Room 3 of the ED, and this is the first time you are meeting the client. Describe how best to demonstrate empathy, respect, and trust using introductions. List what needs to be done and communicated to the client that will aid development of a therapeutic nurse-client relationship.

Case Study 3.5

Abby Chan, aged 30 years, has been married for 12 years and is the mother of a 6-year-old girl. She is admitted to the acute care mental health unit with a possible diagnosis of major depressive disorder. Her husband, John, is a prominent engineer in a downtown firm. Abby tells the nurse that her marriage has not been going well for the past year and she is planning to divorce John. Over the past several months, she has not been sleeping well and has been overeating and having a lot of physical complaints.

　　The nurse, looking at the client, responds to Abby, "You've got a lot of things going on right now. It sounds like a troubling time for you. Tell me about your relationship with your husband."

1.　Identify the communication techniques used by the nurse in response to Abby. Describe the rationale for your identification of the technique.

Case Study 3.6

You are a nurse working on a 24-bed surgical unit in a large city hospital. During the evening shift, a 28-year-old female client is to be admitted with a diagnosis of a bowel obstruction and will be in Room 285A. Jacob is the nurse looking after this room, so you inform him about the admission. Jacob admits the client, Emily Barker, and comments to you later, "Thanks for giving me that admission. She is so attractive." Over the next few weeks, you notice that Jacob is coming in during his days off to care for the client and also asking to switch with other staff for this specific assignment. As a colleague, you are concerned about Jacob's behaviour.

1.　In your assessment of the course of events, what is happening?
2.　How will you approach Jacob about the situation?

CHAPTER SUMMARY

Caring is recognized as central to nursing practice and is fostered through the initiation of the professional-client relationship. This relationship is critical in the establishment of a person-centred approach that is focused on the client's experience of their health–illness continuum. The relationship has been classified as the "caring interaction," and is characterized by traits such as empathy, active listening, presence, genuineness, and respect, which the professional nurse must possess to engage authentically in therapeutic nurse-client relationships.

The nurse-client relationship is characterized by four overlapping phases: pre-interaction, orientation, working, and termination. Pre-interaction is the only phase of the relationship in which the client does not directly participate. During this phase, the nurse is gathering information about client (e.g., their medical record), preparing the physical environment, and thinking about the initial interaction. This process may involve collaboration with other health care providers to prepare for immediate client needs.

In the orientation phase, the parameters of the relationship (e.g., purpose, roles, process rules, and assessment framework) are covered. Here the client and the nurse meet as strangers but work to develop a partnership through communication to address client health needs. In this phase, the nurse begins data collection with the client and builds a sense of trust by introducing themselves. The nurse provides a caring, respectful approach that fosters the client's expression of their feelings and thoughts. At this time, the client's strengths and limitations are assessed, their concerns are identified, and mutually agreed-upon goals are formulated.

Most of the work is done in the working phase. The client's health goals are the focus within an individualized care plan where the client assumes responsibility for completion so that independence is promoted. The final phase is termination, which is discussed at the initial encounter to prepare the client for the relationship closure. A review, evaluation, and summarization of goals is undertaken, and referrals are completed if needed. Also, it is necessary for the nurse to discuss with the client their feelings about termination.

Therapeutic relationships have professional boundaries, which can be physical or psychological. The nurse is responsible for maintaining these boundaries as they help to establish the parameters of the relationship. These boundaries keep the relationship focused on client needs and provide a safe space for the nurse and client to establish rapport and trust where mutual understanding of the client's needs is explored. Nurses are ethically and legally obligated to maintain professional boundaries and can face disciplinary action by their employer or professional nursing organization for failing to do so.

REVIEW QUESTIONS

Read the following three review questions and select the best option to answer each question. State your rationale for choosing your response. For the other four questions, identify your response.

1. During termination of the nurse-client relationship, the client exhibits anger at the nurse. Which of the following responses by the nurse would be *most* appropriate?
    a. "Do not worry. You will feel better once you leave the hospital."
    b. "Anger is a normal emotion. It's okay to feel angry. Let's discuss your concerns about going home."
    c. "You should not be angry. Look at how hard you have worked since admission."
    d. "You are still very angry. Maybe it is best to cancel your discharge."
2. For an effective nurse-client therapeutic relationship, the nurse focuses on which of the following as the *priority*?
    a. The words used to communicate
    b. The client's problems and concerns
    c. The nurse's need for information
    d. The nurse's need to support the client
3. During the orientation (introductory phase) of the nurse-client relationship, the nurse will need to discuss the following topics with the client *except*:
    a. Roles
    b. Termination
    c. Confidentiality
    d. Self-disclosure
4. Identify several differences between a professional nurse-client relationship and a social relationship.
5. Describe why trust is critical in the development of the nurse-client relationship.
6. List several actions by the nurse that would promote the development of trust in the nurse-client relationship?
7. The nurse-client relationship is characterized by four overlapping phases. Explain the phases.

REFERENCES

Arnold, E. C., & Boggs, K. U. (2020). *Interpersonal relationships: Professional communication skills for nurses* (8th ed.). Elsevier.

Ashton, K. S. (2016). Teaching nursing students about terminating professional relationships, boundaries, and social media. *Nurse Education Today, 37*, 170–172. https://doi.org /10.1016/j.nedt.2015.11.007

Baca-Dietz, D., Wojnar, D. M., & Espina, C. R. (2021). The shared decision-making model: Providers' and patients' knowledge and understanding in clinical practice. *Journal of the American Association of Nurse Practitioners, 33*(7), 529–536. https://doi.org/10.1097/ jxx.0000000000000401

Baca, M. (2011). Professional boundaries and dual relationships in clinical practice. *The Journal of Nurse Practitioners, 7*(3), 195–200. https://doi.org/10.1016/j.nurpra.2010.10.003

Benner, P. E., & Wrubel, J. (1989). *The primacy of caring: Stress and coping in health and illness.* Addison Wesley Longman.

Bladh, M. L., & Van Leeuwen, A. M. (2017). Nurse-to-patient etiquette: It's more than good manners. *Nursing, 47*(8), 52–56.

Burkhartzmeyer, H. L., Preston, H. R., Arcand, L. L., Mullenbach, D. L., Nelson, D. E., Lorentz, P. A., & Stevens, S. K. (2021). Speaking to the heart of our patients: An empathic communication education initiative. *The Journal of Continuing Education in Nursing, 52*(7), 319–325. https://doi.org/10.3928/00220124-20210611-06

Canadian Nurses Association. (2017). *Code of ethics for registered nurses* (2017 ed.). https://www.cna-aiic.ca/en/nursing/regulated-nursing-in-canada/nursing-ethics

Canadian Nurses Protective Society. (2021). *InfoLaw: Social media.* https://cnps.ca/article/social-media/

Cannity, K. M., Banerjee, S. C., Hichenberg, S., Leon-Nastasi, A. D., Howell, F., Coyle, N., Zaider, T., & Parker, P. A. (2021). Acceptability and efficacy of a communication skills training for nursing students: Building empathy and discussing complex situations. *Nurse Education in Practice, 50.* https://doi.org/10.1016/j.nepr.2020.102928

Catlin, A. (2013). Considering boundaries in nursing: What the staff nurse needs to know. *Advances in Neonatal Care, 13*(5), 331–334. https://doi.org/10.1097/ANC.0b013e3182a3fef6

Clucas, C., Chapman, H., & Lovell, A. (2019). Nurses' experiences of communicating respect to patients: Influences and challenges. *Nursing Ethics, 26*(7–8), 2085–2097. https://doi.org/10.1177/0969733019834974

College and Association of Registered Nurses of Alberta. (2020). *Professional boundaries: Guidelines for the nurse-client relationship.* http://nurses.ab.ca/docs/default-source/document-library/guidelines/rn_professional-boundaries.pdf?sfvrsn=cc446624-24

College of Nurses of Ontario. (2019). *Therapeutic nurse-client relationship.* cno.org/globalassets/docs/prac/41033-therapeutic.pdf

College of Registered Nurses of Manitoba. (2019). *Professional boundaries for therapeutic relationships.* crnm.mb.ca/uploads/document/document_file_99.pdf?=1438267436

College of Registered Nurses of Newfoundland and Labrador. (2013). *Social media.* crnnl.ca/site/uploads/2021/09/social-media.pdf

College of Registered Nurses of Newfoundland and Labrador. (2014). *The therapeutic nurse-client relationship: Expectations for registered nurses.* crnnl.ca/site/uploads/2021/09/therapeutic-nurse-client-relationship.pdf

College of Registered Nurses of Newfoundland and Labrador. (2019). *Standards of practice: For registered nurses and nurse practitioners.* crnnl.ca/site/uploads/2021/09/standards-of-practice-for-rns-and-nps.pdf

Conroy, T., Feo, R., Boucaut, R., Alderman, J., & Kitson, A. (2017). Role of effective nurse-patient relationships in enhancing patient safety. *Nursing Standard, 31*(49), 53–61. https://doi.org/10.7748/ns.2017.e10801

Covington, H. (2005). Caring presence: Providing a safe space for patients. *Holistic Nursing Practice, 19*(3), 169–172. https://doi.org/10.1097/00004650-200507000-00008

Cussó, R. A., González, J. S., Murillo, D. A., & Salgado, J. G. (2021). A new conceptualization of the nurse-patient relationship construct as caring interaction. *Nursing Philosophy, 22*(2). https://doi.org/10.1111/nup.12335

Deligianni, A., Kyriakidou, M., Kaba, E., Kelesi, M., Rovithis, M., Fasoi, G., Rikos, N., & Stavropoulou, A. (2017). "Empathy equals match": The meaning of empathy as it is perceived by Greek nurse students—A qualitative study. *Global Journal of Health Science, 9*(1). https://doi.org/10.5539/gjhs.v9n1p171

De los Santos, J. A. A., & Labrague, L. J. (2021). Job engagement and satisfaction are associated with nurse caring behaviours: A cross-sectional study. *Journal of Nursing Management, 29*, 2234–2242. https://doi.org/10.1111/jonm.13384

English, W., Gott, M., & Robinson, J. (2021). The meaning of rapport for patients, families, and healthcare professionals: A scoping review. *Patient Education and Counseling, 105*(1), 2–14. https://doi.org/10.1016/j.pec.2021.06.003

Fackler, C. A., Chambers, A. N., & Bourbonniere, M. (2015). Hospital nurses' lived experience of power. *Journal of Nursing Scholarship, 47*(3), 267–274. https://doi.org/10.1111/jnu.12127

Fawcett, J., & Zhang, Y. (2021). Thoughts about power. *Nursing Science Quarterly, 34*(1), 93–95. https://doi.org/10.1177/0894318420965218

Feo, R., Rasmussen, P., Wiechula, R., Conroy, T., & Kitson, A. (2017). Developing effective and caring nurse-patient relationships. *Nursing Standard, 31*(28), 54–63. https://doi.org/10.7748/ns.2017.e10735

Finfgeld-Connett, D. (2007). Meta-synthesis of caring in nursing. *Journal of Clinical Nursing, 17*(2), 196–204. https://doi.org/10.1111/j.1365-2702.2006.01824.x

Flagg, A. J. (2015). The role of patient-centered care in nursing. *Nursing Clinics of North America, 50*, 75–86. https://doi.org/10.1016/j.cnur.2014.10.006

Frankel, M., Rachlin, H., & Yip-Bannicq, M. (2012). How nondirective therapy directs: The power of empathy in the context of unconditional positive regard. *Person-Centered Experiential Psychotherapies, 11*(3), 205–214. https://doi.org/10.1080/14779757.2012.695292

Government of Newfoundland and Labrador. (2008). *Personal health information act.* https://www.gov.nl.ca/hcs/phia/

Granados-Gamez, G., Sáez-Ruiza, I. M., Márquez-Hernández, V. V., Rodríguez-García, M. C., Aguilera-Manrique, G., Cibanal-Juan, M. L., & Gutiérrez-Puertas, L. (2022). Development and validation of the questionnaire to analyze the communication of nurses in nurse-patient therapeutic communication. *Patient Education and Counseling, 105*(1), 145–150. https://doi.org/10.1016/j.pec.2021.05.008

Greene, J., & Ramos, C. (2021). A mixed methods examination of health care provider behaviors that build patients' trust. *Patient Education and Counseling, 104*(5), 1222–1228. https://doi.org/10.1016/j.pec.2020.09.003

Griscti, O., Aston, M., Warner, G., Martin-Misener, R., & McLeod, D. (2017). Power and resistance within the hospital's hierarchical system: The experiences of chronically ill patients. *Journal of Clinical Nursing, 26*(12), 238–247. https://doi.org/10.1111/jocn.13382

Guerrero, J. G. (2019). Nurses towards end-of-life situations: Sympathy vs. empathy. *Open Journal of Nursing, 9*(3), 278–293. https://doi.org/10.4236/ojn.2019.93027

Hall, K. (2011). Building a trusting relationship with patients: Professional boundaries. *Home Healthcare Nurse, 29*(4), 210–217. https://doi.org/10.1097/NHH.06013e318211966a

Hines, M. E. (2017). Advanced holistic nursing practice narratives: A view of caring praxis. *Journal of Holistic Nursing, 35*(4), 328–341. https://doi.org/10.1177/0898010117715849

Jaastad, T. A., Ueland, V., & Koskinen, C. (2022). The meaning of reflection for understanding caring and becoming a caring nurse. *Scandinavian Journal of Caring Science, 36*(4), 1180–1188. https://doi.org/10.1111/scs.13080

Knapp, H. (2015). *Therapeutic communication: Developing professional skills* (2nd ed.). Sage.

Leininger, M. (1995). *Transcultural nursing: Concepts, theories, research, and practice.* McGraw Hill.

Lenzen, S. A., Daniëls, R., van Bokhoven, M. A., van der Weijden, T., & Beurskens, A. (2018). What makes it so difficult for nurses to coach patients in shared decision making? A process evaluation. *International Journal of Nursing Studies, 80,* 1–11. https://doi.org/10.1016/j.ijnurstu.2017.12.005

Lowry, P. (2009). Exploring caring. *Thinking: The Journal of Philosophy for Children, 19*(2–3), 32–41. https://doi.org/10.5840/thinking2009192/311

Manfrin-Ledet, L., Porche, D. J., & Eymard, A. S. (2015). Professional boundary violations: A literature review. *Home Healthcare Now, 33*(6), 326–332. https://doi.org/10.1097/NHH.0600000000000249

Martinez, R. C. (2019). "Lost touch": Situating human-connectedness in technology—caring in the health sciences. *The Journal of Medical Investigation, 66*(1–2), 12–14. https://doi.org/10.2152/jmi.66.12

McKinnon, J. (2018). In their shoes: An ontological perspective on empathy in nursing practice. *Journal of Clinical Nursing, 27,* 3882–3893. https://doi.org/10.1111/jocn.14610

Mikkelsen, K. B., Delmar, C., & Sorensen, E. E. (2019). Fundamentals of care in time-limited encounters: Exploring strategies that can be used to support establishing a nurse-patient relationship in time-limited encounters. *Journal of Nursing Studies and Patient Care, 1*(1), 8–16. https://www.semanticscholar.org/paper/Fundamentals-of-Care-in-Time-Limited-Encounters%3A-be-Mikkelsen-Delmar/86f10acf89b4f8337f34aa80793e14d8f8fd8507

Moudatsou, M., Stavropoulou, A., Philalithis, A., & Koukouli, S. (2020). The role of empathy in health and social care professionals. *Healthcare, 8*(1), 3–9. https://doi.org/10.3390/healthcare8010026

Muscat, D. M., Shepherd, H. L., Nutbeam, D., Trevena, L., & McCaffery, K. J. (2020). Health literacy and shared decision-making: Exploring the relationship to enable meaningful patient engagement in healthcare. *Journal of General Internal Medicine, 36*(2), 521–524. https://doi.org/10.1007/s11606-020-05912-0

Nisa, S. N. U., Hussain, M., Afzal, M., & Gilani, S. A. (2019). Quality of nurse patient therapeutic communication and overall patient satisfaction during their hospitalization stay. *European Academic Research, 7*(3), https://doi.org/10.5455/ijmsph.2017.0211522112016

O'Brien, P. G. (2013). The nurse-client relationship and therapeutic communication. In P. G. O'Brien, W. Z. Kennedy, & K. A. Ballard (Eds.), *Psychiatric mental health nursing: An introduction to theory and practice* (2nd ed., pp. 41–53). Jones & Bartlett Learning.

Ozaras, G., & Abaan, S. (2018). Investigation of the trust status of the nurse-patient relationship. *Nursing Ethics, 25*(5), 628–639. https://doi.org/10.1177/0969733016664971

Patterson, J. (2018). Empathy: A concept analysis. *International Journal of Human Caring, 22*(4), https://doi.org/10.20467/1091-5710.22.4.217

Pavlo, A. J., O'Connell, M., Olsen, S., Snyder, M. K., & Davidson, L. (2019). Missing ingredients in shared decision-making? *Psychiatric Quarterly, 90*(2), 333–338. https://doi.org/10.1007/s11126-019-9624-9

Peplau, H. E. (1991). *Interpersonal relations in nursing.* G. P. Putman.

Peplau, H. E. (1997). Peplau's theory of interpersonal relations. *Nursing Science Quarterly, 10*(4), 162–167. https://doi.org/10.1177/0894318494701000407

Persaud, S., & Thornton, M. (2018). Developing caring behaviors in undergraduate nursing students through simulation. *International Journal for Human Caring, 22*(2), 26–33. https://doi.org/10.20467/1091-5710.22.2.26

Peternelj-Taylor, C. A., & Yonge, O. (2003). Exploring boundaries in the nurse-client relationship: Professional roles and responsibilities. *Perspectives in Psychiatric Care, 39*(2), 55–66. https://doi.org/10.1111/j.1744-6163.2003.t600677.x

Powell, S. K. (2020). Compassion fatigue. *Professional Case Management, 25*(2), 53–55. https://doi.org/10.1097/NCM.0000000000000418

Pratt, H., Moroney, T., & Middleton, R. (2021). The influence of engaging authentically on nurse-patient relationships: A scoping review. *Nursing Inquiry, 28*(2), https://doi.org/10.1111/nin.12388

Registered Nurses' Association of Ontario. (2006). *Nursing best practice guideline: Establishing therapeutic relationships.* https://rnao.ca/sites/rnao-ca/files/Establishing_Therapeutic_Relationships.pdf

Romero-Martin, M., Gómez-Salgado, J., Robles-Romero, J. M., Jiménez-Picón, N., Gómez-Urquiza, J. L., & Ponce-Blandón, J. A. (2019). Systematic review of the nature of nursing care described by using the caring behaviours inventory. *Journal of Clinical Nursing, 28*(21–22), 3734–3746. https://doi.org/10.1111/jocn.15015

Schnellbacher, J., & Leijssen, M. (2009). The significance of therapist genuineness from the client's perspective. *Journal of Humanistic Psychology, 49*(2), 207–228. https://doi.org/10.1177/0022167808323601

Smith, L. L., Taylor, B. B., Keys, A. T., & Gornto, S. B. (1997). Nurse-patient boundaries: Crossing the line. *The American Journal of Nursing, 97*(12), 26–32. https://doi.org/10.2307/3465531

Smythe, E., Hennessy, J., Abbott, M., & Hughes, F. (2018). Do professional boundaries limit trust? *International Journal of Mental Health Nursing, 27*(1), 287–295. https://doi.org/ 10.1111/inm.12319

Steele, D. (2019). Working with an individual patient. In N. L. Keltner & D. Steele (Eds.), *Psychiatric Nursing* (8th ed., pp. 83–96). Elsevier.

Steuber, P., & Pollard, C. (2018). Building a therapeutic relationship: How much is too much self-disclosure? *International Journal of Caring Sciences, 111*(21), 651–657.

Stevens, N., McNiesh, S., & Goyal, D. (2020). Utilizing an SBAR workshop with baccalaureate nursing students to improve communication skills. *Nursing Education Perspectives, 41*(2). https://doi.org/10.1097/01.NEP.0000000000000518

Travelbee, J. (1971). *Interpersonal aspects of nursing* (2nd ed.). F. A. Davis.

Truglio-Londrigan, M., & Slyer, J. T. (2018). Shared decision-making for nursing practice: An integrative review. *The Open Nursing Journal, 12*, 1–14. https://doi.org/10.2174/187443460 1812010001

Turner, K., Locke, A., Jones, T., & Carpenter, J. (2019). Empathy huddles: Cultivating a culture of empathy. *American Association of Neuroscience Nurses, 51*(3), 153–155. https://doi .org/10.1097/JNN.0000000000000444

Wagner, A. L. (2002). Nursing students' development of caring self through creative reflective practice. In D. Freshwater (Ed.), *Therapeutic nursing* (pp. 121–144). Sage.

Watson, J. (2018a). *Unitary caring science: The philosophy and praxis of nursing.* University Press of Colorado.

Watson, J. (2018b). Unitary caring science—Universals of human caring and global micro practices of caritas. *NSC Nursing, 4*(1), 1–7. https://doi.org/10.32549/OPI-NSC-22

Wei, H., & Watson, J. (2019). Healthcare interprofessional team members' perspective on human caring: A directed content analysis study. *International Journal of Nursing Sciences, 6*(1), 17–23. https://doi.org/10.1016/j.ijnss.2018.12.001

Younis, J. R., Mabrouk, S. M., & Kamal, F. F. (2015). Effect of the planned therapeutic communication program on therapeutic communication skills of pediatric nurses. *Journal of Nursing Education and Practice, 5*(8), 109–120. https://doi.org/10.5430/jnep.v5n8p109

CHAPTER 4

Cultural Safety: Communication with Clients from Diverse Cultures

LEARNING OBJECTIVES

After reading this chapter, you will be able to

1. Define *culture* and its related terms
2. Define *bias* and its impact on communication
3. Discuss health inequities within Canada's health care system
4. Recognize the need for cultural safety in health care
5. Describe nurses' role in providing culturally safe care
6. Discuss the connection between culture and communication
7. Discuss communication strategies that enhance care for culturally diverse clients
8. Recognize aspects of a person's culture that influence communication
9. Describe the key components of relational practice

KEY TERMS

Anti-racism	Health inequities
Bias	Heteronormativity
Cultural humility	Interpreter
Cultural safety	LGBTQIA2+
Cultural trauma	Racism
Culture	Relational practice

INTRODUCTION

Canada is a culturally diverse country, and with the global turmoil of war, political and social unrest, and other international events, forced migration is happening, so more persons are seeking asylum. Newcomers include refugees and immigrants who come to Canada from a variety of countries. A refugee is a person fleeing their country of origin because of war or persecution (Statistics Canada, 2019). An immigrant is a person who has chosen to live in Canada, is admitted by the government, and may apply for permanent residency. Moreover, the Canadian government is working to attract more newcomers through changes in its immigration policies and asylum programs.

As of 2021, more than 36 million people live within this country, of which three racialized groups make up 16.1 percent of the total population: South Asian (7.1%), Chinese (4.7%), and Black (4.3%). In addition, 4.9 percent of the population is made up of First Nations, Métis, and Inuit people, who speak more than 70 Indigenous languages and are among the fastest-growing populations (Statistics Canada, 2022). According to Statistics Canada population projections, these racialized populations will continue to increase, shaping the diversity of the country (Statistics Canada, 2022). Also adding to the diversity is a growing LGBTQ2+ community, comprising 4 percent of the population aged 15 years and older (Statistics Canada, 2021).

With such ethnocultural diversity in Canada, federal and provincial governments and health care professionals should take action to achieve a culturally safe health care system. According to the Canadian Nurses Association (CNA, 2018), nurses have a duty to show "respect and value each person's individual culture and consider how culture may impact an individual's experience of health care and the health care system" (p. 1). This chapter defines *culture* and its related terms and describes the role of nurses in building nurse-client relationships with culturally diverse clients through communication. The concept of relational practice as an approach by health care professionals to inquire into the contextual factors of the lived experiences and health care needs of clients is also explained. This chapter identifies barriers to culturally safe care and highlights strategies to increase health professional students' competency and awareness for implementing cultural safety as part of their everyday clinical practice.

CULTURE

In the area of health, two opposing views of culture have been debated: the essentialist view and the constructivist view (Garneau & Pepin, 2015). *Culture* has been commonly defined as a set of learned values, beliefs, assumptions, behaviours, language, customs, and identity shared by a group of people that influences how they view the world and relate to others. These beliefs, customs, and perceptions are passed down through generations and influence their thinking, family roles, and health beliefs and practices (Young & Guo, 2020). This is an essentialist view of culture still found within organizations, educational institutions, and health settings where the interplay of individuals' beliefs and biases impedes their ability to take cultural contexts into account when engaging with others (World Health Organization, 2017). This view of culture contributes to nurses' lack of awareness and understanding of their own cultural values, beliefs, and behaviours as well as those of their clients, affecting the development of the nurse-client relationship. This lack of cultural awareness and knowledge undermines intercultural communication and optimal client care (Tuohy, 2019). Canada's diverse population presents an opportunity for nurses and other health care professionals to change practice and provide direction on the inclusion of culturally safe care to persons who access health care services.

Constructivism, an alternative perspective, views culture as a relational process that is socially constructed through a shared meaning of interactions within the context of relationships (Garneau & Pepin, 2015). Culture is not static but dynamic and changing, both influencing and being impacted by individuals, groups, and contexts. From this standpoint, it "involves people selectively responding to and integrating particular historical, social, political, economic, physical, and linguistic structures and processes" (Hartrick Doane & Varcoe, 2021, p. 233). It is critical for nurses to understand context in clinical practice as it shapes the nurse-client relationship and clients' care experiences (Zou, 2016). To understand and examine health care situations, relational practice enables nurses and nursing students to fully engage with others, ensuring culturally safe person-centred care. This approach will be discussed in more detail later in this chapter.

Culture influences the way persons define *health*, how they care for their health and well-being, and how they make health-related decisions. Cultural differences, language barriers, and barriers to information are identified as major health care obstacles for immigrants and refugees in Canada (Pandey et al., 2022). Similarly, these barriers, along with racism, bias, and stereotyping, have been endured by Indigenous people in Canada's health care system (Berg et al., 2019; Kitching et al., 2020). This is evident in the experience of Joyce Echaquan, a 37-year-old Indigenous woman who—shortly before her death, on September 28, 2020—posted a video to Facebook Live of her discriminatory treatment by health care staff in a hospital in Joliette, Quebec (Godin, 2020). These racial disparities in the quality of care for those who access the health care system are a matter of concern. As a result of such treatment, Indigenous people find it difficult to trust health care providers, causing them to avoid, delay, or reluctantly seek health care services (Breault et al., 2021; Churchill et al., 2020; Wylie & McConkey, 2019).

Case Study 4.1

Joyce Echaquan, an Atikamekw woman, died on September 28, 2020, in the Centre hospitalier de Lanaudière in Saint-Charles-Borromée, Quebec. Before her death, she recorded a Facebook Live (7 minutes) video that showed her screaming in distress and the responses of her health care providers. She was admitted to the hospital on September 26 for complaints of stomach pains. Due to previous

(Continued)

episodes of her falling out of bed, she requested to be restrained to her bed to prevent further occurrences. Even though she voiced concerns about her adverse reaction to morphine, she was administered the medication by hospital staff. During the livestream, two staff members are heard insulting her in French, and while she is moaning in pain, an employee asks her if she is "done acting stupid." Hospital staff comment that Joyce "made some bad choices" and ask what her children would be thinking if they saw her. She responds, "That's why I came here."

Staff are also heard saying she is only "good for sex," the employees are the ones "paying for this," and she is "stupid as hell." She died later that day.

It is evident that Joyce Echaquan was mistreated by her health care providers and did not receive ethical, culturally safe, and competent person-centred care.

1. In this practice situation, what could have been done differently by the health care providers to meet Joyce's health care needs?
2. Reflecting on this situation, what recommendations would you suggest to address the racism experienced by Indigenous clients in the health care system?

Sources: Godin, M. (2020). *Canada outraged by death of Indigenous woman Joyce Echaquan.* https://time.com/5898422/joyce-echaquan-indigenous-protests-canada/; Death of Joyce Echaquan. (2022). *Wikipedia.* https://en.wikipedia.org/wik/Death_of_Joyce_Echaquan

CULTURAL SAFETY

With the increasing cultural, religious, ethnic, and linguistic diversity of Canada's population, providing culturally appropriate client-centred care should be a priority. Cultural humility and cultural safety have replaced the concept of cultural competence in reference to health care, health care systems, and the professionals who provide services to diverse cultures (Curtis et al., 2019). The concept of cultural safety was first described in the 1990s by Māori nurse Irihapeti Ramsden as an approach to address the historical, social, economic, and political processes that contributed to the health inequities of Māori people of New Zealand (Ramsden, 2002). Cultural safety is relevant to health care practitioners as it fosters reflection on their own culture and privilege, and the power that they bring to the health care encounter (Kurtz et al., 2018). The process of critical reflection enhances a nurse's understanding of their own culture, values, and beliefs, which is needed before attempting to understand their client's (Ramsden, 2002). Delivering culturally safe care in a culturally safe environment involves understanding a person in the context of their culture from a relational practice perspective. In this approach, cultural safety helps to "rebalance power dynamics and promote equity in care"

(Tremblay et al., 2020, p. 671). Culturally safe care is defined by the client who receives the care and not by the health care professionals providing care (Brooks-Cleator et al., 2018; Conroy et al., 2017). It entails health care professionals who, from the client's perspective, listen; use clear communication; are ethical, respectful, nonjudgmental, supportive, and knowledgeable; and provide space for cultural practices (Berg et al., 2019; Brooks-Cleator et al., 2018).

These concepts are evident in the codes of the Aboriginal Nurses Association of Canada (ANAC, 2009), the Canadian Association of Schools of Nursing (CASN), the Canadian Nurses Association (CNA), and some professional nursing regulatory practice standards as noted in the following examples:

- College of Registered Nurses of Newfoundland and Labrador (2019) Standard 3: Client Centred Practice (3.9) "Respects diversity and promotes cultural humility and a culturally safe environment for clients and members of the health care team" (p. 7).
- College of Licensed Practical Nurses of Newfoundland and Labrador (2020) Standard 2: Evidence-informed Practice (2.9) "Practice in a culturally safe manner respective of diversity, equity, and inclusion" (p. 5).
- The British Columbia College of Nurses and Midwives (BCCNM, 2022) recently approved a practice standard for all nurses focused on Indigenous-specific racism in the BC health care system. The core concepts and principles relate to cultural safety, cultural humility, and anti-racism. Standard 4: Creating Safe Health Care Experiences (4.1.1) "Treat clients with respect and empathy by acknowledging the client's cultural identity"; (4.2) "Care for a client holistically, considering their physical, mental/emotional, spiritual, and cultural needs" (p. 3).

Student Tip

These ethical principles and documents will guide your development as a professional nurse in providing culturally safe person-centred client care.

In Canada, the concept of cultural safety has been recognized as an approach to improve the health needs of Indigenous people, who, in comparison to non-Indigenous populations, experience significant health inequities and lower quality of health care services (Brooks-Cleator et al., 2018; Nguyen et al., 2020). A predominate outlook of paternalism and the biomedical scientific traditions still endures within the Canadian health care system. Such views hinder how various cultures are acknowledged and accepted within health care settings. In clinical encounters, a cultural safety understanding allows health care professionals to address the power imbalances within the context of the health care experience and to take measures to provide person-centred care. This process helps to facilitate nurse-client relationships based on trust and respect (Curtis et al., 2019). Greenwood et al. (2017) contend that institutions, along with individuals, must embrace cultural safety to build relationships with Indigenous persons and communities.

Several organizations have taken initiatives to address the importance of using a cultural safety approach to reform the health care system. The CNA (2018), in collaboration with the Canadian Indigenous Nurses Association, advocates that all health care clinicians practise from a place of cultural safety. One facility, the University of Victoria School of Nursing, has three cultural safety online modules that reflect on Indigenous people's experiences of colonization and racism with respect to health and health care. These modules, developed by Indigenous persons in collaboration with university faculty and staff, are designed for nurses, nursing instructors and students, and other health and human service workers to learn about the concept of cultural safety and its association with nursing practice. Although each module is designed to stand alone, it is recommended that the modules be worked through in order:

- **Module 1** introduces the relationships between colonial history and health.
- **Module 2** explores power and privilege and the intersections of people's experiences in relation to marginalization, oppression, and dominance.
- **Module 3** explores the intersections of Aboriginal people's experiences in relation to health, health care, and healing.

ANAC (2009), in collaboration with the CASN and CNA, developed a competency framework that calls upon nursing programs to provide students with education on cultural competence and cultural safety. The Truth and Reconciliation Commission of Canada (2015) advocates that all students in medical and nursing programs receive education on cultural competency and cultural safety. The First Nations Health Authority (FNHA, 2022) of British Columbia partnered with the Health Standards Organization and with a committee comprising First Nations client partners and family members, health professionals, policymakers, and academics from BC to develop the BC Cultural Safety and Humility Standard. The Métis Nation British Columbia also provided input into the standard's development. Some of the standard expectations for clients who receive care are as follows:

- Respect and uphold the health-related rights of First Nations, Métis, and Inuit people and communities.
- Commit to establishing a culture of accountability to advance anti-racism and cultural safety and humility.

- Health care providers receive education on cultural safety and humility.
- Health care team uses a holistic approach to First Nations, Métis, and Inuit clients' care plans and models of care.
- First Nations, Métis, and Inuit practitioners are included in clients' care plans.
- Adoption of First Nations, Métis, and Inuit data governance protocols to collect and analyze data for quality improvement initiatives.

Based on these standards, you can see how a cultural safety perspective was adopted within a midwifery practice. Churchill et al. (2020) used a qualitative research design to evaluate the concept of cultural safety from the perspective of Indigenous (n = 9) and non-Indigenous (n = 11) clients at an urban, Indigenous-focused midwifery practice in Toronto, Canada. All of the Indigenous and three of the non-Indigenous clients conceptualized cultural safety as being able to access Indigenous knowledge and protocols. One Indigenous participant stated that cultural safety was about access and "treating cultural things as 'normal,' so it's not a novelty thing that like I was seeing a healer and he was giving me teas to drink.... Like [the midwives] just took it at value that, like, a traditional person gave those to me" (p. 7).

CULTURAL HUMILITY

With the diversity of clients accessing health care services, it is prudent that health care professionals apply cultural humility in all interactions (Kuzma et al., 2019). Hughes et al. (2020) identify cultural humility as the ethical foundation for nurses to use in establishment of an environment that promotes understanding of other cultures. It is impossible for health care professionals to be knowledgeable about all cultures, but it is critical that they respect client differences. This requires that nurses do a self-examination by reflecting on who they are culturally and how their values, beliefs, stereotypes or assumptions, biases, and privileges may impact the development of the therapeutic relationship. Cultural humility fosters supportive relationships based upon listening, respect, empathy, and partnership building (BCCNM, 2022).

According to Foronda (2020), cultural humility involves being flexible and open, egoless (humble), and self-aware, with a focus on others and self. It is a process of critical self-reflection and lifelong learning that contributes to the value of reflective practice for health care professionals, including nurses. Cultural humility shifts the notion from the health care provider as the expert to the client as the expert in knowing self (Ruud, 2018). Since communication is central to nursing practice, it is important that students have a good understanding of their own cultural identity. Having an awareness and recognition of their values, attitudes, biases, and stereotypes is a necessary step in providing a culturally safe nursing practice.

THERAPEUTIC COMMUNICATION

An important consideration in nursing practice is the ability to develop client-centred communication skills, as discussed in chapter 2 of this text. The use of effective communication skills is at the core of building a therapeutic alliance with all clients, regardless of their culture. The concepts of cultural safety and cultural humility are integral components of ethical nursing practice and should be incorporated into care provision. The quality of the nurse-client relationship is affected by the verbal and nonverbal characteristics of communication used by both the client and the nurse. Communication principles related to interactions between clinicians and culturally diverse clients and their families are based on

Exercise 4.1: Cultural Self-Awareness

Purpose: To gain an understanding of your own ethnicity, cultural values, biases, health beliefs, and practices

Procedure
This exercise will be completed as an out-of-class assignment. The next time your class meets, your instructor will facilitate a class discussion on the topic of self-awareness and culture.

1. Identify your own cultural groups (e.g., your family's culture).
2. Think about your own ethnicity, socioeconomic status, sexual orientation, and religious or spiritual beliefs.
3. Thinking about when you were growing up, what factors impacted your socialization (e.g., family, peers, school, media)?
4. What are the values that you acquired from your family?
5. What have you learned from your family regarding health and health care practices?
6. How do these values guide your decision-making and your worldview? Are they something that may affect your practice as a nurse?
7. Does your family have particular customs around events such as births, birthdays, and funerals?
8. How different are these customs compared to those of other people? (Think about your friends, school peers, or people you may work with.)
9. Are you aware of your personal biases and prejudices toward cultures different than your own?

trust, respect, and a building of rapport. This style of communication is collaborative and client-centred, and it includes active listening, the use of appropriate body language, flexibility, and support of client beliefs, values, preferences, and cultural practices (Brooks et al., 2019).

CULTURAL TRAUMA

Cultural trauma is a new term coined by Subica and Link (2022) that reflects an "assault by a dominant group on an individual's culture through force, threats of force, oppressive policies for the purpose of damaging, devaluing, or destroying that culture to advance the dominant group's interests in gaining key resources (e.g., natural, labour) or status/reputation (e.g., colonial empires)" (p. 2). This is evident in the colonial legacy, disrespectful treatment, and systemic racism experienced for generations by Indigenous people in Canada's health care system. Health care professionals working with clients have a lack of awareness of the clients' lived experiences. A trauma-informed framework for care delivery provides a lens for viewing the possibility that every client may have a trauma history (Cannon et al., 2020). Stokes et al. (2017) refer to this phenomenon as "universal trauma-precautions," which is the core of trauma-informed care that requires organizations and health care professionals to provide services and care that are safety-focused for both clients and providers. Health care services delivered in this way encompass the concepts of cultural safety and cultural humility regardless of trauma disclosure. Trauma-informed care provided by nurses entails the establishment and development of the nurse–client relationship as central within a person-centred approach (Goddard et al., 2022). Nurses who use a trauma-informed lens in practice need to be aware of, sensitive to, and responsive to client needs. This involves having awareness of environmental triggers such as touch or procedures that may trigger traumatic memories. As a first step, this begins with nurses asking themselves and their colleagues these three simple questions (Fleishman et al., 2019):

1. **Safety**: Does this cultivate a sense of safety (physical and psychological)?
2. **Respect**: Am I, and others, showing respect?
3. **Trust**: Does this build trust?

This care approach by nurses creates an environment for healing that results in empowerment, resilience, relationship building, and a reduction of trauma triggering (re-traumatization) in the nurse–client relationship (Goddard et al., 2022). In addition, nurses and other health care clinicians need to recognize their own history of trauma; they may be trauma survivors and need to take steps for self-care (Beattie et al., 2019).

Table 4.1: Terms Associated with Culture

Term	Definition
Ethnicity	Membership in a group of people who share common racial, tribal, religious, or cultural origin (Bokor-Billmann et al., 2020)
Ethnocentrism	A perception that one's own values, beliefs, and behaviours are superior (Halter et al., 2019), e.g., expecting others to speak English
Co-culture	A cultural group within the larger culture that has distinct traditions and cultural norms (Beebe et al., 2019), e.g., Amish, LGBTQ2+
Race	A social category or social construction on the basis of certain characteristics, some biological, e.g., skin colour or blood group (Douglas et al., 2014)
Racism	A belief (implied or demonstrated through actions) that a group of people is inferior—based upon skin colour, culture, or spirituality—that leads to discrimination (FNHA, 2021)
Systemic racism (institutional racism)	Established laws, customs, or practices that contribute to racial inequalities that impact health (Phillips-Beck et al., 2020)
Anti-racism	The active practice of taking action to prevent, challenge, eliminate, and change values, structures, policies, programs, practices, legislation, and behaviours that perpetuate racism (Phillips-Beck et al., 2020)
Cultural blindness	Assumption by health care systems that all people are the same and no biases exist and that race or ethnicity does not affect treatment (Tremblay & Echaquan, 2022)

Research Highlight: An Environmental Scan of Indigenous Cultural Safety in Canadian Baccalaureate Nursing and Midwifery Programs

Background

The Truth and Reconciliation Commission (TRC), the Canadian Nurses Association (CNA), the Canadian Indigenous Nurses Association (CINA), and the Canadian Association of Schools of Nursing (CASN) have advocated to include cultural safety competency education in curricula for medical and nursing students and to increase the number of Indigenous practitioners in nursing and midwifery programs.

Purpose of the Study
- To examine nursing and midwifery programs to assess the creation of culturally safe spaces for Indigenous students
- To assess and explore whether TRC recommendations are evident in curricular changes and inclusion of Indigenous content

Method

A digital environmental scan of accredited baccalaureate nursing and midwifery programs (n = 107) was conducted. Data analysis was undertaken using descriptive statistics.

Findings

Of the programs reviewed, one-fifth (n = 19, 17.8%) met all three cultural safety criteria. Fifty-nine schools (55.1%) had designated culturally safe spaces for Indigenous students. Twenty schools (18.7%) had relevant Indigenous coursework, and one-third (n = 36, 33.6%) had some Indigenous-related content integrated throughout their programs. Most schools have made some progress, but more work needs to be done to enhance cultural safety content and Indigenization of the curriculum in nursing and midwifery programs.

Implications for Nursing Education

Nursing and midwifery programs need to make a substantial effort to enhance cultural safety content and to incorporate multiple ways of knowing within program curricula. Nursing and midwifery programs need an increased focus on strengthening the accessibility of their programs for Indigenous students. Providing required course content on Indigenous history and cultural safety assessment to determine their impact on clinical practice is paramount.

Source: Metheny, N., & Fletcher, C. D. (2021). An environmental scan of Indigenous cultural safety in Canadian baccalaureate nursing and midwifery programs. *Canadian Journal of Nursing Research, 53*(4), 417–425. https://doi.org/10.1177/08445621211016143

Self-Reflective Exercise

Reflect on how the implications for nursing education in the research study on cultural safety align with what is occurring within your program of study.

RELATIONAL PRACTICE

Relational nursing practice has been recognized as an approach to meeting the health care needs of clients. It involves using a critical lens to look within the context of relationships to help nurses achieve the core goal of connecting with clients (Emmamally et al., 2020; Zou, 2016). Within this partnership, an exchange between the nurse and the client unfolds through the use of appropriate interpersonal communication skills. Through the establishment of trust, the nurse-client relationship provides a medium for the nurse to learn about the client's lived experiences and the contextual factors that impact the caring interaction. Within this person-centred relationship, the client and nurse come to know each other, which enhances the nurse's understanding of what is needed and how to provide care (Schwind & Manankil-Rankin, 2020).

According to Fyers and Greenwood (2016), relational practice is a way of being that requires a conscious awareness of what's happening in the moment. It enables nurses to work with clients in situations of uncertainty and to understand what they need and how best to respond within the context of the encounter. It is also linked to the concept of cultural safety, requiring health care professionals to recognize cultural diversity and power imbalances and to act (Zou, 2016). Hartrick Doane and Varcoe (2021) contend that a relational nursing practice is shaped by personal values, dominant values in health care settings, and broader social values. The health care professional in clinical situations "requires the skill to integrate and translate multiple forms of knowledge, discern what is most salient, and make the 'best' clinical decisions" (p. 87).

Hartrick Doane and Varcoe (2021) identify five relational capacities (ways of being) that are integral for nurses to develop to enhance their practice: being compassionate, curious, committed, competent, and corresponding. Being compassionate is being able to relate to others and understand what your intention is for doing something. It is how you respond to yourself, others, and the situation, developing compassionate action in your practice. Being curious within the clinical context means not knowing all but being interested and inquisitive and learning how to deal with uncertainty. These attributes help nurses to develop confidence by asking questions of themselves and others, building knowledge, and gaining skills to respond in clinical situations. Being committed as a nurse is about identifying your values and how your actions with clients and others are aligned with those values in your clinical practice. Being competent is having and demonstrating the capacities of being compassionate, curious, and committed in your practice. These characteristics focus you in on clinical situations and orient you to the lived experiences of clients and families in care encounters. Corresponding is about relating to and being present with clients in a meaningful way. This occurs in the nurse-client relationship, where you come to know the client's and family's experience of health/illness along with their concerns. In these relationships you will also learn to enhance your own practice through the process of self-reflection (Hartrick Doane & Varcoe, 2021).

These capacities are not separate entities but are used in an integrated fashion in a given clinical context by the nurse. Developing these capacities is a lifelong practice for nurses in learning the "ways of being" to engage in a person-centred relational practice.

Case Study 4.2

Tim Evans is a 70-year-old male living with his partner, John. He has been on the medical unit in a four-bed room for about a week. Tim was admitted for investigation of dizziness, blurred vision, shortness of breath, and headaches, which he has been experiencing for the past three weeks. He has a central venous port implanted for previous chemotherapy administration for colon cancer, but the port is not currently being used. His medical record indicates a past medical history of cardiopulmonary disease and a second chemotherapy regime for treatment of his cancer that finished six months ago. Tim has had a chest X-ray and a CT scan of his head since admission. You are with Tim when the physician informs him that he has a large tumour on his lung and the CT scan has indicated that the cancer has metastasized to his brain.

1. Using a relational practice approach, in the context of the situation, what does the client need?
2. How can you best respond as a nurse to provide Tim with a person-centred care approach?

CULTURAL CLIENT ASSESSMENT

No matter the practice setting, nurses and students may have opportunities to communicate with culturally diverse clients and their families. They are not expected to have knowledge of all cultures but are expected to use a culturally sensitive approach in all client encounters. An important aspect of relational practice is being more self-aware through the use of self-reflection in clinical practice (Emmamally, 2020). In such situations, the health care provider should be prepared to reflect on their own values, beliefs, and cultural heritage to gain awareness of how these qualities can affect care. As part of the admission process, the nurse, in consultation with the client, completes a cultural health assessment to identify their perceptions, values, beliefs, preferences, and health care needs. This requires that clinicians have the knowledge and skills to communicate using a person-centred approach. Brooks et al. (2019) outline the attributes of culturally sensitive communications:

- Clients and their families are involved in communication and health care decisions.
- Health care professionals prioritize cultural considerations by demonstrating respect for the culture and asking culturally sensitive questions.
- Health care professionals and clients use verbal and nonverbal communication to develop a respectful, trusting relationship.

When meeting a client and their family members at the initial admission intake, introduce yourself and your role. Find out how the client would like to be addressed. To demonstrate respect and establish trust, use their first and last name; if you are unable to pronounce the name, ask the client. If the client is unable to speak English or has limited English proficiency, a professional interpreter is paramount in order to meet the client's cultural and language needs. All health care professionals should be familiar with their agency's policies regarding language access services for culturally diverse clients. As discussed in several chapters in this text, health care providers' verbal and nonverbal communication knowledge and skills are essential in helping to form a connection with the client through the development of the nurse-client relationship. To conduct a cultural assessment, health care professionals need effective communication skills to provide a person-centred care approach. The health care provider should be aware of their own nonverbal behaviour as well as their client's to prevent barriers in nonverbal communication. Nonverbal behaviours and their assigned meanings vary from culture to culture (Li et al., 2017). Some nonverbal behaviours appropriate for health care professionals to use during this procedure are:

- Listen actively and respectfully. Nod to show you are listening.
- Do not interrupt the client. Focus on what is being said.
- Use open and nonthreatening body positioning. (This conveys trust and a sense of value.)
- Use silence.
- Be aware of proxemics (personal space) and their cultural implications. In some cultures, being too close is seen as impolite or threatening. An individual's personal space (bubble) is contextual and varies among cultures (Li et al., 2017). Sit when conversing with client.
- Be mindful of eye contact and its cultural implications. Brief eye contact is considered polite. People in some Indigenous cultures avoid eye contact with authority figures to show respect, as looking in the eye is a sign of disrespect. Do not stare (fleeting eye contact is best).
- Keep your facial expression friendly and open.
- When using touch (greetings/handshake), be aware of cultural implications.

Cultural Assessment Models

There are several nursing models that are used for cultural assessment when caring for culturally diverse clients. Leininger (2002), a nurse, was the first to talk about culturally based nursing care in her culture care diversity and universality theory. Her theory, which is still in use today, led other theorists to include culture and care as concepts in their transcultural care theories, notably the Giger and Davidhizar (1999, 2002) Transcultural Assessment Model.

The model, developed in 1998, suggests that each person is culturally unique, and the assessment framework comprises six dimensions to determine cultural and health care needs. The health care provider, in collaboration with the client and family, can explore all domains to generate information from (1) communication, (2) space, (3) social organization, (4) time, (5) environmental control, and (6) biological variations. See figure 4.1.

Communication

Communication is the essence of nursing and provides connection for rapport and trust building, facilitating development of the nurse-client relationship. During the assessment process, the nurse gathers information through questioning, validation, and observation. According to Giger and Davidhizar (1999), culture and communication influence how language and feelings are expressed or not expressed. The nurse is assessing the language and dialect spoken (e.g., English or language of country of origin, or English as a second language), volume and silence, context of

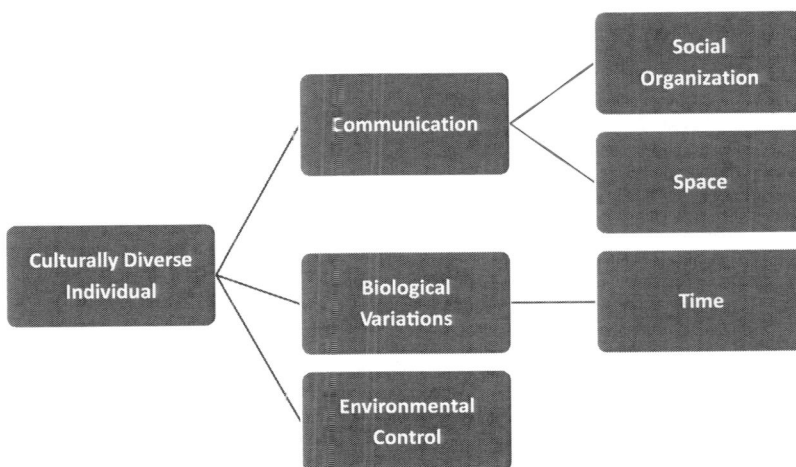

Figure 4.1: Giger and Davidhizar Transcultural Assessment Model (abridged)

Source: Adapted from Giger, J. N., & Davidhizar, R. (1999). *Transcultural nursing: Assessment and interventions* (3rd ed., p. 148). Mosby.

speech or emotional tone, and body language and other nonverbal communication (e.g., gestures, touch, facial expressions, eye contact). The nurse can ask the client directly about the primary language spoken at home and what language they prefer to use while hospitalized. If unsure of what the client has stated, they can seek clarification. When providing information, the health care provider should speak directly to the client, using simple language free from medical jargon. To assess their understanding, the nurse can ask them to repeat information and determine if they have questions.

Space

Proxemics is a term used to describe distance and space when relating verbally or nonverbally to others. Nurses need to be mindful of how clients feel when their space is invaded when the nurse is carrying out specific procedures. They should be cognizant of how clients react when the nurse encroaches on their space and respect their preferences (personal space bubbles). When providing care, health care providers should assess proxemics on an ongoing basis as every client situation is unique. Norms vary concerning personal distance within cultures and also depend on the situation and relationship (Hans & Hans, 2015). In certain situations, physical distance is limited for infection control purposes, which is reflected in facility policy. In some cases, gowns, gloves, and masks are worn, which impacts nonverbal behaviours (e.g., facial expressions) and the use of touch as a communication tool. See chapter 1, which covers strategies for overcoming communication barriers when health care providers wear masks.

Social Organization

Components of social organization may vary by culture with respect to race, ethnicity, family roles, gender roles and function, relationships, clan, work, friends, religion, nutrition, or spiritual beliefs. In some cultures, the family unit or other kinship relationships are considered the most important social organization. Some cultural groups are large and extend beyond the immediate family. In some families, the oldest male adult is considered the head and makes all decisions for the family. The nurse should inquire about religious or spiritual practices. For example, in Islamic culture, the client may read or recite the Koran and pray daily facing Mecca. In Jewish culture, a kosher diet prohibits eating of pork products and mixing meat and dairy products at the same meal. The nurse could ask when assessing family, "Who is involved in family decision-making?" and can inquire about any cultural practices or preferences that may be applicable to health care and would need consideration.

Health care professionals need to be mindful that not all persons who belong to a particular culture will follow the same religious values, beliefs, or family structures and role assignments as others from the same culture (Abualhaija, 2019). Nurses and other health care providers, in providing culturally safe care, need an awareness of their own personal biases or stereotypes toward persons who are culturally diverse. Recognition is the first step in making an effort to overcome biases and provide a culturally safe practice (Sukhera & Watling, 2018).

Time

How time is valued and how it is interpreted as either clock or social time are influenced by family and culture. Time orientation can be past, present, future, cyclical, or seasonal. It is important for the nurse to be aware of how time is viewed by the client in terms of lifespan, growth and development, and other events. Some clients, regardless of their culture, are future-oriented. Others may be more present-oriented and view time as flexible. This will influence their understanding of time with respect to procedures, health screening, and medication administration. For example, in Latino culture, individuals are more present-oriented and view time as flexible. A health care provider who is counselling a client with a major depressive disorder needs to provide clear instructions so that the client is aware of the need to continue their prescribed medications even when symptoms subside.

Environmental Control

Environmental control relates to the amount of control persons feel they have about factors in their environment that affect them. These factors influence individual health beliefs, decisions, and health behaviours. In some cultures, alternative traditional therapies, sacred medicines, or other methods (e.g., coining, used in Asian cultures to rid the body of negative energy) may be used. Nurses can assess the use of other interventions (e.g., traditional healers or folk medicine).

Biological Variations

Nurses need to understand the biological variations between cultures with respect to skin colour, body size, and genetics that predispose some cultures to diseases or disorders, as well as understanding the variations among cultural groups' responses, drug interactions, and metabolism. Colonial impacts and inequities in access to health care services have contributed to the burden of risk factors for specific chronic diseases, such as type 2 diabetes and cardiovascular disease among some Indigenous communities (Anand et al., 2019; Crowshoe et al., 2018; Reading, 2015; Schultz et al., 2021).

When interacting with clients, allow time for them to respond. Once you have obtained information, respect their use of alternative treatments (e.g., dietary customs, cultural rituals, herbal or plant-based medicines) and integrate aspects within the plan of care. Involve the client as an equal partner in setting goals, and per the nursing process, implement and evaluate the plan of care during the client's hospitalization and post-discharge.

An intercultural communication model (LEARN) developed by Berlin and Fowkes (1983) to enhance communication between health care providers and clients in culturally diverse encounters can aid the negotiation of a solution-focused care plan.

> **L:** Listen attentively to client, showing respect and sensitivity, to gain understanding of their health situation with consideration of their cultural beliefs, practices, norms, and values. Use nonjudgmental language and avoid medical jargon. You can ask the client, "What do you think caused your illness?" or "What are your fears of hospitalization?" or "What treatments were used at home?"
>
> **E:** Explain your perception of the health issue and possible causes, incorporating the client's perspective and reason for admission. Review your understanding of the health issue/concern with client.
>
> **A:** Acknowledge differences and similarities in language used in communication in the encounter. Check for validation and understanding from the client's and your perspective. Adapt communication to the client's cultural context. Assess the need to use an interpreter.
>
> **R:** Once data has been obtained and reviewed, recommend treatments that respectfully support the values, knowledge, cultural beliefs, and lifestyle of client (e.g., cultural rituals and health practices such as traditional healers).
>
> **N:** Negotiate an agreement as equal partners in health care decisions/treatments and the implementation and evaluation of the plan of care. Involve family in the decision-making process.

USE OF INTERPRETERS

The health care provider should recognize the need for and can decide to use a professional interpreter when the client does not speak English, speaks English as their second language, or has limited English proficiency. In these situations, communicating without the assistance of an interpreter creates a greater barrier between the health care professionals and the client. The use of a qualified interpreter prevents potential harmful events and promotes client safety in the clinical encounter. Canada has no legislation related to the use of interpreters in health care settings. However, based upon civil rights law, any hospital receiving government funding must have language translation services available for clients. The nurse should have knowledge of the organization's policy on the use of and process for contacting a trained interpreter. In Canada, the Ontario Council on Community Interpreting defines a professional interpreter as a "fluently bilingual individual with appropriate training and experience who is able to interpret with consistency and accuracy and who adheres to the Standards of Practice and Ethical Principles" (n.d.). The ethnic origin, religious background, gender, language, or dialect of the interpreter needs to be considered when seeking services for culturally diverse clients (Yelland et al., 2016). When planning to use an interpreter, it is important to include the client and family members in the decision-making process. However, because of confidentiality protocols, sensitivity, and the complexity of medical information, family members should not be used as interpreters (Squires, 2018). When providing translation services for a client, the health care provider needs to document this information in the client's clinical record and also in their plan of care.

HEALTH INEQUITIES

Health inequities are "differences in health between specific population groups that are systematic, avoidable, and unjust" (Churchill et al., 2021, p. 1). These inequities are determined by income, social status, education, race/racism, colonialism, employment/working conditions, housing, and culture. These social and structural factors contribute to health inequities, which are key elements within the determinants of health. Certain populations and groups of people, like those with lower incomes, those who are living in poverty, those with a disability, immigrants, and those who are marginalized (e.g., Indigenous people, people of colour, people who identify as LGBTQ2+), are challenged to close the gaps in health and health care access to acquire health equity. To address health inequities, governments at all levels need to enact policies to strengthen structural improvements to the social determinants of health (Kirst et al., 2017).

In Canada, Indigenous people have experienced, and continue to experience, health inequities in comparison to the general population. A plethora of studies have documented Indigenous people's significant health inequities (Horrill et al., 2020; Kolahdooz et al., 2015; Wylie et al., 2019). For example, the incidence of cardiovascular disease is at least two times higher among Indigenous people (11.5%) than among non-Indigenous people (5.5%) (Fontaine et al., 2019). Among First Nations, diabetes prevalence is three to five times higher than in other populations. Many communities with families with high rates of type 2 diabetes experience barriers to culturally appropriate self-management programs, which hamper interventions (Crowshoe et al., 2018; Kulhawy-Wibe et al., 2018). These inequities are related to colonial history, which has impacted the social determinants of health for Indigenous people and affected their health and well-being, as evidenced by the Indian Act of 1876, ongoing colonial policies, intergenerational trauma from the residential school system, and racism (Allan & Smylie, 2015; Berg et al., 2019; Goodman et al., 2017;

Wylie et al., 2019). In addition, stigmatization and discrimination experienced by Indigenous clients within the health care system create barriers to those seeking health services (Boyer, 2017; Paradies, 2018).

Indigenous people's colonial legacies and ongoing experiences of discrimination, bias, stereotypes, and racism by health care professionals has led to feelings of distrust and distress in health care settings (Phillips-Beck et al., 2020; Stout et al., 2021; Turpel-Lafond & Johnson, 2021). In Canada, injustices such as the "Indian hospitals," the forced and coerced sterilization of Indigenous women after childbirth, and the treatment and death of Joyce Echaquan are just a few examples of racism toward Indigenous people (Leason, 2021; Lux, 2016; Tremblay & Echaquan, 2022). These behaviours lead to underutilization of health services or avoidance of seeking care, and poor outcomes for Indigenous people (CNA, 2018).

Cultural safety is advocated as an approach to improve health care services for Indigenous people (Brooks-Cleator et al., 2018; Greenwood et al., 2017; Vang et al., 2018; Wylie et al., 2019). An initiative to provide culturally safe programs and community services led to the establishment of the First Nations Health Authority (FNHA), the first province-wide health authority of its kind in Canada. The FNHA is responsible for planning, designing, managing, funding, and delivering services to BC First Nations throughout the province to attain positive health outcomes. The FNHA (2016) has a policy statement on cultural safety and humility entitled "It Starts with Me," meaning that every health care professional is responsible and accountable to "embed cultural safety into the health system across multiple levels" (p. 2).

To address health inequities, some collaborative discussions with Elders and community leaders led to innovative Indigenous health care partnerships that strengthen traditional cultural ways, including health and healing practices (Allen et al., 2020) within some Canadian provinces and territories. For example, the Turtle Lodge International Centre for Indigenous Education and Wellness, located in Sagkeeng First Nation, Manitoba, was founded by Elder Dave Courchene and provides culturally safe care and holistic health practices for Indigenous and non-Indigenous people from all Nations (Cameron et al., 2019).

LGBTQIA2+ POPULATION AND HEALTH INEQUITIES

The acronym LGBTQIA2+ is used to reflect people who identify as lesbian, gay, bisexual, transgender, queer (or questioning), intersex, asexual, and two-spirit, with the + signifying a number of other identities (Loveless, 2021). This population experiences higher rates of health inequities due to stigma, discrimination, violence, and bias related to their sexual orientation and gender identity (House of Commons Standing Committee on Health, 2019; Morris et al., 2019; Waryold & Kornahrens, 2020). Also contributing to these health inequities is the notion of heteronormativity (the idea that everyone is heterosexual) inherent within

Canada's health care system (Schreiber er al., 2021). Research indicates that the LGBTQIA2+ community experiences more mental health issues—such as depression, anxiety, minority stress, and an elevated risk for substance use and suicidality, especially among youth—than heterosexual or cisgender individuals (National Academies of Sciences, Engineering, and Medicine, 2020; Cottrell et al., 2022; Hatchel at al., 2019).

These disparities are also influenced by health care professionals' biases, evidenced by transphobic and homophobic attitudes, discrimination, and hostility experienced by the LGBTQIA2+ community (Henriquez & Ahmad, 2021). These behaviours lead individuals to mistrust health care providers and delay or avoid seeking health services, resulting in suboptimal care and poor health outcomes (Morris et al., 2019). For example, in the following narrative, a study participant speaks of biased judgment from physicians while seeking health care (Henriquez & Ahmad, p. 5):

> I think it's when the doctors are start telling you what you're doing is wrong rather than listening to you. I know friends who have stories [about] the doctor telling them that they're evil or they're sinning." (Participant, gay male)

Such biased behaviours reflect the need for education, directed at all health care professionals, on cultural humility and safety in the provision of care to minority populations. Through a relational practice lens, practitioners can develop person-centred relationships of trust and rapport in providing inclusive and affirming care (Kuzma et al., 2019). Some communication best practices for inclusive care for LGBTQIA2+ people include the following:

- Use inclusive language. Adopt gender-neutral language. Avoid gendered words (e.g., *Mr.* or *ma'am*). Example: "What brings you to the clinic today?"
- Introduce yourself. Example: Hi my name is … and my pronouns are *she/her/hers* (or *he/him/his*). What are yours?"
- When completing an assessment, ask the client respectfully and privately about their name or pronouns. Example: "What name and pronouns would you like us to use?"
- For transgender clients, use open-ended questions, for example, "How do you describe your gender identity?" This approach helps to establish open communication and respect for all at the first interaction (Kyle, 2022; Rosendale et al., 2018).
- Use the terms people use to describe themselves. Example: If a man refers to his "husband," then say, "your husband" when referring to him. Do not say, "your partner" or "your friend."

- When completing an assessment, only ask for information that is required. Use a respectful and sensitive approach in gathering information. Document the client's preferred pronouns, name used, and gender identity.
- Use a welcoming approach, provide privacy, and stress confidentiality with the client.
- When talking to colleagues about the client, use appropriate gender-neutral words, such as *they/them/theirs*.
- If you make a mistake and misgender someone, apologize. Example: "I apologize for using the wrong name or pronoun. I did not mean to disrespect you."

Gender Pronouns

He, him, his, himself
She, her, hers, herself
They, them, theirs, themselves
This is not an exhaustive list.

Source: Egale. (2022). *Egale—pronoun usage guide.* https://egale.ca/awareness/pronoun-usage-guide/

The literature also suggests promoting health equity among the LGBTQIA2+ population in Canada by incorporating content on health care for this population in undergraduate medical, nursing, and other health-focused programs. Other recommendations include institutional-level interventions such as adapting health settings to be more inclusive of clients and staff by using gender-inclusive language on forms, having nondiscrimination policies in place and prominently displayed, having all-gender restrooms, and providing ongoing education for all staff on gender-affirming workplaces (Elertson & McNiel, 2020; Waryold & Kornahrens, 2020).

BIAS IN HEALTH CARE

As a health care professional student, you bring your existing biases into the program and your practice (Persaud, 2019). Biases, also known as stereotypes, can be defined as the evaluation of one group and its members relative to another group. They can be either explicit (aware) or unconscious (outside of one's awareness, implicit) and may include but are not limited to ethnicity, race, gender, gender identity, sexual orientation, social status, religion, or weight (Marcelin et al., 2019; Persaud, 2019). Research suggests that implicit biases and racist attitudes contribute to health inequities (Goodman et al., 2017; Phillips-Beck et al., 2020; Ricks et al., 2022). As a clinician, you should be aware that biases exist in the health care profession as well as in others. Biases undermine work with colleagues and the development of therapeutic relationships, reinforce health inequities, and affect clinical practice (Narayan, 2019). Health care professionals, including nurses, are responsible for providing ethical, unbiased care to all persons. Mindfulness is a recommended strategy for assessment and evaluation approaches to reduce the effects of clinician implicit bias on clients (Burgess et al., 2017; Narayan, 2019; Tudino & Jellison, 2022). One mindfulness technique, STOP, is used to reduce implicit biases by enabling nurses to recognize feelings in the client encounter and taking steps to centre themselves and adjust their response.

STOP Mindfulness Technique

- **Stop** what you're doing.
- **Take** some slow, deep breaths.
- **Observe** your thoughts, feelings, and assumptions.
- **Proceed** with client care/activity.

Self-reflection is also recommended for health care professionals when providing care to clients. Reflecting on feelings in the clinical encounter helps health care professionals acknowledge, refocus, and control implicit biases.

Case Study 4.3

The client, a 55-year-old woman, is admitted to the emergency department at 9:00 AM after being picked up by the local police. They found her wandering in the street, looking very dirty and complaining of pain in her feet and legs. She has a large cut on her lower right leg. The police inform the staff that this woman is homeless. She is thin, is wearing multiple layers of clothing, and appears disheveled and dirty, with matted hair. A nurse informs the attending physician that the client is in Room 10 and states, "This one is a real winner. I wish these clients would have a bath before coming here; they really smell up the place. I would advise you to wear a gown and gloves before doing any assessment."

1. Identify the bias in this situation and discuss how it might affect nursing care.
2. As a health professional student, what would you do to reduce the bias in the situation?
3. Are you aware of your own personal biases or stereotypes toward persons or groups that could impact care to those clients?
4. Identify the strategies that you would use to deal with biases in your clinical practice.

Exercise 4.2: Culturally Diverse Clients

Review the following questions and complete as requested. Your instructor will assign these questions as an individual take-home assignment or an in-class activity.

1. Search the website of your health care facility or health authority to determine the procedures and policies that support culturally safe care services for a client who is LGBTQIA2+.
2. Identify the resources in your community that provide supports for culturally diverse persons.
3. Reflect on the biases that you recognize in yourself when communicating with a client who is Indigenous or from the LGBTQIA2+ community.
4. From your experience as a nursing student, discuss with a classmate your perception of how health care providers communicate with culturally diverse clients.
5. List several approaches to use if you are assigned to care for a client who has limited English proficiency.
6. Search the website of your provincial professional association or college to determine what terminology is used in their standards of practice with respect to cultural safety or humility.

Case Study 4.4

You are admitting a 25-year-old Indigenous male client to the surgical unit. This is the client's first hospitalization; they are being admitted for a pre-booked surgical appendectomy. You note from reviewing the medical record that they were assessed by their family physician. The client is escorted to the unit by the admitting clerk.

1. Identify at least four questions the nurse will ask during their initial interview.
2. List three main priorities of care for the client.
3. What will the nurse do to establish a welcoming environment that is culturally appropriate?

CHAPTER SUMMARY

This chapter explores the concept of culture and its impact on clients who need health services. *Culture* is defined as a set of values, beliefs, behaviours, language, and customs that shape a person's identity and how they negotiate their world. Related terms *cultural blindness*, *cultural safety*, *cultural humility*, *cultural trauma*, *co-culture*, *ethnicity*, and *ethnocentrism* are defined. Communication and language are influenced by culture, which impacts individuals' views of health and health care practices. Relational practice as a way of being in relationships is considered an approach in working with clients who are culturally diverse.

A cultural assessment is an important tool used by the health care providers to determine the clients' needs, and this aids the development of a collaborative nursing care plan. There are several nursing models available for cultural assessment that support the use of a culturally sensitive approach when communicating with the client and their family. To be effective in working with culturally diverse clients, nurses need to understand and adopt the principles of cultural safety and humility in order to build a therapeutic nurse-client relationship. Using the acronym LEARN (Listen, Explain, Acknowledge, Recommend, and Negotiate) supports a culturally safe person-centred approach to care. The issue of health inequities for Indigenous people and the LGBTQIA2+ community is also discussed. Communication approaches for these populations are included to guide health care providers in building a professional, respectful communication encounter.

REVIEW QUESTIONS

Read the following review questions and select the best option to answer each question. State your rationale for choosing your response.

1. A client is newly admitted to the medical unit with a diagnosis of substance use disorder. When working with the client, which should be the health care professional's *initial* action?
   a. Explore with the client the reasons for using substances (e.g., alcohol, street drugs).
   b. Explore with the client the idea that using substances is not the answer to their problem.
   c. Work to establish a nurse-client relationship using relational practice.
   d. Evaluate the nurse's feelings regarding working with the client.
2. What does the term *heteronormativity* mean?
   a. The health care provider conveys an attitude of disrespect for the client
   b. Education of all staff on the topic of heterosexuality and homosexuality in clients

    c.   Ongoing self-reflection on the concept of heterosexuality

    d.   The assumption that everyone is heterosexual and this is superior to all other sexualities

3.   Which of the following is an appropriate question for the health care provider to ask during an initial intake assessment with a client who is transgender?

    a.   "What is your sexual orientation?"

    b.   "What name and pronouns do you prefer?"

    c.   "How long have you been a tranny?"

    d.   "Have you had any sex change surgery?"

4.   Which of the following statements is *true* with regard to cultural safety?

    a.   Cultural safety allows health care professionals to reflect on the impact of their own cultural history/experiences on client care.

    b.   Culturally safe care is defined by those who receive the care and not by the care providers.

    c.   Culturally safe care is client-centred and is applied after disclosure of trauma experience.

    d.   Cultural safety is an important step in ongoing efforts to address Indigenous-specific inequities.

5.   Which of the following is *not* a principle of trauma-informed nursing practice?

    a.   Introduce yourself and your role in every client interaction.

    b.   Use open and nonthreatening body positioning.

    c.   Practice universal trauma precautions.

    d.   To show caring, use touch as a communication tool.

WEB RESOURCES

Egale.ca (Resource for LGBTQIA2+ persons)
https://egale.ca
National Collaborating Centre for Indigenous Health
https://www.nccih.ca/en

REFERENCES

Aboriginal Nurses Association of Canada. (2009). *Cultural competence and cultural safety in nursing education.* https://hl-prod-ca-oc-download.s3-ca-central-1.amazonaws.com/CNA/2f975e7e-4a40-45ca-863c-5ebf0a138d5e/UploadedImages/documents/First_Nations_Framework_e.pdf

Abualhaija, N. (2019). The transformational expedition of cultural competence in nursing. *International Journal of Nursing and Health Care Research, 11*. https://doi.org/10.29011/IJNHR-1127.101127

Allan, B., & Smylie, J. (2015). *First Peoples, second class treatment: The role of racism in the health and well-being of Indigenous peoples in Canada.* Wellesley Institute. https://www.wellesleyinstitute.com/wp-content/upload/2015/02/Summary-First-Peoples-Second-Class-Treatment-Final.pdf

Allen, L., Hatala, A., Ijaz, S., Courchene, D., & Bushie, B. (2020). Indigenous-led health care partnerships in Canada. *CMAJ, 192*(9). https://doi.org/10.1503/cmaj.190728

Anand, S. S., Abonyi, S., Arbour, L., Balasubramanian, K., Brook, J., Castleden, H., Chrisjohn, V., Cornelius, I., Davis, A. D., Desai, D., de Souza, R. J., Friedrich, M. G., Harris, S., Irvine, J., L'Hommecourt, J., Littlechild, R., Mayotte, L., McIntosh, S., Morrison, J., … Toth, E. L. (2019). Explaining the variability in cardiovascular risk factors among First Nations communities in Canada: A population-based study. *The Lancet Planetary Health, 3*(12), e511–e520. https://doi.org/10.1016/s2542-5196(19)30237-2

Beattie, J., Griffiths, D., Innes, K., & Morphet, J. (2019). Workplace violence perpetrated by clients of health care: A need for safety and trauma-informed care. *Journal of Clinical Nursing, 28*(1–2), 116–124. https://doi.org/10.1111/jocn.14683

Beebe, S. A., Beebe, S. J., & Ivy, D. K. (2019). *Communication: Principles for a lifetime* (7th ed.). Pearson.

Berg, K., McLane, P., Eshkakogan, N., Mantha, J., Lee, T., Crowshoe, C., & Phillips, A. (2019). Perspectives on Indigenous cultural competency and safety in Canadian hospital emergency departments: A scoping review. *International Emergency Nursing, 43*, 133–140. https://doi.org/10.1016/j.ienj.2019.01.004

Berlin, E., & Fowkes, W. (1983). A teaching framework for cross-cultural health care: Application in family practice. *Western Journal of Medicine, 139*(6), 934–938.

Breault, P., Nault, J., Audette, M., Échaquan, S., & Ottawa, J. (2021). Reflections on Indigenous health care: Building trust. *Canadian Family Physician, 67*(8), 567–568. https://doi.org/10.46747/cfp.6708567

British Columbia College of Nurses and Midwives. (2022). *Practice Standard: Indigenous cultural safety, cultural humility, and anti-racism.* https://www.bccnm.ca/Documents/cultural_safety_humility/All_PS_cultural_safety_humility.pdf

Bokor-Billmann, T., Langan, E. A., & Billmann, F. (2020). The reporting of race and/or ethnicity in the medical literature: A retrospective bibliometric analysis confirmed room for improvement. *Journal of Clinical Epidemiology, 119*, 1–6. https://doi.org/10.1016/j.jclinepi.2019.11.005

Boyer, Y. (2017). Healing racism in Canadian health care. *CMAJ, 189*(46), e1408–e1409. https://doi.org/10.1503/cmaj.171234

Brooks-Cleator, L., Phillipps, B., & Giles, A. (2018). Culturally safe health initiatives for Indigenous peoples in Canada: A scoping review. *Canadian Journal of Nursing Research, 50*(4), 202–213. https://doi.org/10.1177/0844562118770334

Brooks, L. A., Manias, E., & Bloomer, M. J. (2019). Culturally sensitive communication in healthcare: A concept analysis. *Collegian, 26*, 383–391. https://doi.org/10.1016/j.colegn.2018.09.007

Burgess, D. J., Beach, M. C., & Saha, S. (2017). Mindfulness practice: A promising approach to reducing the effects of clinician implicit bias on patients. *Patient Education and Counseling, 100*(2), 372–376. https://doi.org/10.1016/j.pec.2016.09.005

Cameron, L., Courchene, D., Ijaz, S., & Mauro, I. (2019). The turtle lodge: Sustainable self-determination in practice. *AlterNative, 15*(1), 13–21. https://doi.org/10.1177/1177180119828075

Canadian Nurses Association. (2018). *Position statement: Promoting cultural competence in nursing.* https://hl-prod-ca-oc-download.s3-ca-central-1.amazonaws.com/CNA/2f975e7e-4a40-45ca-863c-5ebf0a138d5e/UploadedImages/documents/Position_Statement_Promoting_Cultural_Competence_in_Nursing.pdf

Cannon, L. M., Coolidge, E. M., LeGierse, J., Moskowitz, Y., Buckley, C., Chapin, E., Warren, M., & Kuzma, E. K. (2020). Trauma-informed education: Creating and pilot testing a nursing curriculum on trauma-informed care. *Nurse Education Today, 85,* https://doi.org/10.1016/j.nedt.2019.104256

Churchill, E., Shankardass, K., Perrella, A. M. I., Lofters, A., Quiñonez, C., Brooks, L., Wilson, D., & Kirst, M. (2021). Effectiveness of narrative messaging styles about the social determinants of health and health inequities in Ontario, Canada. *International Journal of Environmental Research and Public Health, 18*(20), https://doi.org/10.3390/ijerph182010881

Churchill, M. E., Smylie, J. K., Wolfe, S. H., Bourgeois, C., Moeller, H., & Firestone, M. (2020). Conceptualizing cultural safety at an Indigenous-focused midwifery practice in Toronto, Canada: Qualitative interviews with Indigenous and non-Indigenous clients. *BMJ Open, 10.* https://doi.org/10.1136/bmjopen-2020-038168

College of Licensed Practical Nurses of Newfoundland and Labrador. (2020). *Standards of practice for Licensed practical nurses in Canada.* https://www.clpnnl.ca/sites/default/files/2021-03/Standards%20of%20Practice%202020.pdf

College of Registered Nurses of Newfoundland and Labrador. (2019). *Standards of practice for registered nurses and nurse practitioners.* https://www.crnnl.ca/site/uploads/2021/09/standards-of-practice-for-rns-and-nps.pdf

Conroy, T., Feo, R., Boucaut, R., Alderman, J., & Kitson, A. (2017). Role of effective nurse-patient relationships in enhancing patient safety. *Nursing Standard, 31*(49), 53–61. https://doi.org/10.7748/ns.2017.e10801

Cottrell, D. B., Gonzalez, J. D., Atchison, P. T., Evans, S. C., & Stokes, A. (2022). Suicide risk and prevention in LGBTQ+ youth. *Nursing, 52*(2), 40-45. https://doi.org/10.1097/01.NURSE.0000803432.31284.34

Crowshoe, L., Dannenbaum, D., Green, M., Henderson, R., Hayward, M. N., & Toth, E. (2018). Type 2 diabetes and Indigenous peoples: Diabetes Canada clinical practice guidelines expert committee. *Canadian Journal of Diabetes, 42*(1), 5296–5306. https://doi.org/10.1016/j.jcjd.2017.10.022

Curtis, E., Jones, R., Tipene-Leach, D., Walker, C., Loring, B., Paine, S. J., & Reid, P. (2019). Why cultural safety rather than cultural competency is required to achieve health equity: A literature review and recommended definition. *International Journal for Equity in Health*, *18*(174). https://doi.org/10.1186/s12939-019-1082-3

Death of Joyce Echaquan. (2022). *Wikipedia*. https://en.wikipedia.org/wiki/Death_of_Joyce_Echaquan

Douglas, M. K., Rosenkoetter, M., Pacquiao, D. F., Callister, L. C., Hattar-Pollara, M., Lauderdale, J., Milstead, J., Nardi, D., & Purnell, L. (2014). Guidelines for implementing culturally competent nursing care. *Journal of Transcultural Nursing*, *25*(2), 109–121. https://doi.org/10.1177/1043659614520998

Egale. (2022). *Egale—pronoun usage guide*. https://egale.ca/awareness/pronoun-usage-guide/

Elertson, K., & McNiel, P. L. (2020). Answering the call: Educating future nurses on LGBTQ healthcare. *Journal of Homosexuality*, *65*(13), 2234–2245. https://doi.org/10.1080/00918369.2020.1734376

Emmamally, W., Erlingsson, C., & Brysiewicz, P. (2020). Describing healthcare providers' perceptions of relational practice with families in the emergency department: A qualitative study. *Curationis*, *43*(1), a2155. https://doi.org/10.4102/curationis.v43i1.2155

First Nations Health Authority. (2016). *#itstartswithme: FNHA'S policy statement on cultural Safety and humility*. https://www.fnha.ca

First Nations Health Authority. (2021). *Anti-racism, cultural safety & humility framework*. https://www.fnha.ca/Documents/FNHA-FNHC-FNHDA-Anti-Racism-Cultural-Safety-and-Humility-Framework.pdf

First Nations Health Authority. (2022). *British Columbia cultural safety and humility standard*. https://www.fnha.ca/about/news-and-events/news/fnha-and-hso-release-bc-cultural-safety-and-humility-standard

Fleishman, J., Kamasky, H., & Sundborg, S. (2019). Trauma-informed nursing practice. *The Online Journal of Issues in Nursing*, *24*(2). https://doi.org/10.3912/OJIN.Vol24No02Man03

Fontaine, L. S., Wood, S., Forbes, L., & Schulyz, A. S. H. (2019). Listening to First Nations women' expressions of heart health: Mite achimowin digital storytelling study. *International Journal of Circumpolar Health*, *78*(1), 1630233. https://doi.org/10.1080/22423982.2019.1630233

Foronda, C. (2020). A theory of cultural humility. *Journal of Transcultural Nursing*, *31*(1), 7–12. https://doi.org/10.1177/1043659619875184

Fyers, K., & Greenwood, S. (2016). Cultural safety and relational practice: Ways of being with ourselves and others. *Nursing Review*, *16*(4), 22–30.

Garneau, A. B., & Pepin, J. (2015). Cultural competence: A constructivist definition. *Journal of Transcultural Nursing*, *26*(1), 9–15. https://doi.org/10.1177/1043659614541294

Giger, J. N., & Davidhizar, R. (1999). *Transcultural nursing: Assessment and interventions* (3rd ed.). Mosby.

Giger, J. N., & Davidhizar, R. (2002). The Giger and Davidhizar transcultural assessment model. *Journal of Transcultural Nursing*, *13*(3), 185–188. https://doi.org/10.1177/10459602013003004.

Goddard, A., Jones, R., & Etcher, L. (2022). Trauma informed care in nursing: A concept analysis. *Nursing Outlook, 70*(3), 429–439. https://doi.org/10.1016/j.outlook.2021.12.010

Godin, M. (2020). *Canada outraged by death of Indigenous woman Joyce Echaquan.* https://time .com/5898422/joyce-echaquan-indigenous-protests-canada/

Goodman, A., Fleming, K., Markwick, N., Morrison, T., Lagimodiere, L., Kerr, T., & Western Harm Reduction Society. (2017). "They treated me like crap and I know it was because I was native": The healthcare experiences of Aboriginal peoples living in Vancouver's inner city. *Social Science & Medicine, 178,* 87–94. https://doi.org/10.1016/j .socscimed.2017.01.053

Greenwood, M., Lindsay, N., King, J., & Loewen, D. (2017). Ethical spaces and places: Indigenous cultural safety in British Columbia health care. *AlterNative, 13*(3), 179–189. https://doi.org/10.1177/1177180117714411

Halter, M. J., Pollard, C. L., & Jakubec, S. L. (2019). *Varcarolis's Canadian psychiatric mental health nursing: A clinical approach* (2nd ed.). Elsevier.

Hans, A., & Hans, E. (2015). Kinesics, haptics, and proxemics: Aspects of non-verbal communication. *Journal of Humanities and Social Science, 20*(2), 47–52.

Hartrick Doane, G., & Varcoe, C. (2021). *How to nurse: Relational inquiry in action* (2nd ed.). Wolters Kluwer.

Hatchel, T., Polanin, J. R., & Espelage, D. L. (2019). Suicidal thoughts and behaviors among LGBTQ youth: Meta-Analyses and a systematic review. *Archives of Suicide Research, 25*(1), 1–37. https://doi.org/10.1080/13811118.2019.1663329

Henriquez, N. R., & Ahmad, N. (2021). "The message is you don't exist": Exploring lived experiences of rural lesbian, gay, bisexual, transgender, queer/questioning (LGBTQ) people utilizing health care services. *Open Nursing, 7,* 1–10. https://doi.org/10.1177/ 23779608211051174

Horrill, T. C., Lavoie, J. G., Martin, D., & Schultz, A. (2020). Places & spaces: A critical analysis of cancer disparities and access to cancer care among First Nations Peoples in Canada. *The Canadian Journal of Critical Nursing Discourse, 2*(2), 104–123. https://doi .org/10.25071/2291-5796.62

House of Commons Standing Committee on Health. (2019). *The health of LGBTQIA2 communities in Canada: Report of the standing committee on health.* https://www .ourcommons.ca/Content/Committee/421/HESA/Reports/RP10574595/hesarp28/ hesarp28-e.pdf

Hughes, V., Delva, S., Nkimbeng, M., Spaulding, E., Turkson-Ocran, R.-A., Cudjoe, J., Ford, A., Rushton, C., D'Aoust, R., & Han, H.-R. (2020). Not missing the opportunity: Strategies to promote cultural humility among future nursing faculty. *Journal of Professional Nursing, 36,* 28–33. https://doi.org/10.1016/j.profnurs.2019.06.005

Kirst, M., Shankardass, K., Singhal, S., Lofters, A., Muntaner, C., & Quiñonez, C. (2017). Addressing health inequities in Ontario, Canada: What solutions do the public support? *BMC Public Health, 17*(7). https://doi.org/10.1186/s12889-016-3932-x

Kitching, G. T., Firestone, M., Schei, B., Wolfe, S., Bourgeois, C., O'Campo, P., Rotondi, M., Nisenbaum, R., Maddox, R., & Smylie, J. (2020). Unmet health needs and discrimination by healthcare providers among Indigenous population in Toronto, Canada. *Canadian Journal of Public Health*, *111*(1), 40–49. https://doi.org/10.17269/s41997-019-00242-z

Kolahdooz, F., Nader, F., Kyoung, J., & Sharma, S. (2015). Understanding the social determinants of health among Indigenous Canadians: Priorities for health promotion policies and actions. *Global Health Action*, *8*(1). https://doi.org/10.3402/gha.v8.27968

Kulhawy-Wibe, S., King-Shier, K. M., Barnabe, C., Manns, B. J., Hemmelgarn, B. R., & Campbell, D. J. T. (2018). Exploring structural barriers to diabetes self-management in Alberta First Nations communities. *BMC*, *10*(87). https://doi.org/10.1186/s13098-018-0385-7

Kurtz, D. L., Janke, R., Vinek, J., Wells, T., Hutchison, P., & Froste, A. (2018). Health sciences cultural safety education in Australia, Canada, New Zealand, and the United States: A literature review. *International Journal of Medical Education*, *9*, 271–285. https://doi.org/10.5116/ijme.5bc7.21e2

Kuzma, E. K., Pardee, M., & Darling-Fisher, C. S. (2019). Lesbian, gay, bisexual, and transgender health: Creating safe spaces and caring for patients with cultural humility. *Journal of the American Association of Nurse Practitioners*, *31*(3), 167–174. https://doi.org/10.1097/doc.0000000000000131

Kyle, B. L. (2022). Inclusivity and respect: Beyond personal pronouns. *Advances in Neonatal Care*, *22*(2), 95–96. https://doi.org/10.1097/ANC.0000000000001001

Leason, J. (2021). Forced and coerced sterilization of Indigenous women: Strengths to build upon. *Canadian Family Physician*, *67*, 525–527. https://doi.org/10.46747/cfp.6707525

Leininger, M. (2002). Culture care theory: A major contribution to advance transcultural nursing knowledge and practices. *Journal of Transcultural Nursing*, *13*(3), 189–192. https://doi.org/10.1177/10459602013003005

Li, C., Abdulkerim, N., Jordan, C. A., & Son, C. G. E. (2017). Overcoming communication barriers to healthcare for culturally and linguistically diverse patients. *North American Journal of Medicine and Science*, *10*(3), 103–109. https://doi.org/10.7156/najms.2017.10033103

Loveless, G. E. (2021). *The LGBTQIA2+ community: Our pronouns, when and how to use them.* https://sites.austincc.edu/accent/the-lgbtqia2-community-our-pronouns-when-how-to-use-them/

Lux, M. K. (2016). *Separate beds: A history of Indian hospitals in Canada, 1920s–1980s.* University of Toronto Press.

Marcelin, J. R., Siraj, D. S., Victor, R., Kotadia, S., & Maldonado, Y. A. (2019). The impact of unconscious bias in healthcare: How to recognize and mitigate it. *The Journal of Infectious Diseases*, *220*(s2). https://doi.org/10.1093/infdis/jiz214

Metheny, N., & Fletcher, C. D. (2021). An environmental scan of Indigenous cultural safety in Canadian baccalaureate nursing and midwifery programs. *Canadian Journal of Nursing Research*, *53*(4), 417–425. https://doi.org/10.1177/08445621211016143

Morris, N., Cooper, R. L., Ramesh, A., Tabatabai, M., Arcury, T. A., Shinn, M., Im, W., Juarez, P., & Matthews-Juarez, P. (2019). Training to reduce LGBTQ-related bias among medical, nursing, and dental students and providers: A systematic review. *BMC Medical Education, 19*(1), 1–13. https://doi.org/10.1186/s12909-019-1727-3

Narayan, M. C. (2019). Addressing implicit bias in nursing: A review. *American Journal of Nursing, 119*(7). https://doi.org/10.1097/01.naj.0000569340.27659.5A

National Academies of Sciences, Engineering, and Medicine. (2020). *Understanding the well-being of LGBTQI+ populations.* https://nap.nationalacademies.org/catalog/25877/understanding-the-well-being-of-lgbtqi-populations

Nguyen, N. H., Subhan, F. B., Williams, K., & Chan, C. B. (2020). Barriers and mitigating strategies to healthcare access in Indigenous communities in Canada: A narrative review. *Healthcare, 8*(112). https://doi.org/10.3390/healthcare8020112

Ontario Council on Community Interpreting. (n.d.) *What is a professional interpreter?* https://www.occi.ca/faqs

Pandey, M., Kamrul, R., Michaels, C. R., & McCarron, M. (2022). Identifying barriers to healthcare access for new immigrants: A qualitative study in Regina, Saskatchewan, Canada. *Journal of Immigrant and Minority Health, 24*(1), 188–198. https://doi.org/10.1007/s10903-021-01262-z

Paradies, Y. (2018). Racism and Indigenous health. *Global Public Health*, 1–17. https://doi.org/10.1093/acrefore/9780190632366.013.86

Persaud, S. (2019). Addressing unconscious bias: A nurse leader's role. *Nursing Administration Quarterly, 43*(2), 130–137. https://doi.org/10.1097/NAQ.0000000000000348

Phillips-Beck, W., Eni, R., Lavoie, J. G., Kinew, K. A., Achan, G. K., & Katz, A. (2020). Confronting racism within the Canadian healthcare system: Systemic exclusion of First Nations from quality and consistent care. *International Journal of Environmental Research and Public Health, 17*(22), 8343. https://doi.org/10.3390/ijerph17228343

Ramsden, I. M. (2002). *Cultural safety and nursing education in Aotearo and Te Waipounamu* [Master's thesis]. University of Wellington. https://www.croakey.org/wp-content/uploads/2017/08/RAMSDEN-I-Cultural-Safety_Full.pdf

Reading, J. (2015). Confronting the growing crisis of cardiovascular disease and heart health among Aboriginal peoples in Canada. *Canadian Journal of Cardiology, 31*(9), 1077–1080. https://doi.org/10.1016/j.cjca.2015.06.012

Ricks, T. N., Abbyad, C., & Polinard, E. (2022). Undoing racism and mitigating bias among healthcare professionals: Lessons learned during a systematic review. *Journal of Racial and Ethnic Health Disparities, 9*, 1990–2000. https://doi.org/10.1007/s40615-021-01137-x

Rosendale, N., Goldman, S., Ortiz, G. M., & Haber, L. A. (2018). Acute clinical care for transgender patients: A review. *JAMA Internal Medicine, 178*(11), 1535–1543. https://doi.org/10.1001/jamainternmed.2018.4179

Ruud, M. (2018). Cultural humility in the care of individuals who are lesbian, gay, bisexual, transgender, or queer. *Nursing for Women's Health, 22*(3), 255–263. https://doi.org/10.1016/j.nwh.2018.03.009

Schreiber, M., Ahmad, T., Scott, M., Imries, K., & Razack, S. (2021). The case for a Canadian standard for 2SLGBTQIA+ medical education. *CMAJ, 193*(16), e562–565. https://doi .org/10.1503/cmaj.202642

Schultz, A., Nguyen, T., Sinclaire, M., Fransoo, R., & McGibbon, E. (2021). Historical and continued colonial impacts on heart health of Indigenous peoples in Canada: What's reconciliation got to do with it? *CJC Open, 3*(12), s149–s164. https://doi.org/10.1016/j .cjco.2021.09.010

Schwind, J. K., & Manankil-Rankin, L. (2020). Using narrative reflective process to augment personal and aesthetic ways of knowing to support holistic person-centred relational practice. *Reflective Practice, 21*(4), 473–483. https://doi.org/10.1080/14623943 .2020.1777958

Squires, A. (2018). Strategies for overcoming language barriers in healthcare. *Nursing Management, 49*(4), 20–27. https://doi.org/10.1097/01.NUMA.0000531166.24481.15

Statistics Canada. (2019). *Canada in 2041: A larger, more diverse population with greater differences between regions.* https://www150.statcan.gc.ca/n1/daily-quotidien/220908/dq220908a-eng.htm

Statistics Canada. (2021). A statistical portrait of Canada's diverse LGBTQ2+ communities. https:// www150.statcan.gc.ca/n1/en/daily-quotidien/210615/dq210615a-eng.pdf?st=l9lMdmWT

Statistics Canada. (2022). *The Canadian census: A rich portrait of the country's religious and ethnocultural diversity.* https://www150.statcan.gc.ca/n1/en/daily-quotidien/221026/ dq221026b-eng.pdf?st=NXC-AvTW

Stokes, Y., Jacob, J. D., Gifford, W., Squires, J., & Vandyk, A. (2017). Exploring nurses' knowledge and experiences related to trauma-informed care. *Global Qualitative Nursing Research, 4*, 1–10. https://doi.org/10.1177/2333393617734510

Stout, D., Wieman, N., Bearskin, L. B., Palmer, B. C., Brown, L., Brown, M., & Marsden, N. (2021). Gum yan asing Kaangas giidaay han hll guudang gas ga. I will never again feel that I am less than: Indigenous health care providers' perspectives on ending racism in health care. *International Journal of Indigenous Health, 16*(1), 13–20. https://doi.org /10.32799/ijih.v16i1.36021

Subica, A. M., & Link, B. G. (2022). Cultural trauma as a fundamental cause of health disparities. *Social Science & Medicine, 292*. https://doi.org/10.1016/j.socscimed.2021.114574

Sukhera, J., & Watling, C. (2018). A framework for integrating implicit bias recognition into health professions education. *Academic Medicine, 93*(1), 35–40. https://doi.org/10.1097/ ACM.00000000000001819

Tremblay, M.-C., & Echaquan, S. (2022). Fostering cultural safety in health care through a decolonizing approach to research with, for and by Indigenous communities. In L. Potvin & D. Jourdan (Eds.), *Global handbook of health promotion research, vol. 1: Mapping health promotion research.* Springer. https://doi.org/10.1007/978-3-030-97212-7_9

Tremblay, M.-C., Graham, J., Porgo, T. V. Dogba, M. J., Paquette, J.-S., Careau, E., & Witteman, H. O. (2020). Improving cultural safety of diabetes care in Indigenous populations of Canada, Australia, New Zealand and the United States: A systematic rapid review. *Canadian Journal of Diabetes, 44*(7), 670–678. https://doi.org/10.1016/j.jcjd.2019.11.006

Truth and Reconciliation Commission of Canada. (2015). *Truth and reconciliation commission of Canada: Calls to action.* https://www2.gov.bc.ca/assets/gov/british-columbians-our-governments/indigenous-people/aboriginal-peoples-documents/calls_to_action_english2.pdf

Tudino, R. F. & Jellison, W. A. (2022). The effect of mindfulness on increasing self-reported LGBTQ competency level and reducing explicit LGBTQ bias in health care providers. *Psychology of Sexual Orientation and Gender Diversity.* https://doi.org/10.1037/sgd0000608.supp

Tuohy, D. (2019). Effective intercultural communication in nursing. *Nursing Standard, 34*(2), 45–50.

Turpel-Lafond, M. E., & Johnson, H. (2021). This space here. *BC Studies, 209.* https://ojs.library.ubc.ca/index.php/bcstudies/article/view/195283/191064

Vang, Z. M., Gagon, R., Lee, T., Jimenez, V., Navickas, A., Pelletier, J., & Shenker, H. (2018). Interactions between Indigenous women awaiting childbirth away from home and their southern, non-Indigenous health care providers. *Qualitative Health Research, 28*(12), 1858–1870. https://doi.org/10.1177/1049732318792500

Waryold, J. M., & Kornahrens, A. (2020). Decreasing barriers to sexual health in the lesbian, gay, bisexual, transgender, and queer community. *Nursing Clinics of North America, 55*(3), 393–402. https://doi.org/10.1016/j.cnur.2020.06.003

World Health Organization. (2017). *Cultural contexts of health and well-being.* https://www.euro.who.int/__data/assets/pdf_file/0009/334269/14780_World-Health-Organisation_Context-of-Health_TEXT-AW-WEB.pdf

Wylie, L., & McConkey, S. (2019). Insiders' insight: Discrimination against Indigenous Peoples through the eyes of health care professionals. *Journal of Racial and Ethnic Health Disparities, 6,* 37–45. https://doi.org/10.1007/s40615-018-0495-9

Wylie, L., McConkey, S., & Corrado, A. M. (2019). Colonial legacies and collaborative action: Improving Indigenous Peoples' health care in Canada. *The International Indigenous Policy Journal, 10*(5), https://doi.org/10.18584/iipj.2019.10.5.9340

Yelland, J., Riggs, E., Szwarc, J., Casey, S., Duell-Piening, P., Chesters, D., Wahidi, S., Fouladi, F., & Brown, S. (2016). Compromised communication: A qualitative study exploring Afghan families and health professionals' experience of interpreting support in Australian maternity care. *BMJ Quality and Safety, 25*(1). https://doi.org/10.1136/bmjqs-2014-003837

Young, S., & Guo, K. L. (2020). Cultural diversity training: The necessity of cultural competence for health care providers and in nursing practice. *The Health Care Manager, 39*(2), 100–108. https://doi.org/10.1097/HCM.000000000000294

Zou, P. (2016). Relational practice in nursing: A case analysis. *Nursing and Health Care, 1*(1), 1–5. https://doi.org/10.33805/2573-3877.102

CHAPTER 5

Delegation and Documentation

LEARNING OBJECTIVES

After reading this chapter, you will be able to

1. Define *delegation*
2. Explain the nurse's role in delegation
3. Identify the purposes of documentation
4. Describe the legal principles of documentation
5. Recognize different charting formats for written/electronic documentation
6. Explain the guidelines for documentation
7. Discuss electronic health records
8. Discuss the implications for nurses regarding the privacy and confidentiality of client information
9. Explain the nurse's role in the use of social media and social network sites

KEY TERMS

Charting by exception

Confidentiality

Delegation

Documentation

Focus charting

Narrative charting

SOAP (or SOAPIER) charting

Social media

INTRODUCTION

Communication among nurses and other health care providers is key to safe and effective client-centred care. Nurses use the nursing process (assessment, diagnosis, outcomes, planning, implementation, and evaluation) to obtain client information to support their plan of care. In collaboration with other health care professionals, nurses share information with those in the circle of care (see chapter 3) verbally and through documentation. This chapter introduces the components of communication, delegation, and documentation—critical competencies necessary for safe, ethical, and effective nursing practice

DELEGATION

Delegation is a necessary skill for nursing personnel, used in many clinical practice areas to maximize resources and facilitate quality care (Clarke, 2021). Delegation is client-specific and "occurs when either the employer or the nurse transfers authority to an unregulated care provider in a selected situation to perform tasks that are traditionally performed by a nurse" (Canadian Nurses Protective Society [CNPS], 2021, p. 1). Unregulated care providers include, but are not limited to, personal care attendants and home support workers who are not registered or licensed by a regulatory body. The act of delegation involves the decision to delegate and the process of delegating in which the following factors require consideration (CNPS, 2021; British Columbia College of Nurses and Midwives, 2021):

- Awareness of employer policies and nursing professional practice standards
- The client's needs, complexity of health issues, and condition
- The unregulated care provider's job description and competence
- The availability of nurse supervision, competency assessment, and provision of feedback
- Whether the task will be routinely performed
- The anticipated outcome and risk of client harm

Delegation is undertaken in the best interest of the client to achieve optimal client care. The act and process of delegation depend upon the professional or territorial regulatory nursing body standards of practice, delegation documents, employer policies, and the ethical and legal guidelines for regulated nurses in Canada. Nurses have the responsibility to know what is permissible in these documents and follow guidelines for appropriate and safe delegation.

Delegation is identified as a complex nursing skill and a key component of leadership (Crevacore et al., 2022). Effective delegation requires that health care professionals be competent in skills such as communication, critical thinking, prioritization, decision-making, and accountability (Clarke, 2021; Crevacore et al., 2022). New graduate nurses have not fully developed these skills and thus may be hesitant to delegate (Walker et al., 2021). Interventions for nursing students include incorporating delegation into didactic and clinical components of their professional programs (Crevacore et al., 2022; Puskar et al., 2017). Inadequate delegation practices are identified as a factor in missed nursing care and negative client outcomes on clinical units (Puskar et al., 2017; Wagner, 2018). Several researchers suggest that good communication techniques are the foundation for effective delegation between nurses and unregulated care providers and lead to safe quality care (Campbell et al., 2020; Clarke, 2021).

DOCUMENTATION

Documentation is an essential component of communication for health care professionals and is reflective of the care provided to the client. "Documentation whether paper, electronic, audio or visual is used to monitor a client's progress and communicate with other care providers" (College of Nurses of Ontario, 2008, p. 3). In collaboration with the client, the nurse uses the nursing process to obtain information to provide culturally safe, competent care based upon the following:

- **Assessment**: Obtain information through psychosocial assessment, physical examination, interview, and observation.
- **Diagnosis**: Identify concerns/issues and develop nursing diagnosis.
- **Outcome identification**: Identify client outcomes.
- **Planning**: Identify culturally safe interventions in an individualized plan of care.
- **Implementation**: Implement nursing approaches to accomplish practice interventions.
- **Evaluation**: Determine effectiveness of plan in meeting client needs.

The data is documented and incorporated into the client's plan of care, which is updated and evaluated to reflect nursing interventions and client response. The information is communicated to the interprofessional team, client, family members, and others within the client's circle of care. Documentation is considered a critical communication tool of client care, a confirmation that suitable professional care has been provided, and a legal record of accountability (Kilgour, 2015).

The client's medical record contains information on assessments, plan of care, interventions, and outcomes that reflect their health status and treatments. Documentation allows for continuity of care as essential client information is recorded and shared by other health care professionals. Members of the interdisciplinary/interprofessional team can review the chart, identify clinical changes in the client's condition, and recommend treatments and interventions. The medical record presents a clear and accurate picture of health status and interventions, which can be reviewed by all health care providers during the client's hospital admission.

Documentation presents information on all health care professionals who provide client care and their contribution to safe and effective care. It also demonstrates the impact of nursing interventions on client care and responses, and this aids identification of any gaps in or concerns with the provided services. This information has implications for workload management and research, leading to improvement in evidence-based practice and client outcomes.

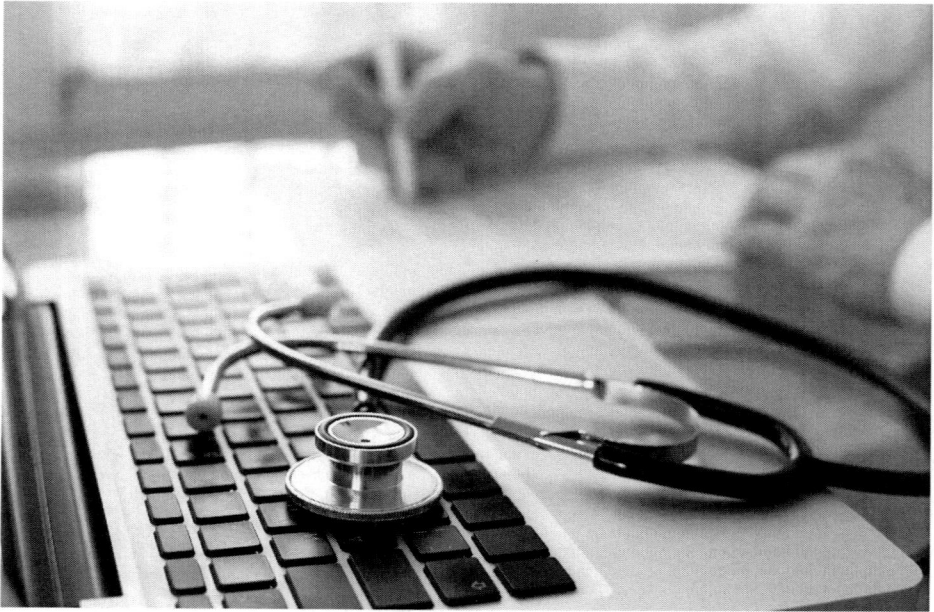

Figure 5.1: Health care professional documenting
Source: Adobe Stock/Song_about_summer

Nurses are responsible and accountable for documenting the care they provide to clients. The client's record is a legal document, so quality documentation skills are critical for legal protection. Practice standards contribute to the regulatory and legislative requirements for nursing documentation in Canada. Nurses should be familiar with their professional association's standards of practice, code of ethics, and documentation principles. This is the standard—along with their health institution's policies, guidelines, and procedures on documentation—that nurses are held accountable to in any legal proceedings in the courts. When a health institution receives a complaint, claim, or notice of legal action, the courts rely on documentation as evidence of care provided by the health care professional. Nurses and other health care providers cannot rely on memory for recalling facts, so documentation of care provided and by whom, and the client's response, is essential. "As many legal proceedings are not commenced or litigated until several years after the provision of the nursing services, the patient's chart often becomes the only reliable source of evidence in regard to the events that occurred and the care that was provided" (CNPS, 2020, p. 1). Nurses do not document for other health care professionals or delegate the task to other colleagues. An exception is made for a designated recorder during an emergency. In the event of a cardiac arrest, a nurse may be the designated recorder, who documents the outcome, care, and treatment given by the team during the arrest situation.

Student Tip

Have you heard the saying "If it isn't documented, it wasn't done"? Courts of law have upheld this statement. During clinical experiences, remember to complete all client documentation. Nurse provincial/territorial regulatory standards, employee policies, and guidelines approved by your educational facility will guide your documentation process.

Table 5.1: Documentation Principles: Paper and Electronic Form

Guideline	Rationale
Write legibly and neatly. Use correct spelling, grammar, and punctuation.	Reflects professionalism. Messy or illegible information is not helpful, may result in client harm.
Maintain accurate, factual, complete, and timely documentation.	Data is based upon the nursing process. Descriptive and objective information, detail about client's care and response to care. Information is recorded during or as soon as possible after interaction/intervention (Nova Scotia College of Nursing [NSCN], 2022a).
Sign/date/time all entries. The date/signature supports the agency policy (e.g., month/day/year). Sign with legal name (spell out), followed by appropriate credential (LPN, RN, RPN, SN). Time should reflect 24-hour military clock.	Signatures and initials need to be identifiable to others. Some health facilities use a master list that matches the provider's initials with a signature and designation linked to their documentation. Students need to include affiliating agency and year of program. In electronic documentation, the user's login password to the computer system is the automatic identifier to their signature.
Correction of documentation mistakes must adhere to agency policy. In a paper-based client record, draw a single line through the word or sentence that is wrong. The error should still be legible. Initial and write "mistaken entry" along with date and time of correction. Continue with the correct documentation.	To protect the integrity of the clinical record, any changes must be made according to agency policy. No removal of chart pages or use of correction products, eraser, felt pens, or markers should hide an error. May be interpreted as modifying documentation and is considered professional misconduct due to falsification of a clinical record.

(Continued)

Table 5.1: Documentation Principles: Paper and Electronic Form (*continued*)

Guideline	Rationale
Organize information in chrono-logical order when charting.	Information not documented in order can lead to misinterpretation. Charting chrono-logically enhances clarity of communica-tion. Helps to identify or reveal changes in client's health status.
For late entries, record information as soon as possible after the event occurs.	May occur because chart was unavailable or provider forgot to document. Make late en-tries according to agency policy. Here is an example of a late entry: 11/02/22 1200 hours Late Entry: I forgot to include this information. On 11/01/22 at 1600 hours. Sling applied to left arm. Hand and fingers warm to touch. Able to move fin-gers without any discomfort or pain. Client helped from bed to chair. Left arm resting on pillow. Elizabeth Snow, LPN
There should be no blank or white space in paper-based documents, as it presents an opportunity for others to add information unknown to the original author.	This is a risk that should be avoided. An ac-cepted practice is to draw a single line com-pletely through the white space, including before and after your signature/credential.
All handwritten entries must be written in blue or black ink. Some agencies record allergies in red ink. Need to follow agency policy.	The use of blue or black ink is considered best for optical scanning technology. Never use gel, felt, or coloured ink pens for docu-mentation on a legal document.
Always read what you have written. Is the message clear, writing legible? Are there any misspelled words?	Verifies that documentation is professional, clear, and concise.
Use hospital- or agency-approved abbreviations and symbols.	Can save time in documentation if all health care team members understand meaning. If used incorrectly, can cause confusion and impact client safety. Policy-approved ab-breviations should be used.
The client's name and identifica-tion (date of birth / room number) should be on all documentation forms.	From a legal perspective, non-identification of clinical forms can lead to errors and af-fect client safety.

Guideline	Rationale
Stick to the facts. Avoid generalizations and bias. Documentation should be concise, accurate, and unbiased. Support documentation by use of objective and subjective data. Biased example: "Patient had not washed his feet for months, which caused his diabetic foot ulcer to get worse. He probably will lose his foot."	Unacceptable to make value judgments. Support with data. Subjective data is what the client tells you: "I have not been sleeping well for about four weeks. I go to bed at 11:30 but toss and turn. Up at 5:30, I don't feel rested." Objective data is what you observe.
Do not use unprofessional words or labels (e.g., Client is *drunk*, acting in a *bizarre* manner). Describe behaviour.	Negative labels are not to be used. Demonstrates lack of respect.
All attempts to contact other health care professionals must be documented, including the date and time of the attempt or contact.	For client issue or concern related to health status, deviation from normal requires intervention. Reflects accountability for safe client care.

Source: Based on Registered Nurses Association of the Northwest Territories and Nunavut. (2015). Documentation guidelines. https://rnantnu.ca/wp-content/uploads/2019/10/Documentation-Guidelines-RNANTNU-Effective-January-19-20151.pdf

Documentation Example

Incorrect Documentation

0630 Hours/11/05/22 Cleint fell out of bed, pulled out foley catheter. Placed back in bed. V/S taken. Doctor called. Urology technician called to replace catherer. Bruise noted on patient's forhead......Tanner Brown, RN.

Correct Documentation

05/11/22 0630 hours On completing unit rounds, found client lying beside his bed with foley catheter (14 FR) by his side. Both of his bed rails were up. Small 5 cm cut (skin broken) on client's forehead. Client is alert but drowsy, vital signs, BP 134/89, P 84, R 24, T 37.2, & PERRLA. Client helped back to bed no complaints verbalized. Dr. Phillips called and informed of incident, will come and assess client. Urology technician called to replace client's foley catheter...Tanner Brown, RN.

(Continued)

Documentation Review

The first documentation note has several spelling errors. The documentation is not objective, and assumptions were made by the nurse (e.g., client fell out of bed, pulled out foley catheter). You document what you see and not what you assume happened. The note also lacks detail: no information is provided on client status or injury, assessment data (e.g., vital signs), or which physician is notified. The second note is the correct way to document. It presents the complete details of the situation.

USING ABBREVIATIONS, SYMBOLS, AND ACRONYMS

The use of abbreviations, symbols, and acronyms can aid the efficiency of documentation if their meaning is understood by everyone. Abbreviations and symbols that are not clear or have multiple meanings can lead to confusion and contribute to errors impacting client safety. For example, what does PT mean? It could be interpreted as *physical therapy* (physio), *patient*, or *prothrombin time*. Consider the documentation for a client who has returned from the postoperative recovery room following an appendectomy.

> 10/04/22 1600 hours Client returned from OR. Vital signs stable as charted on client form. IV of NS running at 125 cc/hr in left arm. Dressing to appendectomy site dry and intact. BS diminished. Client settled in bed and is drowsy. Side rails elevated. ————————John R. Smith, RN——

What does the abbreviation *BS* mean? It could mean bowel sounds, breath sounds, or blood sugar. It is best to write out to clarify meaning or verify agency policy for approved documentation abbreviations.

How you punctuate an abbreviation can also make a difference in its interpretation. For example, a physician writes a medication order on the doctor's order sheet:

> 4IU of Humulin R insulin daily.
> Client received 41 units of insulin by mistake as the order was for 4 international units (IU) of Humulin R insulin.

To prevent a misunderstanding, the physician should have written out the order. Alternatively, in some health facilities an official approved list of abbreviations, symbols, and acronyms for use in the organization is posted on clinical units.

The Institute for Safe Medication Practices (ISMP) Canada has identified a list of *do not use* medication-related error-prone abbreviations, symbols, and acronyms (ISMP, 2021). As a student nurse, it is best to use only approved abbreviations in the client's medical record. If the agency does not have an approved list, make sure you write out the full term so the meaning is clear to others. If using abbreviations from an approved list, it is important that your writing is legible so that others will understand your abbreviations.

FREQUENCY OF DOCUMENTATION

As a student, you may be wondering, how often do I need to document on my assigned client? "The frequency of documentation is influenced by the complexity of a client's health status, the degree of risk involved in a treatment of care, changes to the plan of care, when clients move from one place to another (e.g., admission/transfer, or transport), or from one care provider to another" (College of Registered Nurses of Newfoundland and Labrador [CRNNL], 2021, p. 3). Employer or facility policies may identify the required frequency of documentation as well as the charting method (e.g., FOCUS or SCAP[IER] charting).

Documentation Formats

In Canada about a decade ago, the federal government, along with several provinces and territories, funded the Canada Health Infoway to develop a connected health information electronic medical record. In 2020, a national survey of Canadian nurses reported that 27 percent of nurses are now working in fully electronic systems and are more satisfied than those working in hybrid systems (combination of paper and electronic records systems) (Canadian Nurses Association, 2020).

A variety of documentation tools are used for client documentation, including handover reports, worksheets and Kardexes, care plans, medication administration records (MARs), flowsheets, care maps, clinical pathways, and algorithms. For health care organizations, the tools may be in paper or electronic format. Health care providers may be using a variety of these forms as they carry out their clinical practice duties in the provision of client care.

Narrative Charting

Narrative charting is a common approach where data obtained following the nursing process is written in a paragraph format, highlighting client interventions, outcomes, and responses in chronological order. This is the traditional way of documenting. It is considered time-consuming and at times makes it difficult to find specific information in the client's medical record.

Example of Narrative Charting

08/02/22 1230 hours Client admitted to unit by stretcher from the emergency department (ER) for investigation of bowel obstruction. Client is alert, no complaints of pain. Settled in bed, IV of Ringer's lactate infusing at 125 cc/hr in (R) hand. IV site dry and intact, no redness. Admission assessment completed. Vital signs as charted. 1330 Dr. Walker visited and spoke to client, scheduled for OR in AM for bowel resection. To remain fasting, sign placed on room door. Consent signed and placed in chart. 1400 Client's wife visiting. Aware of scheduled surgery and has no questions. 1500 To x-ray via stretcher for flat abd series. 1600 Returned from x-ray, settled back into bed.
———————————R.J. Chan, LPN——

Focus Charting

Focus charting identifies client-centred concerns or foci. A focus could be a sign or symptom, an acute change in client's condition, a teaching session, or a client behaviour. The focus is the problem, for example, bleeding from surgical site or chest pain. The note is written according to the DAR or DARP framework:

- **Data**: Client assessment data in relation to the focus problem—objective and subjective data following assessment of the concern/issue
- **Action**: Actions or intervention completed
- **Response**: The client's physical and emotional responses to the interventions (evaluation)
- **Plan**: Next steps

Table 5.2: Focus Charting Example

Date/ Time	Focus	Note
15/03/22 1030 hours	**Agitation**	**D**: Client pacing up and down hallway talking to self. Stating in a loud voice, "I'm not staying here. I need to speak to a lawyer." Walking to exit door but is directed back to his room. Speech becomes louder, stating, "I want to leave. Why do you keep me here?" ———
		A: Dr. Crane notified by phone of client's status. Client given Thorazine 50 mg by mouth. Medication administered with no issues. Encouraged to return to his room. ———

Date/ Time	Focus	Note
		R: Client continued to pace back and forth in unit hallway for 15 minutes. No verbalization of loud speech. ———T. Street, RPN—
15/03/22 1100 hours		**R:** Client did return to his room. Presently sitting in chair looking out the window. ———T. Street, RPN—

SOAP Charting

The SOAP charting format for progress notes is known as problem-oriented documentation and focuses on specific client problems. Following assessment, the client's current problems are identified, and a list is created that is linked with the nursing care plan. Written documentation is organized by the acronym *SOAP*:

- **Subjective** data: What client says. How does the client feel? What is the problem of concern? (e.g., "I have this tightness in my chest, like an elephant sitting on my chest.")
- **Objective** data: Information obtained from physical assessment/examination/observation
- **Assessment**: Development of nursing diagnosis based upon subjective and objective data
- **Plan**: Actions to be implemented (health care provider's interventions)

Some health facilities have added an addition to the SOAP format that includes *IER*. The *IER* portion of the SOAPIER acronym is focused on client outcomes and responses:

- **Intervention**: Care and treatment/procedures implemented
- **Evaluation**: How did the client respond to care and treatments/procedures?
- **Revision**: Are revisions needed following evaluation? Implementation plan.

SOAPIER Charting Example

22/11/22 1200 hours   Problem: Chest Pain
S: Client states, "I have tightness in right side of my chest, radiating to left arm. It came on about five minutes ago."

(Continued)

O: Client sitting up in bed, rubbing left arm. Face flushed; sweating noted on forehead.
A: Vital signs BP 140/94, P 100, R 28, T 37.5. Nurse asks client on a scale of 1–10, how would you rate the pain? Client states "8."
P: Initiate chest pain protocol.
I: EKG done stat.
Two chewable aspirin given.
Nitroglycerin spray administered.
Head of bed elevated 45 degrees.
Oxygen 4 L by nasal prongs initiated.
Dr. John notified of client's status.
E: Vital signs BP 130/88, P 90, R 22, T 37.2
Client states, "The pain has lessened somewhat, chest not so tight now. I say it is about a 4 now."
R: Monitor as per chest pain protocol.
————J. Cole, BSN, RN——

Charting by Exception

Charting by exception (CBE) is completed only when abnormal or significant findings are outside of the client's established norms or standards of care. This form of documentation is easy to use at the bedside, eliminates lengthy, repetitive charting, and provides quick access to awareness of changes in the client's health status.

Regardless of the documentation method used in a health organization, always keep in mind the four Cs of documentation for effective communication and to satisfy legal requirements:

- **Clear**: Documentation is clear, unbiased, and accurate. Handwriting is clear and legible.
- **Concise**: Information is thorough and factual and is linked to overall plan of care.
- **Correct**: All assessment findings and nursing actions are noted. Documentation is completed according to agency policy. Charting is done on the correct client. There are no blank spaces.
- **Complete**: All documentation data is included with client interventions/evaluation, including date, time, and signature and designation.

Electronic Documentation

Today health care organizations have moved toward electronic means of providing many aspects of care. Developments in health information technology (IT) have impacted how client information is shared among health care professionals (Campbell & Rankin, 2017). Many hospitals use the electronic health record (EHR), which allows for nursing documentation, order entry, reporting and viewing of laboratory data, diagnostic imaging, and prescribed medications (Tharmalingam et al., 2016). An EHR is "a collection of the personal health information of a single individual, entered or accepted by health care providers, and stored electronically, under strict security" (NSCN, 2022, p. 10).

Nurses working in health facilities access the EHR at computer terminals at the main nursing station or through hand-held devices used at the client's bedside to access or input information. A password, which is linked to the employee as a unique identifier, provides access to the system. The system automatically records the user's name and the entry date and time. For security, it is recommended that nurses change passwords regularly, avoid lending their computer identification or access to anyone, and log off when not using the computer system. Health care organizations with health information technology must have policies to guide users, provide IT support, and maintain security of data management through encryption, virus protection, a well-maintained firewall, backup of client information, and tracking of unauthorized access to client information. In addition, computerized information systems are not necessarily secure, as they are vulnerable to hackers.

Nurses are accountable for all aspects of documentation regardless of format: paper-based or electronic. Documentation is an integral component of effective, ethical, and safe nursing practice. Nurses must have knowledge of and follow agency documentation policies, practice standards, and code of ethics to guide their documentation.

TECHNOLOGY AND NURSING PRACTICE

Technology is impacting how nursing practice is delivered across Canada. Interactions with clients are occurring remotely, using many forms of IT. Virtual nursing practice, also called "telepractice," is not meant to replace face-to-face care but is an option for persons who live in rural and remote locations for whom face-to-face visits with a health care provider at a health facility is not possible. Virtual care technologies may include telephone, text, Messenger, email, video conferencing, or Skype. This type of nursing practice may increase the risk for confidential communication (e.g., client information sent incorrectly to an unintended recipient) and breaches of privacy and confidentiality (CRNNL, 2020). Nurses must increase their competency in the application of these new technologies and have organizational IT support available along with clear policies on the documentation of care and security of client information (e.g., how data are stored, used, and shared). In virtual nursing practice, documentation should meet the standards for documentation as outlined by the provincial regulatory body as well as those of the health facility.

Confidentiality

Confidentiality of client information is a priority for health care professionals. Regardless of the method used to communicate client information (paper or electronic), nurses and students must adhere to the principles of privacy and confidentiality. This is highlighted in provincial or territorial standards of practice and the Canadian Nurses Association Code of Ethics (2017)—for example, the nurse "upholds and protects clients' privacy and confidentiality in all forms of communication including, but not limited to, e-records, verbal, written, and social media" (CRNNL, 2019, p. 7). Also, relevant federal, provincial, and territorial legislation establishes rules on the collection, use, and disclosure of personal health information. Nurses and students should be aware of the legislation in their province or territory related to the disclosure of personal health information.

Tips for Privacy and Confidentiality for Paper/Electronic Documentation

- Ensure all materials that contain personal health information are secure. Follow agency policy for secure disposal of client material (e.g., locked bins, shredding). Students should not write a client's name or location identifier on any clinical documents or assignments.
- Before inputting data, make sure you've retrieved the correct client record.
- Never reveal or allow anyone else access to your personal identification number or password, as these are your electronic signatures.
- Before inputting client data, be aware of monitor location; make sure the computer screen is turned away from passersby.
- Do not leave client information displayed on screen. Complete your entry, exit the client record, and log off before leaving the terminal.
- Only access client information that is required to provide nursing care for that client; accessing client information for purposes other than providing nursing care is a breach of privacy and confidentiality.
- Follow agency policy when sending client information via fax transmission. Always verify the fax number of the recipient.

Social Media

Electronic communication has exploded as more and more people are communicating via social networks. The International Nurse Regulator Collaborative (2016) defines *social media* as "the online and mobile tools that people use to share opinions, information, and experiences, images and video or audio clips, and includes websites and applications for social networking" (para. 2). As a student, you use email and a variety of social network sites like Twitter, Facebook, Instagram, or Snapchat to communicate with your friends, family, and classmates. In some of your theory and clinical classes, you may be using discussion forums or message boards to communicate through postings related to course content and issues in nursing practice. While social media, when used appropriately, has benefits for people worldwide, it also has risks that students and professional nurses need to consider.

Most regulatory organizations for nurses in Canada have guidelines on the use of social media. Nurses are accountable for knowing how their employer's policy, standards of practice, code of ethics, and practice guidelines apply to their use of social media. Six Ps of social media use suggested by the International Nurse Regulator Collaborative (2016) can help you when using social networking sites:

- **Professional**: Project a professional image in online interactions.
- **Positive**: Use positive communication and be respectful of others' comments.
- **Patient/person-free**: Keep posts client- or person-free. Do not post photographs or images, and do not accept client "friend" requests online.
- **Protect yourself**: Protect your professionalism and reputation. Use proper communication channels to talk about workplace issues/challenges/colleagues.
- **Privacy**: Keep your personal and professional lives separate. Client information should not be shared on social networking sites.
- **Pause before you post**: Reduce the risk to offend. Consider the consequences, and do not post comments in haste or anger.

Case Study 5.1

Read the case information below and answer the following questions.

Austin Smith is a 70-year-old retired teacher who lives with his wife, Estell. He is admitted to your hospital with a history of being in a MVA (motor vehicle accident). He has undergone an open reduction of his left femur and a splenectomy and has been transferred to your floor from the surgical step-down unit the second day postop. He has a nasogastric tube for continuous low wall suction and a Foley catheter in place, containing about 150 cc of clear urine. He has a peripheral IV of normal saline with 20 mEq KCl/L at 125 cc/hr in left arm; site is clean, dry, and opsite (transparent film) dressing intact. He has a dressing to his incision site, which is dry and intact. He is ordered morphine 5 mg/IV q2 hr,

(Continued)

PRN. He has a history of major depressive disorder but currently is not prescribed any medications. After he is settled in bed, you make sure his call bell is in place. Before you leave his room, he states, "It hurts when I move, even when I cough. Can I have something to help with the pain?"

1. Use the information from the case history and write a documentation note using the narrative format.
2. Differentiate between objective and subjective data in this case study.
3. Use the information from the case history and write a nurse progress note using the DAR format.
4. After checking Mr. Smith's medication record from the step-down surgical unit, you find out that he can have morphine 5 mg/IV as ordered. You get the medication ready, following the correct process for medication administration, and you return to the client's room. What would be your response to Mr. Smith before you administer the medication as ordered?

Exercise 5.1: Documentation Review

Read the following narrative documentation note and identify the errors that require correction. How many errors can you find?

> 0830 hours Patient transferred from ER this AM. Settled in room. IV running in left arm. Pt unsure of why in hospital. Has history of diabts no c/o of pain. Diagnosis not clear – Some SOB present. Doctor called and ~~notified~~ informed of room location. Blood taken and sent to lab.   Pam, RN
> 0830 Pt alert and unresponsive ———— Pam RN

Exercise 5.2: Social Media

1. List the social networking sites you use. What precautions do you take to protect your privacy while using those sites or platforms?
2. As part of your professional accountability as a student nurse, you need to be aware of social media practice guidelines. Check the website of your regulatory body for this information and review it. Is the information consistent with that presented in this chapter?

CHAPTER SUMMARY

This chapter focuses briefly on the nurses' role in delegation of client specific tasks of care to other care providers. The nurses' role in client documentation is a critical component of safe quality care. Documentation gathered in the nurse-client relationship can be organized in either a paper and/or electronically generated format dependent upon facility. Documentation in a health care facility or setting facilitates communication between health care professionals. During client assessment, subjective and objective data is collected. This information is organized and placed in the client's medical record so others on the interprofessional team can access it. To ensure clear communication and complete accurate documentation of client care, documentation guidelines need to be followed. The agency format for documentation may vary, and some may use narrative, SOAP, or DARP charting.

REVIEW QUESTIONS

Read the following review questions and select the best option to answer each question. State your rationale for choosing your response.

1. A client states, "I am so sick this morning. I have this heavy pain in my stomach and just feel like vomiting." The *best* way for the nurse to document this data would be to write which of the following statements?
   a. "Client is nauseated this morning after finishing breakfast."
   b. "Client is upset that they are feeling so sick this morning."
   c. "Client is sick, nauseated, this morning but did not vomit."
   d. "Client states, 'I am so sick this morning. I have this heavy pain in my stomach and just feel like vomiting.'"

2. Your colleague is going off for an early morning break and asks you to document the findings in a client's chart on an abdominal dressing change they completed. Your response is
   a. "Sure, not an issue, I'll do that. What did the incision look like?"
   b. "I'll do that after I hang this unit of blood in Room 225."
   c. "Sorry, no, it is important that you document the care that you provide."
   d. "I'll do that right now. Tell me, was the incision clean, dirty, or healing?"
3. Charting by exception is used by the health facility for documentation. Using this format, how would you document a routine dressing change to an abdominal incision in the narrative notes?
   a. "Dressing change completed to abdominal incision."
   b. "Dressing change completed to abdominal area by PCA."
   c. "Abdominal dressing changed; client tolerated procedure well."
   d. Not necessary to document this procedure if uneventful and incision healing.

REFERENCES

British Columbia College of Nurses and Midwives. (2021). *Registered nurses and nurse practitioners: Assigning and delegating to unregulated care providers.* https://www.bc.cnm.ca/Documents/learning/RN_NP_assigning_Delegating_ucp.pdf

Campbell, A. R., Layne, D., Scott, E., & Wei, H. (2020). Interventions to promote teamwork, delegation and communication among registered nurses and nursing assistants: An integrative review. *Journal of Nursing Management, 28*(7), 1465–1472. https://doi.org/10.1111/jonm.13083

Campbell, M. L., & Rankin, J. M. (2017). Nurses and electronic health records in a Canadian hospital: Examining the social organization and programmed use of digitised nursing knowledge. *Sociology of Health & Illness, 39*(3), 365–379. https://doi.org/10.1111/1467-9566.12489

Canadian Nurses Association. (2017). *Code of ethics.* https://www.cna-aiic.ca/en/nursing/regulated-nursing-in-canada/nursing-ethics

Canadian Nurses Association. (2020). *Digital health is helping Canadian nurses improve patient care but opportunities for improvement remain.* https://www.cna-aiic.ca/en/blogs/cn-content/2020/05/11digital-health-is-helping-canadian-nurses-improve

Canadian Nurses Protective Society. (2020). *InfoLAW: Quality documentation: Your best defence.* https://cnps.ca/article/infolaw-qualitydocumentation/

Canadian Nurses Protective Society. (2021). *InfoLAW: Delegation to other health care workers.* https://cnps.ca/article/delegation-to-other-health-care-workers/

Clarke, H. (2021). How pre-registration nursing students acquire delegation skills: A systematic literature review. *Nurse Education Today, 106*, 1–7. https://doi.org/10.1016/j.nedt .2021.105096

College of Nurses of Ontario. (2008). *Practice standard: Documentation, revised 2008.* https:// www.cno.org/globalassets/docs/prac/41001_documentation.pdf

College of Registered Nurses of Newfoundland and Labrador. (2019). *Standards of practice: For registered nurses and nurse practitioners.* https://www.crnnl.ca/site/uploads/2021/09/ standards-of-practice-for-rns-and-nps.pdf

College of Registered Nurses of Newfoundland and Labrador. (2020). *Virtual nursing practice.* https://www.crnnl.ca/site/uploads/2021/09/virtual-nursing-practice.pdf

College of Registered Nurses of Newfoundland and Labrador. (2021). *Documentation principles.* https://www.crnnl.ca/site/iploads/2021/documentation-principles.pdf

Crevacore, C., Coventry, L., Duffield, C., & Jacob, E. (2022). Factors impacting delegation decision making by registered nurses to assistants in the acute care setting: A mixed method study. *International Journal of Nursing Studies, 136*, https://doi.org/10.1016/j .ijnurstu.2022.104366

Institute for Safe Medication Practices. (2021). *ISMP's list of error-prone abbreviations, symbols, and dose designations.* https://www.ismp.org/sites/default/files/attachments/2017-11/ Error%20Prone%20abbrevations%202015.pdf

International Nurse Regulator Collaborative. (2016). *Position Statement: Social media use: common expectations for nurses.* https://inrc.com/112.htm

Kilgour, K. N. (2015). Effective documentation. In D. Gregory, C. Raymond-Seniuk, L. Patrick, & T. Stephen (Eds.), *Fundamentals: Perspectives on the art and science of Canadian nursing* (pp. 541–585). Wolters Kluwer.

Nova Scotia College of Nursing. (2022). *Documentation for nurses.* https://cdnl.nscn.ca/sites/ default/files/documents/resources/DocumentationGuidelines.pdf

Puskar, K., Berju, D., Shi, X., & McFadden, T. (2017). Nursing students and delegation. *Nursing Made Incredibly Easy, 15*(3), 6–8. https://doi.org/10.1097/01.NME.0000514216.15640.86

Registered Nurses Association of the Northwest Territories and Nunavut. (2015). Documentation guidelines. https://rnantnu.ca/wp-content/uploads/2019/10/Documentation-Guidelines -RNANTNU-Effective-January-19-20151.pdf

Tharmalingam, S., Hagens, S., & Zeimer, J. (2016). The value of connected health information: Perceptions of electronic health record users in Canada. *BMC Medical Informatics and Decision Making, 16*(93), 1–9. https://doi.org/10.1186/s12911-016-0330-3

Wagner, E. A. (2018). Improving patient care outcomes through better delegation— Communication between nurses and assistive personnel. *Journal of Nursing Care Quality, 33*(2), 187–193. https://doi.org/10.1097/NCQ.0000000000000282

Walker, F. A., Ball, M., Cleary, S., & Pisani, H. (2021). Transparent teamwork: The practice of supervision and delegation within the multi-tiered nursing team. *Nursing Inquiry, 28*(4), https://doi.org/10.1111/nin.12413

CHAPTER 6

Communication with Clients Experiencing Anxiety

LEARNING OBJECTIVES

After reading this chapter, you will be able to

1. Define the terms *stress* and *anxiety*
2. Recognize the levels of anxiety mild, moderate, severe, and panic
3. Define the term *anxiety disorder*
4. Identify assessment procedures for clients with anxiety
5. Identify communication strategies to reduce anxiety
6. Describe anxiety disorders and other related disorders
7. Identify nursing interventions for clients with anxiety
8. Explain the nurse's role in teaching clients about anxiety management

KEY TERMS

Agoraphobia
Alarm
Anxiety disorder
Cognitive behavioural therapy
Diaphragmatic breathing
Exhaustion
Flooding

Generalized anxiety disorder
Panic disorder
Progressive muscle relaxation
Resistance
Social anxiety disorder
Specific phobias
Stress

INTRODUCTION

In all areas of clinical practice, nurses and other health professionals encounter individuals who experience stress and anxiety because of a health issue or concern. Being a client in hospital also provokes anxiety and may interfere with an individual's ability to cope (Alzahrani, 2021). Clients are reported to have higher anxiety levels prior to undergoing an invasive or surgical procedure. Those feelings experienced are related to their fear of the unknown, and uncertainty pre- and post-procedure (Hernández et al., 2021). Research has indicated that anxiety is noted to be high among clients who have cancer or cardiac disorders and those with debilitating chronic conditions (Bolourchifard et al., 2020; Hitchon et al., 2020; Shattuck et al., 2021).

Anxiety disorders are one of the most prevalent mental health problems in Canada (Dozois, 2021). Nurses have a critical role in assessing, managing, and assisting clients and families in coping with anxiety. As the nurse-client relationship is an effective element within professional nursing, counselling interventions for anxiety management based within the context of the "therapeutic relationship" can be employed (Webster et al., 2012). The primary goal for nurses and other health care providers is to assist clients in decreasing their anxiety level. After anxiety is reduced, health care providers are able to help clients examine their coping behaviours and provide guidance for management (Steele, 2019). This chapter presents information on stress, anxiety, and related disorders and highlights the role of health care professionals in assessment, intervention, and education for clients and families with these disorders.

STRESS

Stress is sometimes used interchangeably with the term *anxiety* (Townsend & Morgan, 2020). Stress or a stressor is an external pressure that is placed on an individual, and their ability to cope with the stressor can lead to anxiety. Stress is considered part of everyday activity, and some stressors, such as hospitalizations, illness, or medical treatments, can cause anxiety. If an individual feels overwhelmed due to prolonged stress and is unable to cope, this interferes with daily functioning and may have a prolonged effect on health. Two categories of stress exist: (1) physical, exemplified by trauma, excessive heat, or physical conditions such as infections, hunger, or pain, and (2) psychological, exemplified by divorce, job loss, retirement, or marriage (Halter & Jakubec, 2019).

In groundbreaking work, Hans Selye (1978) was the first to talk about stress and individuals' ability to adapt, demonstrated in the model known as stress adaptation syndrome. Selye's model emphasizes the physiological effects of stress on the body, which are identified by three distinct stages: (1) alarm, (2) resistance, and (3) exhaustion.

Alarm

The body's initial response to a stressor is to stimulate hormonal activity (in the brain) and activate the sympathetic nervous system's "fight or flight" response. The person becomes alert, and their physical and psychological defences are mobilized. The level of anxiety is mild to moderate, and if stressors are not resolved, the individual experiences the next stage (Steele, 2019).

Resistance

In this stage, the person continues to adapt to stress. Coping and defence mechanisms are called into play. Psychosomatic symptoms begin to appear, and the level of anxiety is moderate to severe. The person can be helped with interventions at this time. However, if stressors are prolonged and unresolved, the individual moves to the next stage (Steele, 2019).

Exhaustion

Exhaustion occurs when the stress is overwhelming or the person has lost the ability to cope. Thinking becomes disorganized and illogical. The individual may experience reduced orientation to reality. The level of anxiety is severe to panic. Physical illness and death may occur if exhaustion continues without intervention (Steele, 2019).

ANXIETY

Anxiety is a universal, vague, subjective experienced feeling of uneasiness, apprehension, and doom. Anxiety is a normal response to threatening situations. The feelings associated with anxiety alert individuals to danger and motivate them to be on guard and succeed in the situation (Halter & Jakubec, 2019). All of us become anxious at some point, as this helps us to learn and cope with the challenges of daily life. However, for some individuals, anxiety becomes overwhelming and impedes day-to-day functioning. Anxiety is related to how an individual appraises stressors, which influences their ability to cope.

When working with clients who experience anxiety, it is imperative that health care providers, including nurses, have the knowledge and skill to recognize the physiological, cognitive, and behavioural responses to anxiety. Nurse competency in assessment skills allows early intervention, which helps to alleviate symptoms and prevent behaviour from escalating further and impacting overall health. See table 6.1, which highlights the physiological and behavioural responses to anxiety for individuals whose level ranges from mild to panic.

Because the signs and symptoms of anxiety are varied, it is important for the nurse in assessment to determine the level and stage of anxiety that the client is experiencing, in order to provide appropriate interventions. If anxiety occurs and the individual can manage, no intervention is necessary. However, panic is the most extreme, and this level is considered an emergency and requires immediate intervention. The nurse is concerned with the client's safety at this time, and the goal is to reduce or relieve anxiety. Acute panic can lead to exhaustion and death (Halter & Pollard, 2019a).

Table 6.1: Anxiety Levels and Responses

Anxiety Level	Physiological	Cognitive	Emotional/Behavioural
Mild	Vital signs normal Little muscle tension Pupils normal, constricted	Awareness of environmental and internal stimuli	Fidgeting Some restlessness Alert Irritability
Moderate	Narrow perceptual field Selective inattention Vital signs increased	May need guidance Some ability to solve problems	Difficulty with concentration Headache, voice tremors
Severe	Hyperventilation Tachycardia Dizziness	Confusion Unable to concentrate Distorted perceptions	Loud, rapid speech Sense of impending doom Sweaty palms
Panic	Vitals signs elevated Dilated pupils	Unable to focus Hallucinations or delusions may be present	Emotional paralysis Unable to speak Severe shakiness Feelings of terror Chest pain Fear of dying Palpitations

Source: Based on Halter, M. J., & Pollard, C. L. (2019a). Anxiety and related disorders. In M. J. Halter, C. L. Pollard, & S. L. Jakubec (Eds.), *Varcarolis's Canadian psychiatric mental health nursing: A clinical approach* (pp. 200–243). Elsevier.

It is important to note that some individuals who experience anxiety may have an anxiety disorder or medical disorder, so a detailed assessment is necessary to determine the underlying cause. Anxiety may be also caused or exacerbated by medications or the use or misuse of other substances. Once a detailed history is completed, the information obtained will guide appropriate intervention.

ANXIETY DISORDERS

Anxiety disorders are the most common of all mental health problems, and it is estimated that one in ten Canadians is affected by these disorders. A survey on COVID-19 and mental health in Canada reported that 13 percent of Canadians aged

18 years and older screened positive for anxiety and 15 percent screened positive for depression (Public Health Agency of Canada, 2021). According to the *Diagnostic and Statistical Manual of Mental Disorders*, fifth edition (DSM-5; American Psychiatric Association [APA], 2013), anxiety disorders share a common feature of anxiety and fear. These disorders differ from "transient fear or anxiety, often stress-induced, by being persistent, typically lasting longer than 6 months" (p. 189). These disorders include (1) generalized anxiety disorder (GAD), (2) social anxiety disorder (social phobia), (3) specific phobias, (4) panic disorder, and (5) agoraphobia.

Generalized Anxiety Disorder

A person with this disorder has a persistent, unrealistic worry or apprehension that has been occurring for at least six months. The individual finds it difficult to control the worry. These feelings cause significant impact in social, occupational, or interpersonal functioning. The person has problems with memory, concentration, and sleep disturbances. The disorder is not attributed to a particular medical condition or a drug of use or misuse. Onset is usually in childhood or adolescence but may also occur in young adulthood (APA, 2013).

Social Anxiety Disorder

The essential feature of this disorder is an intense fear or anxiety of social or performance situations in which the individual is observed by others (e.g., eating or drinking in public, meeting unfamiliar people, asking questions in a classroom, singing in a church choir). The fear is out of proportion to the actual threat posed by the social situation (APA, 2013). Individuals with social anxiety may experience overwhelming anxiety, which causes them to change careers or programs of study. In some instances, individuals may self-medicate with alcohol or other drugs to help alleviate the anxiety (Halter & Pollard, 2019b).

Specific Phobias

This disorder is identified by fear of specific objects or situations (e.g., heights, flying, seeing blood). The phobic object or situation triggers immediate fear or anxiety, and the individual works to avoid the object or situation. Exposure to the object or situation can cause overwhelming symptoms of panic, shortness of breath, and palpitations. The feelings or avoidance associated with the object or situation causes significant impact in the individual's social, interpersonal, and occupational functioning (APA, 2013). See table 6.2 for the clinical names of some common phobias.

Table 6.2: Clinical Names for Common Phobias

Classification	Feared Object/Situation
Acrophobia	Heights
Ailurophobia	Cats
Belonephobia	Needles
Claustrophobia	Closed spaces
Hematophobia	Blood
Pyrophobia	Fire
Zoophobia	Animals

PANIC DISORDER

Panic disorder (PD) is characterized by recurrent unexpected panic attacks, which are manifested by intense apprehension, fear, or terror and feelings of severe discomfort that peak in minutes. The symptoms are not triggered by exposure to an anxiety-provoking situation but can come on suddenly, last several minutes, and then subside. Individuals experiencing a panic attack often believe they are having a heart attack. During this time, four or more of the following symptoms must be present to determine the presence of a panic attack (APA, 2013):

- Palpitations, pounding heart, or accelerated heart rate
- Sweating
- Trembling or shaking
- Sensations of shortness of breath or smothering
- Feelings of choking
- Chest pain or discomfort (client may state it feels like an elephant on their chest)
- Nausea or abdominal distress
- Feeling dizzy, unsteady, light-headed, or faint
- Chills or heat sensations
- Paresthesia (numbness or tingling sensations)
- Derealization (feelings of unreality) or depersonalization (feelings of being detached from oneself)
- Fear of losing control or "going crazy"
- Fear of dying

Self-Reflective Exercise

Think about a time when you felt anxious. Make some notes as you recall what your thoughts and feelings were at that time. Where were you when you felt this way? Is there anything that may have triggered the anxiety? Were you aware of anything that you did that may have helped during that situation? Then think about a time when you were relaxed. What do you notice that is different in that situation?

Agoraphobia

The outstanding feature of this disorder is the intense fear or anxiety of being in a real or anticipated exposure to a place or situation. The individual is afraid of being caught in a situation where escape is impossible, and panic symptoms occur. For a diagnosis, an individual must have symptoms in at least two of the following five places or situations (APA, 2013):

- Using public transportation (e.g., planes, buses, taxis)
- Being outside of the home alone
- Standing in line or being in a crowd
- Being in enclosed places (e.g., elevators, movie theatres)
- Being in open spaces (e.g., bridges, open markets)

Persons with this disorder could have an extreme case where they become incapacitated and cannot leave their home. This disorder is more common in women than in men (Townsend & Morgan, 2020).

LAZARUS AND FOLKMAN'S MODEL OF COPING

Psychologists Lazarus and Folkman (1984) introduced a new perspective to the field of anxiety. They suggested that stress is a transaction "between an individual and their environment" (p. 21). The person's appraisal of an event is related to their personal and cognitive assessment of the situation. An appraisal of the situation by the individual, their available supports, and their beliefs and values influence coping. Lazarus and Folkman, in their process model of coping, described two approaches to coping:

- Problem-focused coping is centred on the individual's appraisal of the stressful event and the attempts to manage following their assessment of the situation. For example, a client is scheduled for a colonoscopy but is not sure about having the procedure because of a fear of bowel perforation. Collaboration with the nurse—who provided information and some teaching with the use of DVDs, family supports—and nurse presence during the procedure helped with coping.

- Emotion-focused coping involves supporting clients to help them with their emotional responses to the stressful event or threat. The nurse and client discuss the feelings related to the procedure and focus on the intervention as routine and necessary for recovery. Assessment and support by the nurse are ongoing both pre- and post-procedure.

Research Highlight: Preoperative Anxiety in Ambulatory Surgery—The Impact of an Empathic Patient-Centred Approach on Psychological and Clinical Outcomes

Background

Anxiety is a psychological reaction to a stressful situation. Surgery or other invasive procedures tend to cause an increase in clients' anxiety. High levels of anxiety can lead to poor client outcomes and prolonged recovery. Strategies for health care professionals have been suggested to reduce preoperative anxiety in inpatient and outpatient clients. These client-centred interventions are associated with best practice outcomes.

Purpose of the Study

To examine the outcome of a preoperative nursing client-centred intervention on the preoperative anxiety and post-surgical recovery of clients undergoing procedures in an ambulatory day surgery

Method

Clients (n = 104) undergoing ambulatory surgery were randomly assigned to either an intervention group (IG) or a control group (CG). Prior to their surgical procedure, the IG participated in a nurse-facilitated empathic person-centred interview. The CG received standardized information on surgical procedures. The State-Trait Anxiety Inventory questionnaire was used to assess anxiety pre- and post-interview and after the procedure. Post-surgery, wound healing, recovery, and client satisfaction were evaluated.

Findings

Prior to the intervention, anxiety, sociodemographic, and clinical characteristics for both groups were similar. After client-centred intervention, in comparison to the CG, the IG demonstrated lower levels of preop anxiety and pain ($p < 0.001$), better surgical recovery ($p < 0.01$), greater levels of daily activity ($p < 0.001$), and greater satisfaction. The IG group also demonstrated better wound healing.

Practice Implications

This empathic client-centred approach is applicable as a nurse-focused intervention for the care of clients undergoing surgical procedures in the context of a variety of health care settings. This study provides support for this practice intervention in the promotion of best client surgical outcomes.

Source: Adapted from Pereira, L., Figueiredo-Braga, M., & Carvalho, I. P. (2016). Preoperative anxiety in ambulatory surgery: The impact of an empathic patient-centered approach on psychological and clinical outcomes. *Patient Education and Counseling, 99*(5), 733–738. https://doi.org/10.1016/j.pec.2015.11.016

ANXIETY ASSESSMENT

Nurses' assessment and observation skills are critical in helping clients with anxiety. The initial step in the therapeutic nurse-client relationship is the nurse's approach. Support and reassurance offered by the nurse help to promote trust, with the priority goal of reducing the client's anxiety. There are several screening tools that can be used for assessment of anxiety symptoms. The most administered tool is the Hamilton Rating Scale for Anxiety (HAM-A). This basic screening tool helps the nurse to elicit specific anxiety symptoms that the client may not disclose unless asked. The symptom inventory in the rating scale (0 = Not present, 1 = Mild, 2 = Moderate, 3 = Disabling, 4 = Severe) has 14 items that are used to measure psychological distress and physical complaints associated with anxiety. A score of 14–17 indicates mild anxiety, 18–24 moderate anxiety, and 25–30 severe anxiety (Thompson, 2015). By asking specific questions and using observations, the nurse rates the client's anxiety level. Having this information enables the nurse and the health care team to institute appropriate intervention strategies.

In situations where the client is experiencing anxiety, the best approach for the health care professional is to use a variety of appropriate therapeutic communication techniques. The initial intervention is to determine the level of distress, assess, and focus on decreasing the client's anxiety. Keep in mind that, as noted in chapter 4, culture can affect how anxiety is manifested. It is important for health care professionals to identify the source of anxiety that contributes to the client's symptoms and feelings. Severe anxiety impacts the person's ability to focus and interact with the environment. The nurse's goal is to intervene early to prevent the client's anxiety from escalating into a panic attack. However, if the client is experiencing a panic attack, the nurse should act quickly and use a variety of environmental and communication interventions to provide support and safety (Steele, 2019).

Exercise 6.1: Role Play

Purpose: To gain awareness about the behavioural responses of anxiety as assessed by the clinician through the use of the HAM-A

Procedure
1. Break into groups of two.
2. Go online and a print copy of the HAM-A (https://www.mcgill.ca/psy/files/psy/ham-a.pdf).
3. One student will role-play the anxious client and display some of the behavioural manifestations of anxiety as indicated on the form. The other student will role-play the nurse and administer the HAM-A. Switch roles and repeat the exercise. Total your scores from the HAM-A and compare results.
4. Share your responses with the class. Were there any differences in the scores among the class? How could you use what you have learned in this exercise in your clinical practice?

Nurse Interventions for Panic Attack

- Maintain a calm, nonthreatening approach.
- Use active listening.
- Stay with the client.
- Use an empathic approach.
- Provide reassurance.
- Assess vital signs.
- Reduce environmental stimuli (quiet environment, dim lights).
- Take control and focus on client (safety).
- Speak clearly, in short, simple, clear sentences.
- Give one (brief) direction at a time.
- Communicate to the client that they are safe.
- If the client is hyperventilating, if available, provide a brown paper bag and focus on breathing with the client.
- Demonstrate and tell the client how to breathe (abdominal breathing exercises).
- Do not use touch as a communication technique; touching can increase feelings of panic.
- Assess nonverbal body cues.

- Keep in mind proxemics—do not invade client's "personal bubble." Invading their space can make them more anxious.
- Walk with the client if necessary to decrease anxiety.
- Later, when anxiety has abated, explore cause of panic attack.
- When anxiety is decreased, provide food and fluids.
- Physician may use anxiolytics (antianxiety agents) as part of the treatment plan. Administer as ordered and assess for effectiveness and for any adverse effects.

For clients who experience anxiety, some of the nursing interventions noted for panic attacks are appropriate. The nurse should also be aware that anxiety is contagious and should not become anxious themselves but focus on the client. All clients who feel anxious due to upcoming surgery, an invasive procedure, or a diagnosis require support and reassurance by the nurse. The research study by Pereira et al. (2016) investigating preoperative anxiety, highlighted in this chapter, confirms that an empathic approach, along with other therapeutic communication techniques discussed in chapter 2, is relevant for use in client anxiety situations. The following are some sample questions that the nurse would focus on when working with clients experiencing anxiety:

- "Tell me about your anxiety level today."
- "When you are feeling anxious, what happens to you?"
- "What are you concerned about or afraid might happen?"
- "Are there situations or places you avoid because they upset you?"
- "When you experience panic attacks, is there something that triggers them? How long do they last?"
- "What helps when these attacks occur?"

An important detail nurses and other health care providers need to consider when working with clients experiencing anxiety is to assess their previously used coping mechanisms and their support systems (e.g., family, friends, pets). Once the client's anxiety level has decreased, it is an appropriate time to provide information about surgical procedures or tests that have contributed to the client's anxiety. During the process of intervention and management, nurses can provide psycho-education for the client and their family members. The type of information provided may include intervention techniques to control breathing, stress reduction strategies, relaxation techniques, education about medications and medical management, and education on anxiety disorders for family members. All client and family teaching should be documented in the clinical record. The documentation should include the teaching information provided, along with the client's and family's response to the intervention.

INTERVENTIONS FOR ANXIETY DISORDERS

Management for anxiety disorders is a multipronged approach, and use of anxiolytics (antianxiety medications) and nonpharmacological interventions can be used.

Relaxation Techniques

Several relaxation techniques, including diaphragmatic breathing, progressive muscle relaxation, guided imagery, and visualization are nursing interventions useful in reducing symptoms of anxiety. Some of these procedures require nurse certification before use in clinical practice.

Diaphragmatic Breathing

Also known as "abdominal breathing," diaphragmatic breathing (DB) is an effective intervention for use with clients who are experiencing anxiety (Jerath et al., 2015). In this approach, the client is instructed to take a deep breath through the mouth and inhale to slowly fill the lungs using the abdominal muscles while relaxing the muscles of the diaphragm. The nurse can demonstrate the technique to the client and instruct them to place their hand on their abdomen, inhale slowly and deeply through the nose to the count of five, and exhale to the count of five. The client repeats the exercise for 5–10 rounds of deep breaths until their anxiety level has decreased.

Progressive Muscle Relaxation

This technique, also known as systematic muscle relaxation, was developed by Jacobsen in 1934, can be practised anywhere, and requires no technology or equipment (Harorani et al., 2020). The premise of the technique is that the release and tension of muscles can reduce stress and anxiety. The nurse will instruct the client to tense a group of muscles (e.g., "Clench your right hand into a fist and just think about the tension in your right hand. Hold the contraction for 10–15 seconds while breathing in and release the tension for about 20 seconds while breathing out"). The nurse can instruct the client to start with the arms and then move to other parts of the body (e.g., face, eyes, cheeks, legs, feet). The client can complete the procedure while lying down or sitting; a quiet environment is best. Once the client has practised the technique, guidance from the nurse is no longer required; however, there are DVD recordings and exercises accessible on YouTube Canada. This information can benefit clients who will continue to use progressive muscle relaxation when discharged to their home from the health care facility.

Guided Imagery and Visualization

This is a mind-body intervention that helps to alleviate anxiety and promote a sense of well-being in the client (Cole, 2021). In this technique, the client uses their own imagination and mental processing to visualize an object, place, event, or situation that is pleasant. This could be the image of walking through the forest, listening to birds in the trees, or sitting underneath a palm tree lying on a beach. During the process of visualization, clients are instructed to close their eyes and focus on their breathing. The client should stay focused on the pleasant images until fully relaxed, then slowly open their eyes and return to their present environment. Guided imagery and visualization can be easily incorporated into client care activities as it requires no technology or equipment. There are audio and video recorded guided imagery relaxation sessions that clients can purchase at retail centres, and exercises are also available on YouTube Canada.

Health teaching is an important role for nurses when working with all clients. For clients who have issues related to the management of stress and anxiety, it is important that nurses have the knowledge of these treatments to provide guidance and recommendations as part of their clinical role. One of the most effective treatments for anxiety disorders is cognitive behavioural therapy (CBT). Other recommendations the nurse can offer clients to help with anxiety include walking, swimming, or some other form of exercise.

COGNITIVE BEHAVIOURAL THERAPY

Cognitive behavioural therapy is a commonly used, effective therapeutic tool to treat clients with anxiety disorders (Bogucki et al., 2021). The goal of CBT is to change the client's behavioural reaction to anxiety-provoking situations. An important function for the nurse is to educate the client on the role that the client's thoughts and beliefs play in activating anxiety. One approach is to teach the client deep breathing or relaxation techniques to cope with anxiety. In CBT, cognitive restructuring is used to help clients examine and challenge the thoughts that trigger their anxiety symptoms (Halter & Pollard, 2019b). As a result of therapy, the client, in collaboration with the nurse, works to replace the negative thoughts with more supportive and positive thinking, leading to reduced anxiety. In CBT, homework assignments that focus on problem-solving are used, which helps the client to identify specific strategies and techniques to mitigate anxiety (Townsend & Morgan, 2020). There are also several forms of behavioural therapy that are used with clients who have phobias. The most common forms of interventions are (a) modelling, (b) systematic desensitization, and (c) flooding or implosion therapy (Halter & Pollard, 2019b).

Modelling can be used by the nurse or therapist in helping the client respond to difficult situations in appropriate ways. In this approach, for example, the nurse could use role play to demonstrate responses for a client who has claustrophobia (fear of closed spaces). Following role-play sessions, the nurse rides in an elevator with the client, who has avoided elevators for years.

In systematic desensitization, the client is gradually introduced to a feared object or situation through real or imagined exposure. For example, a client who has a fear of bees (apiphobia) is shown pictures of bees, moving on to looking at a toy bee, holding it, and then visiting an apiary with the therapist. While working to achieve these situations, the client applies relaxation techniques to reduce anxiety.

Flooding is a therapeutic process where the client is confronted with the object or situation intensely and rapidly. The client is exposed to the object or situation, either in an imagined or real situation, for a prolonged time. During flooding, clients are prevented from escaping or avoiding the object/situation. For example, a client who has a common phobia called zoophobia (fear of animals) is exposed to several breeds of dogs in a confined space. The sessions are guided by the client's response until the object or situation no longer provokes anxiety.

PHARMACOLOGICAL INTERVENTIONS

Sometimes in treatment of anxiety disorders, clients are prescribed a combination of therapies including pharmacotherapy. Several classifications of medications have been found to be effective in the treatment of anxiety disorders. Anxiolytics, for example, benzodiazepines (e.g., alprazolam [Xanax] or lorazepam [Ativan]), are the most commonly prescribed. These benzodiazepines are recommended because of their quick onset of action. However, due to the potential for dependence, short-term use is advocated. Other classes of medications that are also used to treat anxiety disorders include beta blockers, antihistamines, anticonvulsants, and antidepressant medications (Halter & Pollard, 2019a). The nurse has an important role in client and family teaching related to the use of medications, adverse effects, and interactions. It is also important for the nurse to assess the client's intake of caffeine, colas, chocolate, and other substances that can contribute to an increase in anxiety symptoms.

Summary of Nursing Interventions for Anxiety Management

- Listen attentively.
- Convey empathy.
- Utilize attending cues (e.g., nodding, saying "Go on").
- Provide a quiet and calm environment.
- Provide effective management of anxiety and related symptoms.
- Use nursing presence—stay with client during extreme periods of anxiety.
- Explore the client's perceptions of anxiety symptoms.
- Correct any misconceptions about anxiety.
- Explore with client their past coping strategies.
- Encourage the client to express anxiety-associated worries, thoughts, and feelings.
- Assess current support systems.
- Teach client to recognize the symptoms of anxiety.
- Teach interventions that may help client to decrease anxiety (e.g., diaphragmatic breathing, guided imagery, progressive muscle relaxation).
- Involve client in going for walks or playing recreational games.
- Educate the client and family about antianxiety agents and other prescribed medications.
- Encourage the client to establish a routine for daily activities.
- Make referrals for the client to therapy support groups as appropriate.
- Provide client with telephone numbers for mental health crisis lines for crisis situations.

Source: Adapted from Webster, S., Gallagher, S., Brown, P., Evans, J., Flynn, M., & Lopez, V. (2012). The perceptions of nurses in their management of patients experiencing anxiety. *Journal of Nursing Education and Practice, 2*(3), 38–45. https://doi.org/10.5430/jnep.v2n3p38

Case Study

You, the nurse, are at the front desk of the primary health clinic when a young woman and her husband appear. The husband states that his wife, Betty, is having a heart attack. He asks you to help her. The client complains of being short of breath, dizzy, and light-headed. She states, "I have chest pain, and I do not want to die." Her hands are trembling and profusely sweating. You call the physician and place the client on the cardiac monitor in Room 2. You note no signs of cardiac symptoms, as the cardiac monitor shows no irregularity. You stay with Betty and tell her you're now going to check her vital signs, blood pressure, temperature, and pulse.

(Continued)

1. It is determined that the client is not experiencing a cardiac event. You suspect the client is experiencing a panic attack. What questions would give you more specific information to support that assumption?
2. Using therapeutic communication, what specific approach would you use in your interactions with client and her husband?
3. What additional assessment data should you obtain?
4. If the client is experiencing a panic attack, what interventions should you implement?
5. Following the health assessment, new data is obtained about the client's situation. She has been married to her husband, Daniel, for 10 years, and they have five children. The client reports fears of an inability to care for her children. She admits to being afraid to drive the car or ride on the city bus. Recently, the client has been having headaches, trouble sleeping at night, and a fear of dying. After the physician assesses the client and collaborates with you, they decide that the plan of care is alprazolam (Xanax) 0.5 mg twice a day, anxiety management techniques, and cognitive restructuring. You will explain what is meant by anxiety management techniques and cognitive restructuring. What would be your responses in this clinical situation?

Exercise 6.2: Anxiety Disorders

1. Identify interventions that the nurse employs to decrease stimulation for a hospitalized client with a panic disorder.
2. How would these strategies differ if someone has mild or severe anxiety?
3. Describe the difference between social anxiety and phobia disorders.

CHAPTER SUMMARY

Anxiety is a universal phenomenon and is considered a normal reaction to a situation or object and necessary for survival. Nurses encounter clients with anxiety in all health care settings, so it is important that they have knowledge of anxiety and its related disorders. The nurse uses a person-centred approach and a focus on building the nurse-client relationship to assess, explore, and implement appropriate interventions. Showing empathy and establishing rapport are important when interacting with clients with anxiety. Clients experience stress when they are faced with hospitalization, surgical procedures, chronic illness, a diagnosis, or some other health issue. These stressors trigger an emotional response in individuals, which leads to anxiety ("fight or flight"). Levels of anxiety range from mild to moderate, severe, and panic. The client may report symptoms of restlessness, trembling or shaking, dread, and apprehension. Physiological signs of anxiety may include increased heart rate, blood pressure, depth and rate of respirations, and perspiration.

Anxiety disorders include (1) generalized anxiety disorder, (2) panic disorder, and (3) social anxiety disorder (social phobia). Agoraphobia is demonstrated by a fear or anxiety that is out of proportion to the actual danger posed by the real or anticipated exposure to the situation. Clients may have a fear of being in enclosed places (e.g., cinema). Specific phobias are a very common disorder where the individual has a marked fear or anxiety of a specific situation or object (e.g., heights, flying). The nursing intervention for these clients is aimed at decreasing the fear and increasing the ability to function in the presence of the phobic stimulus. Treatment approaches for clients with anxiety or anxiety-related disorders consist of psychological treatments and pharmacological therapies. Assisting those persons through an anxiety attack is an important intervention for nurses and other health care providers. During panic attacks, the nurse remains calm, takes control, provides reassurance, stays with the client, and reduces environmental stimuli. The nurse helps clients to identify the source of their anxiety and uses psychoeducation to teach the client ways to cope. Some of these interventions may include guided imagery, progressive muscle relaxation, breathing exercises, and relaxation techniques. The nurse's role includes providing education on anxiety management, medications, and diet to both the client and their family members.

REVIEW QUESTIONS

Read the following review questions and select the best option to answer each question. State your rationale for choosing your response.

1. A client is admitted to the unit with a diagnosis of anxiety. In care planning, which nurse action is *most* important?
    a. Suggest to the admitting physician that an anxiolytic medication be prescribed.
    b. Identify whether the client wishes to order a room telephone to connect with family while hospitalized.
    c. Consider ways to decrease environmental stimuli that could cause increased anxiety in the client.
    d. Choose a room near the nursing station so the client can be observed for the potential of panic attacks.

2. Which of the following is a physiological response to a panic level of anxiety?
    a. Inability to focus
    b. Dilated pupils
    c. Little muscle tension
    d. Delusions
3. The *most* appropriate nursing action for a client experiencing a panic attack is to
    a. Teach the client about cognitive behavioural therapy to decrease anxiety
    b. Use touch as a communication tool to demonstrate caring
    c. For safety concerns, stay with the client and show presence
    d. Explain the irrational nature of the client's behaviour that triggered the attack
4. All of the following therapies are considered interventions for use with clients experiencing anxiety *except*
    a. Cognitive behavioural therapy
    b. Progressive muscle relaxation
    c. Transcranial magnetic stimulation
    d. Diaphragmatic breathing
5. During an interaction with a newly admitted client, the nurse noticed that the client jumped up and started to pace around the room. In this situation, what is the nurse's *best* course of action?
    a. Change the subject of the conversation.
    b. Administer anxiolytic medication as ordered.
    c. Leave the room and return when client is ready to talk.
    d. Share their observations with the client: "It appears you are anxious."

REFERENCES

Alzahrani, N. (2021). The effect of hospitalization on patients' emotional and psychological well-being among adult patients: An integrative review. *Applied Nursing Research, 61,* https://doi.org/10.1016/j.apnr.2021.151488

American Psychiatric Association. (2013). *Diagnostic and statistical manual of mental disorders* (5th ed.).

Bogucki, O. E., Craner, J. R., Berg, S. L., Wolsey, M. K., Miller, S. J., Smyth, K. T., Johnson, M. W., Mack, J. D., Sedivy, S. J., Burke, L. M., Glader, M. A., Williams, M. W., Katzelnick, D. J., & Sawchuk, C. N. (2021). Cognitive behavioral therapy for anxiety disorders: Outcomes from a multi-state multi-site primary care practice. *Journal of Anxiety Disorders, 78.* https://doi.org/10.1016/j.janxdis.2020.102345

Bolourchifard, F., Savadishafi, M., & Pazoklan, M. (2020). Examining the effect of nursing counseling on anxiety and depression in the elderly patients undergoing open heart surgery. *Archives of Pharmacy Practice, 11*(S1), 100–104.

Cole, L. (2021). The impact of guided imagery on pain and anxiety in hospitalized adults. *Pain Management Nursing, 22*(4), 465–469. https://doi.org/10.1016/j.pmn.2021.02.007

Dozois, D. J. A. (2021). Anxiety and depression in Canada during the COVID-19 pandemic: A national survey. *Canadian Psychology, 62*(1), 136–142. https://doi.org/10.1037/cap0000251

Halter, M. J., & Jakubec, S. L. (2019). Understanding responses to stress. In M. J. Halter, C. L. Pollard, & S. L. Jakubec (Eds.), *Varcarolis's Canadian psychiatric mental health nursing: A clinical approach* (pp. 65–78). Elsevier.

Halter, M. J., & Pollard, C. L. (2019a). Anxiety and related disorders. In M. J. Halter, C. L. Pollard, & S. L. Jakubec (Eds.) *Varcarolis's Canadian psychiatric mental health nursing: A clinical approach* (pp. 200–243). Elsevier.

Halter, M. J. & Pollard, C. L. (2019b). Relevant theories and therapies for nursing practice. In M. J. Halter, C. L. Pollard, & S. L. Jakubec (Eds.), *Varcarolis's Canadian psychiatric Mental health nursing: A clinical approach* (pp. 45–64). Elsevier.

Harorani, M., Davodabady, F., Masmouei, B., & Barati, N. (2020). The effect of progressive muscle relaxation on anxiety and sleep quality in burn patients: A randomized clinical trial. *Burns, 46*(5), 1107–1113. https://doi.org/10.1016/j.burns.2019.11.021

Hernández, C. R., Gómez-Urquiza, G. L., Pradas-Hernández, L., Roman, K. V., Suleiman-Martos, N., Albendín-García, L., & Cañadas-De la Fuente, G. A. (2021). Effectiveness of nursing interventions for preoperative anxiety in adults: A systematic review with meta-analysis. *Journal of Advanced Nursing, 77*. https://doi.org/10.1111/jan.14827

Hitchon, C. A., Zhang, L., Peschken, C. A., Lix, L. M., Graff, L. A., Fisk, J. D., Patten, S. B., Bolton, J., Sareen, J., El-Gabalawy, R., Marriott, J., Bernstein, C. N., & Marrie, R. A. (2020). Validity and reliability of screening measures for depression and anxiety disorders in rheumatoid arthritis. *Arthritis Care & Research, 72*(8), 1130–1139. https://doi.org/10.1002/acr.24011

Jerath, R., Crawford, M. W., Barnes, V. A., & Harden, K. (2015). Self-regulation of breathing as a primary treatment for anxiety *Applied Psychology and Biofeedback, 40*, 107–115. https://doi.org./10.1007/s10484-015-9279-8

Lazarus, R. S., & Folkman, S. (1984). *Stress, appraisal, and coping.* Springer.

Pereira, L., Figueiredo-Braga, M., & Carvalho, I. P. (2016). Preoperative anxiety in ambulatory surgery: The impact of an empathic patient-centered approach on psychological and clinical outcomes. *Patient Education and Counseling, 99*(5), 733–738. https://doi.org/10.1016/j.pec.2015.11.016

Public Health Agency of Canada. (2021). *Symptoms of anxiety and depression during the COVID-19 pandemic.* https://www.canada.ca/en/public-health/services/publications/diseases-conditions/symptoms-anxiety-depression-covid-19-pandemic.html

Selye, H. (1978). *The stress of life* (Rev. ed.). McGraw-Hill.

Shattuck, S. M., Diarratou, K., Zhou, A. N., & Polenick, C. A. (2021). Social contact, emotional support, and anxiety during the COVID-19 pandemic among older adults with chronic conditions. *Clinical Gerontologist, 45*(1), 36–44. https://doi.org/10.1080/07317115.2021.1957051

Steele, D. (2019). Anxiety-related, obsessive-compulsive, trauma- and stressor-related, somatic, and dissociative disorders. In N. L. Keltner & D. Steele (Eds.), *Psychiatric nursing* (8th ed., pp. 307–329). Elsevier.

Thompson, E. (2015). Hamilton rating scale for anxiety (HAM-A). *Occupational Medicine, 65,* 601. https://doi.org/10.1093/occmed/kqv054

Townsend, M. C., & Morgan, K. L. (2020). *Psychiatric mental health nursing: Concepts of care in evidence-based practice.* F. A. Davis.

Webster, S., Gallagher, S., Brown, P., Evans, J., Flynn, M., & Lopez, V. (2012). The perceptions of nurses in their management of patients experiencing anxiety. *Journal of Nursing Education and Practice, 2*(3), 38–45. https://doi.org/10.5430/jnep.v2n3p38

CHAPTER 7

Communication with Clients Experiencing Anger and Aggression

LEARNING OBJECTIVES

After reading this chapter, you will be able to

1. Define and differentiate between the terms *anger, aggression,* and *violence*
2. Discuss predisposing factors that contribute to maladaptive expressions of anger, aggression, and violence
3. Identify how anger, aggression, and violence interfere with communication
4. Describe the assessment process for clients who display anger, aggression, and violence
5. Identify the therapeutic approach for clients who demonstrate anger, aggression, and violence
6. Explain how personal bias toward clients who demonstrate anger, aggression, and violence impacts development of the nurse-client therapeutic relationship
7. Discuss the components of de-escalation for intervention in management of anger, aggression, and violence

KEY TERMS

Aggression

Anger

De-escalation

Restraints

Seclusion

Violence

INTRODUCTION

Workplace violence is an increasing global concern (Thompson et al., 2022). Nurses and other health care providers are not immune to expressions of anger and aggression exhibited by clients, family members, and visitors in health care and community settings (Somani et al., 2021). According to the Canadian Nurses Association and Canadian Federation of Nurses Unions (2017), workplace violence directed at nurses is more common in health care than in any other private sector industry. This chapter will introduce the concepts of anger, aggression, and violence as displayed by clients within health care. Nurses and other health care providers are on the front lines of health care and need knowledge of the precipitating factors that contribute to client anger, aggression, and violence. They also need the communication and assessment skills to recognize and intervene therapeutically with clients to interrupt the escalation of anger into aggression and violence (Thompson et al., 2022). Recognizing client anger and the need for early intervention is important to ensure the safety of clients and health care providers. Interventions to effectively combat workplace violence against nurses is explained in this chapter, and information on one such intervention, de-escalation—suggested as the first line of defence for health care professionals experiencing anger, aggression, and/or potential workplace violence—is discussed (Robbins, 2019).

ANGER

Anger is a normal emotion or feeling common to everyone in response to a particular situation that they may find stressful or frustrating. Nurses in the health care industry often encounter situations where anger is an issue for clients. Clients who enter a health care facility experience stress due to being in an unfamiliar environment, facing long wait times, receiving a specific diagnosis, waiting for surgery or a diagnostic procedure, receiving bad news, or generally not feeling well (e.g., experiencing pain) (Granek et al., 2019). Clients can also experience anger due to feeling unheard or uninvolved in their health care decisions (Dunkley et al., 2018). This stress may lead to anger and feelings of frustration, agitation, aggression, or violence that is directed at health care professionals (Havaei, Astivia, & MacPhee, 2020). These clients feel vulnerable and disempowered as they try to make sense of their loss of control, which leads to stress and anxiety, which triggers anger.

These feelings of anger may be alleviated therapeutically by the nurse within the realms of the nurse-client relationship through the building of trust and rapport. In relationship development, the nurse engages with the client to understand the feelings behind their anger. Using communication skills, the nurse can validate the client's feelings of anger, explore the reasons for those feelings, and work together with the client to resolve the issue. However, it may be difficult for nurses to be therapeutic when they are verbally attacked or criticized by clients. In these situations, nurses may perceive these behaviours as a personal attack and disconnect from clients. In some cases, nurses become angry, defensive, and judgmental, and label the client as hostile or difficult (Gerhart et al., 2015). Such behaviours are barriers to the nurse being therapeutic. It is crucial that nurses learn not to take the anger personally but focus on what is happening with the client (Funk et al., 2021). To be therapeutic, nurses need knowledge and skill in assessment, therapeutic communication, self-awareness, and reflection.

Not all persons who experience anger respond with aggression and violence (Hull, 2019). *Anger* is defined as a multidimensional construct that occurs on a continuum from mild irritation or annoyance to outright rage and violence (Chen et al., 2021). Individuals who are angry express it in different ways. Some express their anger verbally (e.g., talking to others or yelling, swearing); some suppress it and remain silent; some act out and direct it toward others (e.g., kicking, throwing things); while some might turn their anger inward and harm themselves (e.g., cutting themselves). If nurses are clinically astute, they have an awareness of the client's nonverbal behaviours that are indicative of their emotional state and know it is best practice to intervene early and appropriately to prevent potential harm.

Case Example

The client, named Quinn, is admitted for treatment of bipolar 1 disorder. They have a history of alcohol use and are exhibiting agitation (pacing, loud speech). The nurse enters the room to complete an admission intake. Quinn invades the nurse's space and loudly shouts, "Get out of here! I will not speak to a nurse. Send the doctor in here right now!"

Self-Reflective Exercise

Think of a recent situation that made you feel angry.

1. What do you think caused you to feel angry?
2. Is this typical of situations that cause you to become angry?
3. What symptoms did you experience?
4. How did you deal with the situation?
5. Did you deal with it successfully and in an effective way?
6. How could you use what you learned from doing this exercise in your clinical practice?

BEHAVIOURS ASSOCIATED WITH ANGER

Nurses working in all clinical areas need knowledge and awareness of behaviours that are associated with clients who experience anger. Awareness helps with assessment, approach, and early intervention. Individuals vary in how they express anger, but some of the typical behaviours observed in clients include (but are not limited to) the following (Townsend & Morgan, 2020):

- Restlessness, pacing, agitation
- Loud speech—yelling and shouting (swearing)
- Defensiveness—not listening
- Lack of eye contact or intense eye contact
- Clenched fists
- Screaming
- Hitting the wall or furniture
- Facial flushing
- Irritability

Clinical engagement, an aspect of relational practice (see chapter 4) with an emphasis on client-centred care, is a critical component of the nurse's role when working with clients experiencing anger and aggression. Nurses who observe or are the target of these behaviours should use verbal de-escalation to therapeutically engage the client and explore their experience of anger (Jubb & Baack, 2019; Sheldon, 2014).

Communication Approaches for Use with Clients Experiencing Anger

- Remain calm.
- Practise active listening (focus on the client).
- Do not interrupt.
- Identify the client's concern.
- Speak clearly, using a normal tone and volume.
- Address the client by name.
- Show respect and dignity for the client's feelings.
- Avoid being judgmental.
- Demonstrate empathy.
- Sit down at eye level with the client.
- Use open-ended questions and validation.
- Reflect or restate what has been said.
- Give the client adequate personal space (proxemics).
- Be aware of the use of touch.
- Ensure your verbal and nonverbal body language are congruent.
- Do not argue with the client.
- Observe for anger-escalation signs and cues in client's verbal/nonverbal behaviours.
- Teach the client how to communicate needs and concerns in a positive manner.
- If the situation changes, the client's behaviour is escalating, or there is a threat of physical harm, seek assistance immediately (prioritize safety).

During the encounter, the nurse is assessing the client and exploring the client's feelings and reasons for anger. Are there specific things happening that have triggered their anger? What client needs are not presently being met? It is important that the nurse acknowledge and validate the client's feelings, even asking simply, "I can see you are upset. What can I do to help you?"

These responses demonstrate the clinician's focus on using a relational practice lens to offer an empathic approach showing respect for and validation of the client's feelings. Therapeutic communication is key in helping the client to a "calmer place" where anger can be released in a healthy and appropriate way. These actions encourage clients to express their feelings and concerns, reducing the risk of them acting aggressively. However, in some situations, health care providers have done everything right, but the client's behaviour has escalated into aggression and violence nonetheless (Hull, 2019).

Nurse Communication Response Examples: Angry Client

- "I can see you are frustrated; how can I help?"
- "I want to make sure that I understand why you are upset this morning. Is it because the laboratory technician took so long to get your blood? Is that correct?"
- "I'll check that right now. I'll see what is holding up the doctor with your discharge prescription."
- "I can see that you are having a lot of pain. I'll get you something right now to help."

Case Example

Jodie is admitted to the assessment unit for psychiatric evaluation where they start threatening to kill anyone who comes close. You, as the nurse, attempt to offer an oral antipsychotic medication. Jodie refuses to take the medication (throwing the cup across the room) and accuses you of giving them poison. Jodie starts to pace around the room, swinging their arms, and shouts at you in a loud voice, "The devil is telling you to give me that poison. Why are you working with the devil?"

DE-ESCALATION

De-escalation is defined as the use of techniques, including verbal and nonverbal communication, aimed at defusing anger and preventing aggression in clients (Gaynes et al., 2017; Jubb & Baack, 2019). De-escalation also includes a range of interventions consisting of ongoing assessment, nonconfrontational limit-setting, and actions to maintain a safe clinical environment (Brewer et al., 2017; Hallett & Dickens, 2017). Medication administration can also be used as a component of de-escalation strategies (Rabenschlag et al., 2019). The critical focus for the nurse when using de-escalation with a client who is angry and agitated is to try to understand the issue from their perspective and ask what can be done to help. During the interaction, communication should be clear, supportive, and not demanding. The focus is on the client, so the nurse may state (calling client by name), "I would really like to help you feel better. What has helped in the past when you felt this way?" The nurse should have an awareness of their own verbal and nonverbal behaviour to ensure it is relaxed, nonthreatening, assertive, and empathic.

In these situations, safety is important for the client and staff, as well as for other clients. Focus on remaining calm and securing the environment, which could include moving the client to a calmer location, moving furniture, or getting other clients out of the area. The following are some strategies to guide interventions (Bowers, 2014; Jubb & Baack, 2019; Sheehan, 2012):

- Do not go into a room alone with the client.
- Keep a distance from client—stay at least four feet away.
- Make sure you have access to the door in case you need to exit quickly.
- Do not turn your back away from the client.
- Only one primary person should speak to the client at any one time (one-on-one communication).
- When speaking to the client at a distance, do not stand in a doorway or directly in front of the client as this could be interpreted as confrontational.
- Remain calm, speak softly, and listen (focus on client).
- Be aware of your own body language. It should be open and congruent.
- Do not use a lot of gestures. Keep your hands where the client can see them.

AGGRESSION AND VIOLENCE

Aggression and violence are one way that individuals express anger (Ladika, 2018). Aggression is an emotion that involves actions or behaviours that can result in harm, hurt, or injury to another person or object. Aggressive behaviours are classified as verbal or physical attacks. Violence is the intent to harm and can be directed to persons or objects (Hull, 2019). Nursing observation and assessment skills are critical in identifying clients who are anxious and agitated. This information enables clinicians to intervene early to prevent the situation from escalating to verbal and physical aggression and violence (Flores, 2008). Three risk factors to consider in client assessment for potential violence include (1) a history of violence, (2) diagnosis, and (3) current behaviour (Mavandadi et al., 2016). The assessment provides an opportunity to obtain information about past and current behaviour related to aggression and violence. Some diagnoses that are closely correlated with aggressive behaviour are substance-related disorders, head trauma, bipolar disorder, dementia, and major depressive disorder (Scott & Resnick, 2017).

A brief assessment tool, the Brøset Violence Checklist (BVC), is recommended for nursing staff to use in therapeutic approaches with clients who are exhibiting anger. This quick, reliable tool can be used as an assessment of risk for potential violence in clients admitted to any health care setting. It has 63 percent accuracy in predicting violence and a 92 percent accuracy in predicting that violence will not occur (Almvik et al., 2000). The behaviours assessed and rated by the nurse are confusion, irritability, boisterousness, physically threatening, verbally threatening, or attacking objects. Clients are assigned one point for each behaviour observed. A score of one to two is considered moderate risk; and a score greater than two represents a high risk. This tool enables the nurse to determine who may be at risk for violence on the next shift (Abderhalden et al., 2004; Almvik et al., 2000; Almvik & Woods, 1999).

Research Highlight: Implementation of the Brøset Violence Checklist on an Acute Psychiatric Unit

Background

Workplace aggression and violence in inpatient psychiatric settings has increased, but it is difficult to determine its frequency because of underreporting. Violence in the workplace is demonstrated by threatening behaviours, and verbal and physical abuse directed at staff. Research is needed to determine if the BVC is an accurate instrument for predicting client violence.

Purpose of the Study

The study aims were to determine the relationship between BVC scores and incidence of violence within 24 hours among a population of clients admitted to an adult inpatient psychiatric unit, to compare scores among clients requiring nursing interventions for violence, and to assess the impact of scores on length of stay (LOS) and readmission rates.

(Continued)

Method
Using a retrospective cohort design, 20 registered nurses were trained on use of the BVC tool. Nurses completed the checklist on client admission and on all clients every day until they were discharged or transferred.

Findings
Statistical logistic regression analysis indicates 3.4 times greater risk of violence for every additional point on admission BVC (odds ratio = 3.4, 95% confidence interval = [2.29, 5.08], $p < .0001$). Clients requiring high-level interventions by nursing staff for violence had higher mean BVC scores on both day one and day two of admission. Pearson correlation was significant for positive association between BVC on admission and LOS ($p < .001$). Findings did not establish a link between BVC scores and readmission rates.

Implications for Practice
Health care professionals continue to experience workplace violence. Preventative tools are needed to predict occurrence of violence to support clinical practice safety for health care providers and clients. This study shows that the BVC is an effective tool useful in reducing the number of violent episodes through early identification of and intervention into client disruptive behaviour.

Source: Sarver, W. L., Radziewics, R., Coyne, G., Colon, K., & Mantz, L. (2019). Implementation of the Brøset violence checklist on an acute psychiatric unit. *Journal of the American Psychiatric Nurses Association, 25*(6), 476–486. https://doi.org/10.1177/1078390318820668

The nurse's goal in assessment is to determine the potential risk of aggression and violence in clients with anger. The nurse is observant of any changes in the client's behaviour that would indicate they are escalating. This entails a plan for preventing aggression and violence, managing environmental triggers (e.g., noise), and helping the client to verbally de-escalate (Matthew et al., 2012). Through therapeutic engagement, the nurse focuses on alleviating the client's feelings of anger with a collaborative management plan. If the client becomes aggressive and a dangerous situation is identified, the nurse still needs to attempt to de-escalate the situation. This includes verbal de-escalation to communicate to the client that the nurse is there to help. Some communication strategies that can be used are the following:

- Ask open-ended questions such as "What is upsetting you?"
- Acknowledge the client's emotions—tell them you will help them maintain control. For example, "I am here to keep you safe" or "You are in a safe environment."
- Respond in a genuine, professional manner.

- Convey empathy.
- Be flexible not authoritarian.
- Reassure the client that the aim is to work on a collaborative solution.
- Encourage communication.
- Maintain eye contact (this shows interest). Do not stare (fleeting eye contact is best).
- Do not threaten or make false promises.
- Avoid power struggles.
- Offer choices and options (if available).

However, if the client does not settle with verbal de-escalation strategies and the behaviour continues, other de-escalation management interventions can be used to help with agitation symptoms. Pharmacological measures can be offered to the client to help "calm" them without over-sedation (Roppolo et al., 2020). Medications such as anxiolytics (antianxiety), antipsychotics, and mood stabilizers can be used to alleviate symptoms (Hull, 2019). If the situation allows, the client needs to be involved in the decision-making regarding the type and route of medication administration (e.g., oral or intramuscular [IM]). Offering oral medications is considered the first-line strategy as it promotes client autonomy and health care provider safety (Burke et al., 2021). If the client refuses these options and their behaviour becomes more threatening (e.g., physically acting out, aggressive body language), then immediate intervention is needed to maintain safety.

In this situation, the client is not able to maintain control and becomes violent. It is necessary to employ physical restraints to maintain the safety of the client and health care providers and to administer IM medication (Burke et al., 2021). Health care providers and nursing students should be aware of policies and procedures for managing a violent/aggressive situation relevant to their health care facility or agency.

In health care settings, there may be instances where verbal de-escalation is not successful and the use of restraints or seclusion—which are considered restrictive practices—may be utilized (Mooney & Kanyeredzi, 2021). Seclusion involves placing the client in a safe room alone to decrease agitation and external stimulation. Chemical (medication), environmental (seclusion), or physical restraints are coercive approaches that are used to restrict the client's movements, decrease agitation, and promote a culture of safety (Hull, 2019). The care of clients in seclusion or restraints requires a physician's order and one-to-one monitoring by a health care provider. When caring for the client, facility policies and protocols for restraints and seclusion should be followed (Hull, 2019; Roppolo et al., 2020). Health care professionals need to ensure all requirements (e.g., protocol monitoring) and other forms of documentation during client restraint and/or seclusion practices are completed. In most health care facilities, restraints and seclusion are used as a last resort, supporting the principles of least restrictive environment to manage aggressive or violent incidents

(Registered Nurses' Association of Ontario, 2012; Riahi et al., 2016). Following an aggressive or violent episode and the use of seclusion or restraints, best practice would be a debriefing with staff and the client (Allikmets et al., 2020).

In working with clients who are experiencing anger and aggression, a trauma-informed care approach (see chapter 4) should be utilized. This acknowledges that both staff and clients may have a trauma history and utilization of organization policies and restrictive practices may re-traumatize clients and health care providers. In using this approach, nurses and other health care providers engage with clients through therapeutic relationships to understand and address their experience of trauma to prevent re-traumatization (Polacek et al., 2015). The use of restrictive practices such as seclusion and restraints can adversely impact the health and well-being of both clients and health care providers. Participant narratives from two research studies investigating the impact of seclusion and restraint use in health care provide support of its negative impact:

> This guy was put in seclusion, and it took five of us to hold him down … and they administered an injection.… I knew it had to be done, but it's not a nice thing … I reckon it's very degrading for the person who has to receive it, it's very sort of embarrassing, you know, it's inhumane, you're just powerless really. (Nurse) (Mooney & Kanyeredzi, 2021, p. 1707)

> I just remember being really distressed. Makes you more, made me more determined that, I'm really on my own. And seems no matter where you get put for care, ultimately, there is no help. [It] just feels totally like, abandoned, helpless." (Client) (Askew et al., 2020, p. 276)

It is recommended that health care organizations integrate trauma knowledge into policies, programs, and practices in order to promote trauma-informed practice. Such organizational change facilitates healing and recovery-centred engagement for clients and well-being for all staff (Barnhill et al., 2019).

Student Tip

If a client is agitated or hostile, for safety concerns, follow these principles (Burke et al., 2021; Jubb & Baack, 2019):

- If in a closed area, make sure you have access to the door in case you need to exit quickly.
- Do not turn your back to the client.
- Do not go into a room alone with client. Go with another person.

- Do not wear anything that can be grabbed and used as a weapon (e.g., stethoscope).
- Stay at least two armlengths away from the client. If a violent outburst occurs, it provides you with space to escape if needed.
- Do not let the client get between you and the door; this blocks access to the exit.

With an increase in workplace violence in health care settings, de-escalation training should be available so staff are able to learn de-escalation skills. Some health care agencies, as a condition of employment, require staff to complete a nonviolent crisis intervention course that teaches de-escalation as well as restrictive and nonrestrictive interventions. This education course is offered globally and in Canada through the Crisis Prevention Institute (CPI). The CPI link https://institue.crisisprevention.com/cpi/training will direct you to its website. CPI's website provides current information that may be of interest to you as a health professional student, such as case studies and a library with resources for those working in health care.

NURSE SAFETY

Nurses have the right to a respectful and safe workplace free from violence. However, many nurses do expect to experience violence and aggression and feel it is an occupational hazard of working in health care (Jubb & Baack, 2019). Workplace violence (WV) within health care settings in Canada is on the rise, and health care workers have a four-fold higher rate of exposure than that seen in other professions (House of Commons, 2019). There is a risk of health care providers experiencing WV in all health care and community settings. The Canadian Federation of Nurses Unions (2020) used an online survey to assess nurses' (n = 7153) perceptions of their work environment and found that WV was a major issue in all provinces and territories in the country. Reports of verbal abuse by clients or their families was most common: one in five participants (21.2%) experienced it daily. Although less prevalent, physical abuse from clients and their families was noted to occur from daily (7.9%) to once a month (12.2%), and a few times a year (29.2%). In a similar study, Havaei, MacPhee, & Ma (2020) used an online survey to examine workplace violence among nurses (n = 4462) in British Columbia. Participants reported emotional abuse, threats of assault, and physical assault as the most common types of workplace abuse.

Workplace violence has adverse effects on the health and well-being of health care providers. WV is related to increased reports of burnout, anxiety disorders, physical injuries, job dissatisfaction, and absenteeism (Mento et al., 2020,

Somani et al., 2021). WV also affects the delivery of health care, impacting care outcomes and client safety (Havaei, MacPhee, & Ma, 2020). Health care organization recommendations to decrease WV include the following (Somani et al., 2021):

- Education and staff training for WV management
- Standardized reporting system for WV
- Workplace violence prevention policy and safety procedures for staff
- Implementation of an admission alert system to identify high-risk clients
- Security locks, panic buttons
- Input from health care personnel for environmental changes

An important recommendation for all health care professionals to combat WV is the development of self-care strategies. It is imperative that students in the health professions care for themselves so that they can best care for others.

Case Study 7.1

Harry is admitted to the medical unit for reassessment of type 2 diabetes. They have not been looking after themselves for the past five months and not following their diet or taking insulin as prescribed by the family doctor. Harry has vascular neuropathy, impaired function, and sensation in all four extremities. You are the nursing student assigned to this client. After getting a verbal report from the primary nurse, you are informed that the client was caught smoking in their room, has been arguing with the staff nurses, and is known to raise their voice when angry. The facility has a no-smoking policy. Upon entering the room, you note that the client is sitting up in bed, smoking a cigarette. You inform Harry that it is against hospital policy to smoke in the facility. The client responds, "Listen, nurse, I have been here for a short while, and no one is going to tell me that I can't smoke in my room. Who do you think you are? I am going to tell you a thing or two; you don't tell me what to do." The client's voice is loud, and they are staring and pointing a finger at you.

1. What would be your most therapeutic nursing intervention in response to the client's outburst?
2. Identify verbal intervention strategies to use with the client at this time.
3. What can you do to assess the client's emotions?
4. Identify several communication techniques to use for the development of client rapport.

Case Study 7.2

Brighton, age 25, is admitted for psychiatric evaluation after getting into a verbal fight with their partner in a downtown bar. While they were arguing, Brighton broke several chairs and tables, so the police were called. Brighton is found hiding outside in the alley and is brought to the emergency department by the police. Following assessment, Brighton is admitted to the general admission unit. On the unit, they spend most of the time in their room alone but come out and get into an argument with other clients on the unit in the dining area. When Brighton is out of their room, staff nurses observe them pacing up and down the corridor with their hands clenched. When approached by the nursing staff, the client states, "Leave me alone." After lunch, the client retreats to the lounge to watch TV. Upon entering the lounge, Brighton grabs the remote from another client and changes to a sports channel. Two other clients, who were watching a movie, complain, and Brighton shouts (in a loud voice), "You were watching TV all day, and now it is my turn. I am putting it on this channel, and if you don't like it, you can all go to hell!" The nurse enters the lounge.

1. Describe the cues that Brighton's behaviour was escalating in this situation.
2. Where might the nurse have intervened earlier to diffuse the client's anger?
3. Identify verbal and nonverbal intervention strategies to use with the client at this time.
4. How should the nurse position themselves in the TV room, and how can they ensure their safety while speaking with Brighton?

Exercise 7.1: Therapeutic Communication

Review the two case examples presented in this chapter. Identify how you, as the nurse, would communicate with clients Quinn and Jodie in these scenarios. Discuss your approach for de-escalation for each client.

CHAPTER SUMMARY

This chapter focuses on the concepts of anger, aggression, and violence faced by nurses and other health care providers in their workplace as exhibited by clients and their family members. Anger is a normal, healthy emotion that alerts us to potential threats and helps people deal with stressful situations in a positive way. Clients admitted to hospital or visiting a health care facility may experience anger due to many factors that impact their care experience. In these situations, clients may express anger appropriately or direct it at others. Health care professionals play an important role in the assessment of the client's emotional state and use management strategies to understand their feelings of anger. Anger, if not assessed and managed, may lead to aggression or violent behaviour. Early intervention is key in the management of anger, aggression, or violence. In assessment, nurses need to know and be aware of symptoms and behaviours exhibited by clients with anger to apply therapeutic interventions. Three types of intervention strategies are de-escalation (verbal), pharmacological, and physical (seclusion and restraints). The first line of defence in aggressive situations is de-escalation, to communicate and prevent escalation of client behaviour. Depending upon the clinical situation, these approaches may be used separately or in combination, indicated by the client's needs. The critical issue in managing aggression and violence in the health care system is safety for clients, health care providers, and staff. Workplace violence is a serious problem in health care in Canada, impacting the health and well-being of health care professionals and clients. Intervention strategies such as educational programs for staff on violence management, organizational changes (e.g., violence reporting policies), and work-life balance supports can have a positive effect.

REVIEW QUESTIONS

Compassion fatigue (burnout) is a phenomenon that occurs in staff working in health care settings. Self-care strategies can help health care professionals to combat compassion fatigue. As a professional health care student, it is important for you to identify and use self-care strategies in your career development.

1. List several self-care strategies that help promote health care professionals' physical and psychological well-being.
2. Identify those that you use in your own self-care.

REFERENCES

Abderhalden, C., Needham, I., Miserez, B., Almvik, R., Dassen, T., Haug, H.-J., & Fischer, J. E. (2004). Predicting inpatient violence in acute psychiatric wards using the Brøset-Violence-Checklist: A multicentre prospective cohort study. *Journal of Psychiatric and Mental Health Nursing, 11*(4), 422–427. https://doi.org/10.1111/j.1365-2850.2004.00733.x

Allikmets, S., Marshall, C., Murad, O., & Gupta, K. (2020). Seclusion: A patient perspective. *Issues in Mental Health Nursing, 41*(8), 723–735. https://doi.org/10.1080/01612840.2019.17 10005

Almvik, R., & Woods, P. (1999). Predicting inpatient violence using the Broset violence checklist (BVC). *The International Journal of Psychiatric Nursing Research*, *4*(3), 498–505.

Almvik, R., Woods, P., & Rasmussen, K. (2000). The Brøset Violence Checklist: Sensitivity, specificity, and interrater reliability. *Journal of Interpersonal Violence*, *15*(12), 1284–1296. https://doi.org/10.1177/088626000015012003

Askew, L., Fisher, P., & Beazley, P. (2020). Being in a seclusion room: The forensic psychiatric inpatients' perspective. *Journal of Psychiatric and Mental Health Nursing*, *27*(3), 272–280. https://doi.org/10.1111/jpm.12576

Barnhill, J., Fisher, J. W., Kimel-Scott, K., & Weil, A. (2019). Trauma-informed care: Helping the healthcare team thrive. In M. R. Gerber (Ed.), *Trauma-informed approaches: A guide for primary care* (pp. 197–213). Springer.

Bowers, L. (2014). A model of de-escalation. *Mental Health Practice*, *17*(9), 36–37.

Brewer, A., Beech, R., & Simbani, S. (2017). Using de-escalation strategies to prevent aggressive behaviour. *Mental Health Practice*, *21*(2), 22–28. https://doi.org/10.7748/mhp.2017.e1221

Burke, C. J., Hardy, J., & Isaacs, E. D. (2021). Caring for the agitated patient: A tiered approach. *Clinics in Integrated Care*, *7*. https://doi.org/10.1016/j.ihtcar.2021.100063

Canadian Federation of Nurses Unions. (2020). *Outlook on nursing: A snapshot from Canadian nurses on work environments pre-COVID-19.* https://nursesunions.ca/wp-content/uploads/2020/12/CFNU_outlook_ENfinal_web.pdf

Canadian Nurses Association & Canadian Federation of Nurses Unions. (2017). *Workplace violence.* https://nursesunions.ca/campaigns/violence/

Chen, X., Luo, L., Jiang, L., Shi, L., Yang, L., Zeng, Y., Li, F., & Li, L. (2021). Development of the nurse's communication ability with angry patients scale and evaluation of its psychometric properties. *Journal of Advanced Nursing*, *77*(6), 2700–2708. https://doi.org/10.1111/jan.14788

Dunkley, C., Borthwick, A., Bartlett, R., Dunkley, L., Palmer, S., Gleeson, S., & Kingdon, D. (2018). Hearing the suicidal patient's emotional pain. *Crisis*, *39*(4), 267–274. https://doi.org/10.1027/0227-5910/a000497

Flores, N. (2008). Dealing with an angry patient. *Nursing*, *38*(5), 30–31. https://doi.org/10.1097/01.NURSE.0000.317577.17161.5e

Funk, L., Spencer, D., & Herron, R. (2021). Making sense of violence and victimization in health care work: The emotional labour of "not taking it personally." *International Review of Victimology*, *27*(1), 94–110. https://doi.org/10.1177/0269758020953760

Gaynes, B. N., Brown, C. L., Lux, L. J., Brownley, K. A., Van Dorn, R. A., Edlund, M. J., Coker-Schwimmer, E., Weber, R. P., Sheitman, B., Zarzar, T., Viswanathan, M., & Lohr, K. N. (2017). Preventing and de-escalating aggressive behavior among adult psychiatric patients: A systematic review of evidence. *Psychiatric Services*, *68*(8), 819–831. https://doi.org/10.1176/appi.ps.201600314

Gerhart, J. I., Sanchez Varela, V., Burns, J. W., Hobfoll, S. E., & Fung, H. C. (2015). Anger, provider responses, and pain: Prospective analysis of stem cell transplant patients. *Health Psychology*, *34*(3), 197–206. https://doi.org/10.1037/hea0000095

Granek, L., Ben-David, M., Shapira, S., & Ariad, S. (2019). "Please do not act violently towards the staff": Expressions and causes of anger, violence, and aggression in Israeli cancer patients and their families from the perspectives of oncologists. *Transcultural Psychiatry, 56*(5), 1011–1035. https://doi.org/10.1177/1363461518786162

Hallett, N., & Dickens, G. L. (2017). De-escalation of aggressive behaviour in healthcare settings: Concept analysis. *International Journal of Nursing Studies, 75*, 10–20. https://doi.org/10/1016/j.ijnurstu.2017.07.003

Havaei, F., Astivia, O. L., & MacPhee, M. (2020). The impact of workplace violence on medical-surgical nurses' health outcome: A moderated mediation model of work environment and burnout using secondary data. *International Journal of Nursing Studies, 109.* https://doi.org/10.1016/j.ijnurstu.2020.103666

Havaei, F., MacPhee, M., & Ma, A. (2020). Workplace violence among British Columbia nurses across different roles and contexts. *Healthcare, 8*(2), 98. https://doi.org/10.3390/healthcare8020098

House of Commons. (2019). *Violence facing health care workers in Canada.* https://www.ourcommons.ca/DocumentViewer/en/42-1/HESA/report-29/page-36

Hull, M. B. (2019). Anger, aggression, and violence. In M. J. Halter, C. L. Pollard, & S. L. Jakubec (Eds.), *Varcarolis's Canadian psychiatric mental health nursing: A clinical approach* (2nd ed., pp. 512–529). Elsevier.

Jubb, J. M., & Baack, C. J. (2019). Verbal de-escalation for clinical practice safety. *American Nurse Today, 14*(1), 5–7. https://www.myamericannurse.com/verbal-de-escalation-safety/

Ladika, S. (2018). Violence against nurses: Casualties of caring. *Managed Care, 27*(5), 32–34. https://pubmed.ncbi.nlm.nih.gov/29763407/

Matthew, J. M., Sayles, K., & DaSilva, M. (2012). The patient with anger. In L. Damon, J. M. Matthew, J. L. Sheehan, & L. A. Uebelacker (Eds.), *Inpatient psychiatric nursing: Clinical strategies and practical interventions* (pp. 1–23). Springer.

Mavandadi, V., Bieling, P. J., & Madsen, V. (2016). Effective ingredients of verbal de-escalation: Validating an English modified version of the "De-escalating Aggressive Behaviour Scale." *Journal of Psychiatric and Mental Health Nursing, 23*(6–7), 357–368. https://doi.org/10.1111/jpm.12310

Mento, C., Silvestri, M. C., Bruno, A., Mustcatello, M. R. A., Cedro, C., Pandolfo, G., & Zoccali, R. A. (2020). Workplace violence against healthcare professionals: A systematic review. *Aggression and Violent Behavior, 51.* https://doi.org/10.1016/j.avb.2020.101381

Mooney, M., & Kanyeredzi, A. (2021). "You get this conflict between you as a person and you in your role that changes you": A thematic analysis of how inpatient psychiatric healthcare staff in the UK experience restraint, seclusion, and other restrictive practices. *International Journal of Mental Health Nursing, 30.* https://doi.org/10.1111/inm.12926

Polacek, M. J., Allen, D. E., Damin-Moss, R. S., Schwartz, A. J. A., Sharp, D., Shattell, M., Souther, J., & Delaney, K. R. (2015). Engagement as an element of safe inpatient psychiatric environments. *Journal of the American Psychiatric Nurses Association, 21*(3), 181–190. https://doi.org/10.1177/1078390315593107

Rabenschlag, F., Cassidy, C., & Steinauer, R. (2019). Nursing perspectives: Reflecting history and informal coercion in de-escalation strategies. *Frontiers in Psychiatry, 10*, https://doi .org/10.3389/fpsyt.2019.00231

Registered Nurses' Association of Ontario. (2012). *Promoting safety: Alternative approaches to the use of restraints.* https://rnao.ca/bpg/guidelines/promoting-safety-alternative-approaches -use-restraints

Riahi, S., Thomson, G., & Duxbury, J. (2016). An integrative review exploring decision-making factors influencing mental health nurses in the use of restraint. *Journal of Psychiatric and Mental Health Nursing, 23*(2), 116–128. https://doi.org/10.1111/jpm.12285

Robbins, K. C. (2019). De-escalation in health care. *Nephrology Nursing Journal, 46*(3), 345–346.

Roppolo, L. P., Morris, D. W., Khan, F., Downs, R., Metzger, J., Carder, T., Wong, A. H., & Wilson, M. P. (2020). Improving the management of acutely agitated patients in the emergency department through implementation of project beta (Best practices in the evaluation and treatment of agitation). *JACEP Open, 1*(5). https://doi.org/10.1002/ emp2.12138

Sarver, W. L., Radziewicz, R., Coyne, G., Colon, K., & Mantz, L. (2019). Implementation of the Brøset Violence Checklist on an acute psychiatric unit. *Journal of the American Psychiatric Nurses Association, 25*(6), 476–486. https://doi.org/10.1177/1078390318820668

Scott, C. L., & Resnick, P. J. (2017). Clinical assessment of aggression and violence. In R. Rosen & C. L. Scott (Eds.), *Principles and practice of forensic psychiatry* (3rd ed., pp. 623–631). Routledge.

Sheehan, J. L. (2012). Managing violence. In L. Damon, J. M. Matthew, J. L. Sheehan & L. A. Uebelacker (Eds.), *Inpatient psychiatric nursing: Clinical strategies and practical interventions* (pp. 363–374). Springer.

Sheldon, L. K. (2014). Anger, anxiety, and difficult communication styles. In L. K. Sheldon & J. B. Foust (Eds.), *Communication for nurses: Talking with patients* (3rd ed., pp. 199–220). Jones & Bartlett Learning.

Somani, R., Muntaner, C., Hillan, E., Velonis, A. J., & Smith, P. (2021). A systematic review: Effectiveness of interventions to de-escalate workplace violence against nurses in healthcare settings. *Safety and Health at Work, 12*(3), 289–295. https://doi.org/10.1016/j .shaw.2021.04.004

Thompson, S. L., Zurmehly, J., Bauldoff, G., & Rosselet, R. (2022). De-escalation training as part of a workplace violence prevention program. *The Journal of Nursing Administration, 52*(4), 222–227. https://doi.org/10.1097/NNA.0000000000001135

Townsend, M. C., & Morgan, K. I. (2020). *Psychiatric mental health nursing: Concepts of care in evidence-based practice* (9th ed.). F. A. Davis.

CHAPTER 8

Communication with Clients Experiencing Communication Difficulty

LEARNING OBJECTIVES

After reading this chapter, you will be able to

1. Discuss barriers to communication for persons with verbal, visual, auditory, and cognitive impairments
2. List ways for effective communication with persons who have communication difficulties related to impairments in verbal, visual, auditory, or cognitive functioning
3. Identify the safety strategies health care providers implement for clients with visual, auditory, and cognitive impairment
4. Describe appropriate assistive tools for clients with communication difficulties
5. Identify organizations and community supports for persons with communication deficits

KEY TERMS

Aphasia

Communication impairment

Conductive hearing loss

Deafblindness

Dysarthria

Macular degeneration

Presbycusis

Sensorineural hearing loss

Vision loss

INTRODUCTION

Effective communication is critical to the practice of nursing, as well as for other health care disciplines. Health care professionals, including nurses, work in a variety of community and clinical settings and care for clients with health issues that present barriers to clinician-client communication. Some of these obstacles are due to the presence of a medical illness or disorder that leads to verbal, visual, hearing, and cognitive impairment. These situations provide a challenge for both the health care provider and the client in the initiation of a person-centred approach to care. Nurses and clients experience frustration, anxiety, and discomfort when communication is unsuccessful (Sirch et al., 2017). In addition, ineffective nurse-client communication increases the risk to client safety and the risk of inadequate health care outcomes (James et al., 2022). Nurses need knowledge of these conditions and therapeutic communication strategies to overcome barriers in health care delivery for this population. This chapter presents an overview of specific conditions—decreased cognition and verbal, visual, and hearing impairments—that hinder communication. Communication strategies for facilitation of the therapeutic nurse-client relationship for clients with communication difficulty are discussed.

EPIDEMIOLOGY OF HEARING AND VISION LOSS

Hearing loss is a major public health issue and is considered the third-most common physical condition affecting Canadians. One in ten Canadians report some degree of hearing loss, and in the population of those 65 years of age and older, one in three has hearing loss (Canadian Hard of Hearing Association, 2020). In Canada, it is estimated that 19 percent of adults (4.6 million) have mild hearing loss in the speech-frequency range (0.5, 1, 2, and 4 kHz), while 35 percent (8.4 million) have a high degree of hearing loss in the range of 3, 4, 6, and 8 kHz, which is where age-related hearing loss begins (Ramage-Morin et al., 2019). The top four assistive devices used by Canadians with hearing loss are hearing aids or cochlear implants, closed captioning, telephone-related devices, and visual alarms. About one-quarter of Canadians with hearing difficulty (23%) lip-read (Statistics Canada, 2019).

It is estimated that 1.5 million Canadians have a visual impairment and about 5.59 million have an eye disease (e.g., cataracts, glaucoma, macular degeneration, diabetic retinopathy) that may lead to sight loss. About 500,000 Canadians are blind or partially sighted. Normal visual acuity is 20/20, and to be considered legally blind by law, visual acuity is 20/200 (or 6/60) or less in both eyes after correction and/or the visual field is 20 degrees or narrower (Canadian National Institute for the Blind [CNIB], 2021). Some clients who visit a health facility may have a dual sensory loss referred to as deafblindness that involves a loss of hearing and vision (CNIB, 2021). This disorder is identified by its broad categories: congenital and acquired (Simcock, 2017).

COMMUNICATION IMPAIRMENT

A communication impairment is an inability to communicate one's needs to others. The impairment involves the incapability of receiving, comprehending, sending, writing, or reading, which leads to problems in both expressive and receptive communication (Belva et al., 2012). These include impairments of hearing, vision, speech or language, and/or cognition. Clients with communication-related difficulties are at risk of being disengaged by health care providers and experiencing poor health outcomes such as adverse events and dissatisfaction with their care (Crotty & Doody, 2015; Hemsley et al., 2016; Shukla et al., 2018). These client difficulties interfere with the establishment and development of the therapeutic nurse-client relationship.

Other barriers identified for clients with communication impairments relate to health care providers' negative attitudes, stigmas, and stereotyping (Hemsley et al., 2001). Another factor impacting the ability to communicate with these clients within the health care setting is the lack of knowledge and skills of nurses who may not take time to communicate (Hemsley et al., 2012; Sharpe & Hemsley, 2016). Making the effort and taking the time to communicate facilitates clinician-client communication, leading to an understanding of client needs. The physical environment is also considered a barrier to communication between these clients and health care professionals. The noise levels in hospital environments, crowded client rooms, and poor lighting play a role in impeding effective, respectful communication (Crotty & Doody, 2015; Richardson, 2014).

TYPES OF HEARING LOSS

According to the World Health Organization (WHO, 2021), a person is considered to have hearing loss when they have a hearing threshold of 20 decibels (dB) or more in both ears. Hearing loss may be mild (20–34.9 dB), moderate (35–49.9 dB), moderately severe (50–64.9 dB), severe (65–79.9 dB), or profound (80–94.9 dB); can occur across the lifespan from infancy to older adulthood; and can affect one or both ears (Olusanya et al., 2019). Hearing loss is classified as either sensorineural (most common), caused by damage to the inner ear, or conductive, caused by the inability of sound to travel along the pathway from the outer to the middle and inner ear or an interference with this process (Lasak et al., 2014; Olusanya et al., 2019). Mixed hearing loss refers to a combination of conductive and sensorineural loss, where a problem occurs in both the outer or middle and the inner ear. Hearing loss can occur during the prenatal and perinatal period, childhood and adolescence, or adulthood and older age (WHO, 2021). In older adults, age-related hearing loss (sensorineural) leads to a condition called presbycusis, caused by degeneration of ear structures (Hao et al., 2018). Hearing loss is associated with lower quality of life and mortality for individuals due to its social and health consequences (Mick et al., 2018; Ramage-Morin et al., 2019; WHO, 2021).

It is important for health care professionals to have knowledge and use correct terminology when interacting with clients with hearing loss. Using incorrect terminology demonstrates a lack of respect, can upset the client or family, and can hinder the development of the nurse-client relationship. The term *hearing impairment* is often used by health professionals, but it is best to avoid it, as it has a negative connotation (Ekstrom, 2000). The following are recommended terms to use:

- *Hard of hearing* refers to persons with hearing loss ranging from mild to severe. These individuals usually communicate through spoken language and may use lip-reading, hearing aids, cochlear implants, or other assistive devices (WHO, 2021).
- The terms *deaf* and *Deaf* (with an upper-case D): *deaf* refers to people who have profound hearing loss, which indicates little or no hearing, and who use spoken language. They often use lip-reading and may benefit from a hearing aid. People who call themselves *Deaf* usually use sign language as their first language. They consider themselves "culturally" Deaf, meaning deafness is not a disability but a difference in human experience. They usually have profound deafness and may use some lip-reading but prefer to communicate in sign language (Middleton et al., 2010; WHO, 2021).
- *Deafblindness* refers to dual sensory loss of vision and hearing. This usually occurs in the older population (65+), and individuals may be completely deaf and blind or have some residual hearing and/or vision (Alfaro et al., 2020; Guthrie et al., 2016).

VISION LOSS

Vision loss is recognized as a major public health concern and is defined as partial or complete impaired vision that cannot be corrected by eyeglasses, contact lenses, medication, or surgical intervention (WHO, 2019). About 3 percent of Canadians aged 15 years and older have some form of vision loss, which limits their activities of daily functioning and poses implications for health and social care services (Jaiswal et al., 2021; Statistics Canada, 2016). Vision impairment causes serious limitations, which lead to a loss of independence impacting physical, cognitive, psychological, and social functioning (Swenor et al., 2020). Age is considered a major risk factor for vision loss. With aging, vision in the older adult often decreases gradually. The five major causes of age-related vision loss in Canada are age-related macular degeneration, cataract, diabetic retinopathy, glaucoma, and refractive error (McGrath, 2021). The Canadian population is aging: by 2030 seniors will number 9.5 million (Government of Canada, 2014), and it is expected that by 2032 the number of people with vision loss will greatly increase, requiring increased health care services (Cruess et al., 2011).

ASSESSMENT OF COMMUNICATION ABILITIES

Nurses have an important role, during the admission process or when meeting the client for the first time in a health care situation, to assess for communication difficulties. Having awareness of the client's communication abilities helps to address communication barriers in the hospital setting and facilitates a person-centred plan of care to ensure quality, safe care. Health care organizations have a legal obligation to accommodate persons with communication difficulties. Health care professionals should have knowledge of relevant policies and procedures within their facility that relate to client accommodation. Nurses are obligated to pass on information about a client's communication needs to all health team members and also during the handover report. Following this practice helps team members provide a positive health care experience for clients. Assessment also provides information for the referral process, which is needed to involve other specialists or therapists in the client's "circle of care" (e.g., audiologist, dietitian, speech language therapist).

CLIENTS WITH HEARING LOSS

As part of the admission interview, nurses should assess clients for functional hearing ability. Once the nurse determines the presence of a hearing issue, steps can be taken to maximize the client's ability to communicate. Anyone can acquire a hearing loss at any time of life, so the assessment should include the age of onset, degree of hearing loss, family history of hearing loss, current medical conditions, and any prescribed medications. At this time, the nurse should assess the person's lived experience of living with hearing loss (Aquino-Russell, 2006). To explore with the client, they might ask, "What is it like for you?" This knowledge can enhance the nurse's understanding of how the client relates to others and their own personal strategies of living with a different sense of hearing. These perspectives can be integrated into the client's health care plan.

During the admission process, health care providers can observe for any nonverbal sign of a hearing difficulty, such as leaning forward, turning the head toward the speaker, or cupping the ear when asked questions (Funk et al., 2018). The nurse can ask questions: "Can you tell me about any concerns you have with your hearing?" If hearing issues are revealed, the nurse can use follow-up questions: "What can we do to enable our communication to be helpful?" or "What strategies for communication might be helpful?" or "Do you use assistive listening devices such as a hearing aid, telephone attachment, or another means to communicate?"

In 2017, 319,000 Canadians with hearing difficulty did not use a hearing aid but needed one. Sixty-six percent stated they did not use one because of cost (Statistics Canada, 2019). Nurses need to educate and empower clients with hearing loss about appropriate accommodations that can be provided during their hospital stay or clinic visit. In communication, people who are Deaf use American Sign Language as their first or preferred language.

AMERICAN SIGN LANGUAGE

The language of Deaf people is sign language. Within Canada, there are two sign languages that are recognized by governmental and other agencies: American Sign Language (ASL) and Langue des signes québécoise (LSQ); there is also a regional dialect, Maritime Sign Language (MSL). These sign languages are recognized internationally, and ASL is the third-most widely used language after English and Spanish (Canadian Association of the Deaf, 2015; Shuler et al., 2014). Sign language has a different structure from English; it is abbreviated and more pictorial (using gestures and facial expressions) than grammatical English (Ekstrom, 2000). It has its own grammar, syntax, and vocabulary, but does not have a written form, instead using signs, body language, and facial expressions in its constructs of communication (Richardson, 2014).

Interpreters are utilized frequently as an accommodation for persons who are Deaf or hard of hearing and use one of several sign languages. Health care professionals should ask clients if they need accommodation services. The client preference to use an interpreter should take precedence as this will aid successful communication and contribute to better health outcomes (Chong-hee Lieu et al., 2007). Nurses should be aware of whether their facility has an interpretation policy and a process to arrange for the services of a certified sign language interpreter. In instances where an accommodation is required, family members or friends should not be used due to issues of confidentiality and lack of skill in signing for medical information (Chong-hee Lieu et al., 2007; Shuler et al., 2014).

DEAF CULTURE

Nurses who work with clients with hearing loss must become knowledgeable of the differences between Deafness as a culture and being deaf (Chong-hee Lieu et al., 2007; Shuler et al., 2014). People who are Deaf or hard of hearing see themselves as a community with a common, unique culture. The community is considered a subculture of the larger hearing community that developed in Canada in response to the marginalization of persons who are Deaf. Their sense of cultural identity is bound by their recognition as a Deaf culture with social norms, common experiences, and a distinct sign language (Richardson, 2014). It is important for health care providers not to assume that all Deaf persons are proficient in sign language. Best practice is to ask and confirm with the client their preferred mode of communication. Some may prefer one method or a combination of ways to communicate. These may include lip-reading, written communication, visual aids, or sign language (Malebranche et al., 2020). If sign language is preferred, an interpreter should be available. All facilities in Canada that provide health care services are required to provide interpreter services. Clients who are Deaf have a legal right to access a certified sign language interpreter.

Case Example

Client Toni Becker is at the pre-admission clinic for their admission work-up to prepare for right-hand surgical repair in three days' time. The client is to be admitted to the hospital one day before the scheduled procedure. The client wears a hearing aid and is able to lip-read.

Nurse: (*Looks at client and smiles*) Good morning, Toni Becker. Welcome to the clinic. Please have a seat. I am Hunter Snow, your nurse, and I will be completing your pre-admission work-up. Before I begin, I'd like to ask, what is your preferred way to communicate?

Client: (*Looking at nurse*) It is okay if we talk. I have a new battery in my hearing aid, and I can lip-read as well.

Nurse: (*Sitting with an open posture, looking at client*) Thanks, we can do that. If you have any questions during our interaction, please let me know. First, I want to take some blood. Is that okay with you? Once that is done, I will go over your surgical preparation information. The admission process should take about 40 minutes. Which arm do you wish me to use for taking the blood?

In the case example, the nurse used a number of strategies in the admission work-up:

- Pleasant, welcoming approach
- Introduced self
- Called client by name
- Explained purpose of the encounter (time/information)
- Assessed how client communicates
- Sought permission before procedure
- Sat in chair facing client

Strategies for Communicating with Clients Who Have Hearing Difficulty

- Sit facing the client (with face and mouth clearly visible).
- Establish eye contact. Keeps hands and hair away from face. Do not chew gum.
- Begin conversation by getting the client's attention. Call them by name or tap overbed table/desk.
- Speak clearly at a normal pace—no shouting.
- Do not speak directly into the client's ear.
- Explain procedures (e.g., dressing change) in simple terms.
- Introduce one idea at a time.
- Allow extra time for them to process and respond to information.
- Assess their understanding. You may need to repeat information.
- Maintain a quiet environment (no distractions). Turn off the radio and television. Close the door or curtain room barrier.
- Ask how they prefer to communicate and what you might do to enable communication.
- Use communication tools (pen/paper, whiteboards, computer, hearing aid, sign language) as needed.
- Avoid standing or sitting in front of windows or bright lights (glare) as this presents a barrier to communication.
- In a group situation, only one person should speak at any one time.
- Arrange for an interpreter if necessary.
- If the client uses a hearing aid, check to make sure it is on and working properly. Also check hearing aid batteries.
- If the client wears glasses, they should be clean and in place.
- Use gestures, facial expressions, and pictures to reinforce verbal information.
- Assess the need for other services (e.g., audiologist).

CLIENTS WITH VISION DIFFICULTY

During the admission process, a vision assessment should be completed routinely by the health care provider. If a person has a visual impairment, onset may be at birth or during another developmental period. It may occur gradually or suddenly because of injury, eye disease, or age-related vision loss. The five major causes of visual impairment for persons in Canada are macular degeneration, cataract, diabetic retinopathy, glaucoma, and refractive error (Cruess et al., 2011). Unlike physical impairment, visual impairment is rarely obvious when you meet the client at the initial encounter. Nurses interacting with clients in the hospital or clinic setting during an admission interview should ask, "Do you have any issues with your vision that I should know about?" If any concerns are revealed, then other questions can be asked: "Can you describe the difficulties you are experiencing?" Clients should be asked about their support network, family or friends, and community supports (e.g., Canadian National Institute for the Blind). The level of visual impairment will guide the intervention process while the client is receiving health care services. When interacting, take time to communicate, listen, and not rush the client. Persons who have severe impairment may not be able to see visual cues, nonverbal signals, facial expressions, and furniture placement. As these factors impact the therapeutic relationship, the nurse needs to work with the client to maximize their communication. Nurses can use words to express what the client cannot see in the message. Using Braille communication or providing information in different font styles, large print, or audio format (e.g., smartphone applications that read text aloud) can assist the client. Always identify yourself when you enter the client's presence and let them know when you leave the room.

When caring for clients with progressive eye disease such as macular degeneration, it is useful to determine what assistance is required for activities of daily living. Persons with this condition retain some peripheral vision, so when interacting, sit at a 45-degree angle from them rather than face to face. Nurses need to be aware of potential safety risks in the environment when caring for clients with vision difficulties. Strategies to make the environment user-friendly include turning on night-lights, placing personal care items within easy reach, checking for room obstacles, and keeping visual assistance devices (e.g., glasses, magnifiers) close at hand (Moore, 2001).

ENVIRONMENTAL HAZARDS

Depending upon the degree of visual difficulty, clients may be at an increased risk of accidents and falls. Persons with low vision or blindness who are admitted to a health facility are challenged by their new surroundings. Nurses and other health care providers have an important role in maintaining a safe environment by providing care interventions. During the admission process, you should orient the client to the room by describing the size and placement of furniture and equipment, as well as orienting the client to the bathroom. Furniture positions should not be changed once a person is oriented to their room (Moore, 2001). Use accurate and specific language when giving directions or explaining the layout of a room. For example, "The bathroom door is on your left."

When helping the client to their room, offer your arm for them to hold just above the elbow instead of taking their arm. Provide information and advance notice of changes in the ground surface (e.g., going from tiled to carpeted floor). If the client is assigned to a semi-private or four-unit bedroom and the other persons are present, get them to introduce themselves. This technique helps the client to recognize the sound of a person's voice. For a client with some vision, make sure the room has adequate lighting and provide a night-light. In providing respectful care, ask clients whether they would like assistance with activities of daily living (e.g., walking, bathing). If you are assisting with meals, you can give instructions according to the face of a clock in describing food placement on their tray. For example, cereal is at 9 o'clock, the coffee mug is at 10 o'clock, and the breakfast plate is at 11 o'clock. Open juice containers if asked to do so. Let client guide what assistance is necessary, but continue to promote independence.

Orient the client to the nursing call system and ensure that it is within easy reach and the client is aware of its placement in the room. The assigned room should be kept free of any unnecessary hospital equipment to prevent client falls or injury. If equipment is being used as part of the treatment plan, inform the client of its placement in the room.

Strategies for Communicating with Clients with Vision Difficulty

- Knock before entering client's area (knock on door or overbed table). Identify yourself using your full name, status, and your role in their care.
- Always identify yourself clearly when entering the client's room and inform them when you leave. Do not assume they will recognize your voice.
- Face the client directly when speaking and use their name; tap or knock their overbed table or bed to gain their attention.
- If the client wears communication aids (glasses or hearing aid), make sure their glasses are clean and in place and their hearing aid is on and working (check batteries).
- Speak in a normal, natural tone of voice while making eye contact.
- Ask the client to describe their level of vision and what assistance they require.
- Ask the client whether they would like assistance with activities of daily living (do not make assumptions). Help promote independence by letting them do as much of the care as they are able.
- In a group atmosphere, introduce the other people present.
- Maintain a quiet environment as much as possible (avoid distractions).
- Be aware of your own position to the client. Do not stand in front of a window (glare).
- All staff should narrate their actions (e.g., "Hi, Mrs. Chang, it's Kerry Jackson, your nurse. I'm here to check your blood pressure in your right arm. Is that okay?").

- Check to make sure the best possible lighting is available to aid residual vision.
- If assisting with meals or explaining the position of objects, use the analogy of the face of a clock (e.g., "The sink is in front of you at 12 o'clock").
- For safety, do not move furniture in the client's room. Clients with visual impairment have a mental picture of where familiar items are placed and can easily reach them.
- Use verbal and nonverbal communication techniques as appropriate (e.g., assess the use of touch—you do not want to startle the client).
- Use other means of communication depending on client's level of vision and preference (e.g., Braille or other assistive devices; printed materials should be bold and large print; magnification lens).
- Describe procedures or treatments in advance so the client is aware of what to expect and has time to ask questions.
- Provide information in simple narrative terms and offer supplements (e.g., print, audio, electronic) to support client-nurse interactions.
- When walking with the client, walk slightly in front (pace should be neither too fast nor too slow).
- Never channel communication to client through a third person (e.g., another client, family member); always address the client.
- If an interpreter is necessary to aid communication, seek the client's permission.

IMPAIRED VERBAL COMMUNICATION SECONDARY TO STROKE

Clients who have a cerebrovascular accident, also known as a stroke, have communication impairments that affect their ability to produce speech and to process, express, and comprehend language due to damage to a particular area of the brain (Carragher et al., 2021). These factors impact the person's ability to engage with their health care provider and influence development of the therapeutic relationship (Bright & Reeves, 2020).

Communication impairments, including aphasia and dysarthria, are prevalent in clients who have experienced a stroke (Mitchell et al., 2021). These communication issues can also occur in individuals who have a head injury, brain tumour, infections, or dementia. *Aphasia* is a communication disorder due to an acquired impairment of language caused by damage to a specific area of the brain. Aphasia affects the person's quality of life and impacts functioning across relationships, life roles, and activities (Berg et al., 2020). Aphasia can present as either an expressive or receptive impairment. A person who has *expressive aphasia* can understand what is being said but is unable to express thoughts or feelings in words, while *receptive aphasia* causes difficulties in receiving and processing written and oral messages. A client with *global aphasia* has difficulty with expressive language and the reception of messages. *Dysarthria* is characterized by difficulty controlling the muscles used for speech (Mitchell et al., 2021).

According to health care professionals, communication difficulties with clients who have post-stroke aphasia disrupt care and impede the provision of client-centred care (Carragher et al., 2021). These professionals suggest that an environment lacking resources for client-provider communication contributes to the limiting or avoidance of client engagement (Carragher et al., 2021; Hersh, 2016). Nurses are part of an interprofessional team (along with, for example, a dietitian, a speech-language pathologist) that provides a collaborative approach for meeting the communication needs of these clients (Dondorf et al., 2016). In a metasynthesis of the literature on the perspectives of persons with communication impairment after stroke, Bright and Reeves (2020) found that therapeutic relationship development is dependent upon the clinician's communication behaviours. Clients identified nurse behaviours that contribute to a sense of connection, such as making the client feel valued and heard, showing respect, being genuine and supportive, using verbal and nonverbal behaviours, taking time, and including the client as a communication partner and in care decisions.

The communication practices reported by clients that led to a therapeutic disconnection were being talked over, being treated as a "task" or "just a number," being ignored or excluded in conversations, and nurses' use of infantilizing communication. These negative communication practices reinforced the clients' sense of isolation and frustration, contributing to feelings of disempowerment. Several authors advocate for communication programs to support and improve communication between nurses and persons with aphasia (Chu et al., 2018; Clancy et al., 2020; van Rijssen et al., 2019).

Strategies for Communication with Clients Who Have Aphasia

- Sit or stand on the unaffected side of the client.
- Use SOLER principles as discussed in chapter 2.
- If the client wears glasses or uses a hearing aid, make sure they are in place.
- Maintain a quiet environment.
- Build rapport.
- Be patient—demonstrate a caring presence.
- Use attentive listening skills.
- Observe the client's nonverbal cues.

- Use short, simple sentences.
- Encourage and support the client's ability to speak.
- Speak slowly in a normal tone of voice.
- Use closed-ended questions.
- Break down information into small bits of information.
- Augment the message with gestures or pictures (e.g., picture boards, whiteboards).
- Do not overload the client with information.
- Verify client understanding. Do not rush them; wait for a response.
- If the client misunderstands, do not raise your voice.
- Repeat information.
- Do not interrupt or complete the client's sentence.
- Use touch if appropriate.
- Make sure the client is oriented to the call bell system and it is within reach.

Exercise 8.1: Sensory Loss: Vision

Purpose: To help you better understand the experience of a person who has low vision or total vision loss

Procedure
1. Pair up with another student. One student should wear a sleep mask or glasses with semi-opaque lenses. If you have your own glasses, they can be covered with plastic wrap folded multiple times over your lenses.
2. The student with unimpaired vision should guide the student with "impaired vision" around the building. The guider should offer the back of their arm to the other student (client) just above the elbow and walk one step ahead. The guider leads the client during a 10-minute walk, describing the landscape and pointing out barriers along the route.
3. Switch roles and complete step 2 again.
4. In class, share your observations and answer the following questions.

Discussion
1. What did you find challenging about completing this exercise?
2. Describe how you felt about the experience.
3. What did you learn about yourself by completing this exercise?
4. How can you apply this knowledge to you own clinical practice when working with clients with vision loss?

IMPAIRED COGNITIVE FUNCTIONING

Persons with impaired cognition have a variety of levels of interference (mild, moderate, severe) in their thought and communication processes. The role of the nurse is to support and maintain the person's optimum level of functioning and enhance quality of life. In interactions, appropriate verbal and nonverbal communication used by the health care provider decreases client anxiety and encourages their participation in the interpersonal process. Clients with specific disorders such as major depressive disorder, substance abuse, schizophrenia, delirium, and dementia will have problems with cognitive processing. Persons who have experienced trauma (brain injury) or stroke will have problems with cognition that also hinder communication. For more information on cognitive impairment, see chapter 9, which covers the topic of communicating with clients with neurocognitive disorders.

Case Study 8.1

Mr. John Rossi is a 76-year-old male who is blind and was admitted to the medical unit for investigation of left cardiac failure. He was assigned to a private room next to the nursing station. While he is lying in bed, with his wife sitting in the room, a health care provider enters and shouts, "I am here to check your vital signs!" The client is startled and begins to ask a question, then realizes the health care professional has left the room.

1. Is this the correct, professional approach for this client?
2. If you were the nurse in this situation, what would be your approach?
3. What would be your goals when communicating with this client?
4. How would you address the issue with his wife?

Case Study 8.2

Jude Bowers is a 25-year-old animal groomer who is admitted to the hospital with a possible kidney infection. The client was born without hearing to parents who could hear. She attended regular school with her brother, John. Her parents sent her to a local school where she learned to read and write as well as lip-read. Jude likes her job as a pet groomer at the local pet store. She is difficult to understand when speaking as she sometimes mumbles and often, to be understood, repeats her words. During the admission process, a complete blood count and a mid-stream urine are ordered for analysis. The physician orders a regular chest X-ray, which is scheduled for the afternoon.

1. How will you communicate the information to the client?
2. Identify your approach in explaining the collection of the urine sample.
3. List several principles for effective communication with a person experiencing hearing loss.
4. What did you learn from doing this case study that you can use within your clinical practice?

CHAPTER SUMMARY

This chapter discusses the communication needs of clients with communication difficulties. Health care providers who use a person-centred approach and effective communication skills convey a message of caring in their engagement of those who have impaired communication. Effective and appropriate communication strategies for persons who are experiencing sensory loss of hearing and sight foster the best client health care outcomes. In working with this population, health care professionals need a broad knowledge of these disorders and of the specialized assistive technologies that are used to enhance communication. It is important that they have the skills to be proactive in promoting client safety. Clients with these issues who seek health care services appreciate the support from nurses who treat them as people and are able use their skills to adapt to the clients' preferred methods of communication. Health care professionals' competency in assessment, communication, and referral for clients with communication difficulties helps to facilitate a supportive environment and successful nurse-client relationships.

REVIEW QUESTIONS

Read the following three review questions and select the best option to answer each question. State your rationale for choosing your response. For the other four questions, identify your response.

1. A client is admitted to the medical unit following a stroke resulting in aphasia and dysarthria. Which communication strategy would be *most* helpful for this client?
   a. Providing a language interpreter to converse with client
   b. Providing a private room near the nursing station so nurses can always have time to interact
   c. Speaking to the client and providing written material to supplement information
   d. Listening attentively, allowing time, and not interrupting

2. A client has visited the walk-in clinic with complaints of problems with their hearing for about three months. Following an assessment and examination by the physician, a diagnosis of presbycusis is made. The client asks you, the clinic nurse, what that means. Your response is
   a. "A wax build-up in the inner ear that impacts communication"
   b. "A problem with sound wave connection within the tympanic membrane"
   c. "A sensorineural hearing loss due to degeneration of ear structures"
   d. "A conductive hearing loss due to degeneration of ear structures"
3. A 30-year-old client who is Deaf comes to the emergency department with a swollen right leg. You are unable to get a certified ASL interpreter. To begin the assessment, which of these communication strategies would you use? Select all that apply.
   a. Ask the client how best to communicate with them.
   b. Exaggerate your lip movements when speaking as this aids lip-reading.
   c. Sit and face the client directly to collect information.
   d. Establish eye contact. Keep your hands and hair away from your face and mouth.
4. Identify safety strategies health care professionals use for clients with a visual impairment.
5. Describe the difference between sensorineural and conductive hearing loss.
6. List several nurse communication strategies for clients with hearing difficulty.
7. Identify nurse communication strategies for clients with aphasia.

WEB RESOURCES

Canadian Deafblind Association
https://www.cdbanational.com
Canadian National Institute for the Blind (CNIB)
https://www.crwdp.ca/en/partners/canadian-national-institute-blind-cnib

REFERENCES

Alfaro, A. U., Guthrie, D. M., McGraw, C., & Wittich, W. (2020). Older adults with dual sensory loss in rehabilitation show high functioning and may fare better than those with single sensory loss. *Plos One, 15*(8), e0237152. https://doi.org/10.1371/journal .pone.0237152

Aquino-Russell, C. E. (2006). A phenomenological study: The lived experience of persons having a different sense of hearing. *Nursing Science Quarterly, 19*(4), 339–348. https://doi.org/10.1177/0894318406292827

Belva, B. C., Matson, J. L., Sipes, M., & Bamburg, J. W. (2012). An examination of specific communication deficits in adults with profound intellectual disabilities. *Research in Developmental Disabilities, 33*(2), 525–529. https://doi.org/10.1016/j.ridd.2011.10.019

Berg, K., Isaken, J., Wallace, S. J., Cruice, M., Simmons-Mackie, N., & Worrall, L. (2020). Establishing consensus on a definition of aphasia: An e-Delphi study of international aphasia researchers. *Aphasiology.* https://doi.org/10.1080/02687038.2020.1852003

Bright, F. A. S., & Reeves, B. (2020). Creating therapeutic relationships through communication: A qualitative metasynthesis from the perspectives of people with communication impairment after stroke. *Disability and Rehabilitation, 44*(12), 2670–2682. https://doi.org/10.1080/09638288.2020.1849419

Canadian Association of the Deaf. (2015). *Language.* http://cad.ca/issues-positions/language/

Canadian Hard of Hearing Association. (2020). *Hearing loss toolkit.* https://www.chha.ca/hearing-loss-toolkit/

Canadian National Institute for the Blind. (2021). *Blindness in Canada.* https://www.cnib.ca/en/sight-loss-info/blindness/what-blindness?region=A1

Carragher, M., Steel, G., O'Halloran, R., Torabi, T., Johnson, H., Taylor, N. F., & Rose, M. (2021). Aphasia disrupts usual care: The stroke team's perceptions of delivering healthcare to patients with aphasia. *Disability and Rehabilitation, 43*(21), 3003–3014. https://doi.org/10.1080/09638288.2020.1722264

Chong-hee Lieu, C., Sadler, G. R., Fullerton, J. T., & Stohlmann, P. D. (2007). Communication strategies for nurses interacting with deaf patients. *MESSURG Nursing, 16*(4), 239–245. https://www.researchgate.net/publication/5936730_Communication_strategies_for_nurses_interacting_with_deaf_patients#:~:text=Options%20to%20assist%20in%20communication,Sign%20Language%20or%20video%20interpreters

Chu, C. H., Sorin-Peters, R., Sidari, S., De La Huerta, B., & McGilton, K. (2018). An interprofessional communication training program to improve nurses' ability to communicate with stroke patients with communication disorders. *Rehabilitation Nursing, 43*(6), E25–E34. https://doi.org/10.1097/rnj.0000000000000041

Clancy, L., Povey, R., & Rodham, K. (2020). "Living in a foreign country": Experiences of staff-patient communication in inpatient stroke settings for people with post-stroke aphasia and those supporting them. *Disability and Rehabilitation, 42*(3), 324–334. https://doi.org/10.1080/09638288.2018.1497716

Crotty, G., & Doody, O. (2015). Therapeutic relationships in intellectual disability nursing practice. *Learning Disability Practice, 18*(7), 25–29. https://doi.org/10.7748/ldp.18.7.25.e1660

Cruess, A. F., Gordon, K. D., Bellan, L., Mitchell, S., & Pezzullo, M. L. (2011). The cost of vision loss in Canada. 2. Results. *Canadian Journal of Ophthalmology, 46*(4), 315–318. https://doi.org/10.1016/j.jcjo.2011.06.006

Dondorf, K., Fabus, R., & Ghassemi, A. E. (2016). The interprofessional collaboration between nurses and speech-language pathologists working with patients diagnosed with dysphagia in skilled nursing facilities. *Journal of Nursing Education and Practice, 6*(4), https://doi.org/10.5430/jnep.v6n4p17

Ekstrom, I. A. (2000). Getting your message through to your hard of hearing or deaf patients or families. *Plastic Surgical Nursing, 20*(3), 181–194. https://doi.org/10.1097/00006527-200020030-00012

Funk, A., Garcia, C., & Mullen, T. (2018). Understanding the hospital experience of older adults with hearing impairment. *American Journal of Nursing, 118*(6), 28–34. https://doi.org/10.1097/01.NAJ.0000534821.03997.7b

Government of Canada. (2014). Government of Canada—Action for seniors report. https://www.canada.ca/en/employment-social-development/programs/seniors-action-report.html

Guthrie, D. M., Declercq, A., Finne-Soveri, H., Fries, B. E., & Hirdes, J. P. (2016). The health and well-being of older adults with dual sensory impairment (DSI) in four countries. *PLOS One.* https://doi.org/10.1371/journal.pone.0155073

Hao, W., Wang, Q., Li, L., Qiao, Y., Gao, Z., Ni, D., & Shang, Y. (2018). Effects of phase-locking deficits on speech recognition in older adults with presbycusis. *Frontiers in Aging Neuroscience, 10*(397). https://doi.org/10.3389/fnagi.2018.00397

Hemsley, B., Balandin, S., & Worrall, L. (2012). Nursing the patient with complex communication needs: Time as a barrier and a facilitator to successful communication in hospital. *Journal of Advanced Nursing, 68*(1), 116–126. https://doi.org/10.1111/j.1365-2648.2011.05722.x

Hemsley, B., Georgiou, A., Hill, S., Rollo, M., Steel, J., & Balandin, S. (2016). An integrative review of patient safety in studies on the care and safety of patients with communication disabilities in hospital. *Patient Education and Counseling, 99*(4), 501–511. https://doi.org/10.1016/j.pec.2015.10.022

Hemsley, B., Sigafoos, J., Balandin, S., Forbes, R., Taylor, C., Green, V. A., & Parmenter, T. (2001). Nursing the patient with severe communication impairment. *Journal of Advanced Nursing, 35*(6), 827-835. https://doi.org/10.1046/j.1365-2648.2001.01920.x

Hersh, D. (2016). Therapy in transit: Managing aphasia in the early period post stroke. *Aphasiology, 30*(5). https://doi.org/10.1080/02687038.2015.1137555

Jaiswal, A, Santhakumaran, S., Walker, S., Sukhai, M. A., Packer, T., & Kessler, D. (2021). A scoping review of vision rehabilitation services in Canada. *British Journal of Visual Impairment, 41*(1). https://doi.org/10.1177/02646196211029344

James, T. G., Coady, K. A., Stacciarini, J. M., McKee, M. M., Phillips, D. G., Maruca, D., & Cheong, J. (2022). "They're not willing to accommodate Deaf patients": Communication experience of Deaf American sign language users in the emergency department. *Qualitative Health Research, 32*(1), 48–63. https://doi.org/10.1177/10497323211046238

Lasak, J. M., Allen, P., McVay, T., & Lewis, D. (2014). Hearing loss: diagnosis and management. *Primary Care: Clinics in Office Practice, 41*(1), 19–31. https://doi.org/10.1016/j.pop.2013.10.003

Malebranche, M., Morisod, K., & Bodenmann, P. (2020). Deaf culture and health care. *CMAJ*, *192*(50), e1809. https://doi.org/10.1503/cmaj.200772

McGrath, C., Karsan, I., Corrado, A. M., Lyons, T. A., & Blue, M. (2021). The impact of combined age-related vision loss and dementia on the participation of older adults: A scoping review. *PLOS One*, *16*(10), https://doi.org/10.1371/journal.pone.0258854

Mick, P., Parfyonov, M., Wittch, W., Phillips, N., & Pichora-Fuller, K. M. (2018). Associations between sensory loss and social networks, participation, support, and loneliness. *Canadian Family Physician*, *64*(1), e33–e41. https://www.cfp.ca/content/64/1/e33.short

Middleton, A., Niruban, A., Girling, G., & Myint, P. K. (2010). Communicating in a healthcare setting with people who have hearing loss. *BMJ*, *341*, c4672. https://doi.org/10.1136/bmj.c4672

Mitchell, C., Gittins, M., Tyson, S., Vail, A., Conroy, P., Paley, L., & Bowen, A. (2021). Prevalence of aphasia and dysarthria among inpatient stroke survivors: Describing the population, therapy provision and outcomes on discharge. *Aphasiology*, *35*(7), 950–960. https://doi.org/10.1080/02687038.2020.1759772

Moore, L. W. (2001). Macular degeneration in older adults. *Geriatric Nursing*, *22*(2), 96–99. https://doi.org/10.1067/mgn.2001.115206

Olusanya, B. O., Davis, A. C., & Hoffman, H. J. (2019). Hearing loss grades and the international classification of functioning, disability and health. *Bulletin of the WHO*, *97*(10), 725–728. https://doi.org/10.2471/BLT.19.230367

Ramage-Morin, P. L., Banks, R., Pineault, D., & Atrach, M. (2019). Unperceived hearing loss among Canadians aged 40 to 79. *Statistics Canada Health Reports*, *30*(8), 11–20. https://www.doi.org/10.25318/82-003-x201900800002-eng

Richardson, K. J. (2014). Deaf culture: Competencies and best practices. *The Nurse Practitioner*, *39*(5), 20–28. https://doi.org/10.1097/01.NPR.0000445956.21045.c4

Sharpe, B., & Hemsley, B. (2016). Improving nurse-patient communication with patients with communication impairments: Hospital nurses' views on the feasibility of using mobile communication technologies. *Applied Nursing Research*, *30*, 228–236. https://doi.org/10.1016/j.apnr.2015.11.012

Shukla, A., Nieman, C. L., Price, C., Harper, M., Lin, F. R., & Reed, N. S. (2018). Impact of hearing loss on patient-provider communication among hospitalized patients: A systematic review. *American Journal of Medical Quality*, *34*(3), 284–292. https://doi.org/10.1177/1062860618798926

Shuler, G. K., Mistler, L. A., Torrey, K., & Depukat, R. (2014). More than signing: Communicating with the deaf. *Nursing Management*, *45*(3), 20–27. https://doi.org/10.1097/01.NUMA.0000444299.04190.94

Simcock, P. (2017). One of society's most vulnerable groups? A systematically conducted literature review exploring the vulnerability of deafblind people. *Health and Social Care in the Community*, *25*(3), 813–839. https://doi.org/10.1111/hsc.12317

Sirch, L., Salvador, L., & Palese, A. (2017). Communication difficulties experienced by deaf male patients during their in-hospital stay: Findings from a qualitative descriptive study. *Scandinavian Journal of Caring Sciences*, *31*(2), 368–377. https://doi.org/10.1111/scs.12356

Statistics Canada. (2016). *Canadian survey on disability: Seeing and hearing disabilities, 2012.* https://www150-statcan.gc.ca/n1/daily-quotidien/160229/dq160229c-eng.htm

Statistics Canada. (2019). *Canadians with a hearing disability.* https://www150.statcan.gc.ca/n1/pub/11-627-m/11-627-m2019025-eng.htm

Swenor, B. K., Lee, M. J., Varadaraj, V., Whitson, H. E., & Ramulu, P. Y. (2020). Aging with vision loss: A framework for assessing the impact of visual impairment on older adults. *The Gerontologist, 60*(6), 989–995. https://doi.org/10.1093/geront/gnz117

van Rijssen, M., Veldkamp, M., Meilof, L., & van Ewjik, L. (2019). Feasibility of a communication program: Improving communication between nurses and persons with aphasia in a peripheral hospital. *Aphasiology, 33*(11), 1393–1409. https://doi.org/10.1080/02687038.2018.1546823

World Health Organization. (2019). *World report on vision 2019.* https://www.who.int/health-topics/blindness-and-vision-loss#tab=tab_1

World Health Organization. (2021). *Deafness and hearing loss.* https://www.who.int/news-room/fact-sheets/detail/deafness-and-hearing loss#:text=A

CHAPTER 9

Communication with Clients Experiencing Neurocognitive Disorders

LEARNING OBJECTIVES

After reading this chapter, you will be able to

1. Define *neurocognitive disorders*
2. Identify the major neurocognitive disorders
3. Identify behaviours associated with neurocognitive disorders
4. Differentiate between delirium and dementia
5. Describe symptoms of delirium and dementia
6. Identify therapeutic communication strategies and interventions for persons with cognitive issues
7. Analyze nursing interventions for persons related to their cognitive function
8. Describe assessment strategies for persons with neurocognitive disorders
9. Describe the treatment options for persons with neurocognitive disorders
10. Identify the challenges families experience in caring for family members with dementia

KEY TERMS

Agnosia

Alzheimer's disease

Amnesia

Delirium

Dementia

Neurocognitive disorders

INTRODUCTION

Neurocognitive disorders have a significant impact on Canadians. According to the Public Health Agency of Canada (PHAC, 2017), more than 402,000 seniors (65 years and older) are living with dementia. However, with a growing and aging population, the number of Canadians living with dementia will dramatically increase, contributing to an overall cost to the health care system of $16.6 billion by 2031. This chapter presents an overview of the most common neurocognitive disorders and associated behaviours that hinder individuals' abilities to complete activities of daily living and to communicate. It also identifies strategies for the assessment and enhancement of communication processes to provide effective nursing interventions in person-centred care. Treatment approaches nurses and other health care providers can use in caring for persons with neurocognitive disorders are discussed. In addition, this chapter identifies the role that health care professionals play in offering guidance and support to families or primary caregivers who are caring for a family member diagnosed with a neurocognitive disorder.

NEUROCOGNITIVE DISORDERS

Neurocognitive disorders are brain diseases that impact a person's cognition, perception, memory, reasoning, learning, judgment, and decision-making. These disorders are described as ranging from minor to major with respect to the level of impairment. The *Diagnostic and Statistical Manual of Mental Disorders*, 5th edition (American Psychiatric Association, 2013) identifies two major neurocognitive disorders, delirium and dementia.

DELIRIUM

Delirium is characterized as a syndrome comprising a disturbance in consciousness, impaired cognition that develops over a short period of time (hours to days), and difficulty maintaining concentration and attention (Mossello et al., 2018). Delirium is considered the most common of the neurocognitive disorders and is reported to be a complication of hospitalization, especially in older adults. This disorder occurs in 6 to 30 percent of the general hospital population and 7 to 52 percent of postsurgical clients, and it occurs most frequently in those over 65 years of age (50%) (Inouye et al., 2014). The causes of delirium are multifactorial, and several risk factors have been identified. Delirium is considered a medical emergency and is associated with increased morbidity and mortality. However, delirium is preventable, reversible, and treatable if recognized (Weldingh et al., 2022). Several researchers report that delirium occurrence is under-reported and is not always recognized by registered nurses in clinical settings due to their lack of knowledge of and the complexity of presenting symptoms, and inability to differentiate between delirium, dementia, and depression (Harrison Dening, 2019; Pryor & Clarke, 2017). Delirium increases the risk of complications due to prolonged hospitalizations. Clients may acquire hospital-based infections, experience falls, and develop pressure ulcers (Seeganna & Antai-Otong, 2016).

The presentation of delirium is classified into three types (Lahariya et al., 2016; Seeganna & Antai-Otong, 2016):

- **Hyperactive:** Client is restless, agitated, and hypervigilant. Hallucinations and delusions may be evident.
- **Hypoactive:** Client is drowsy, lethargic, and sleepy. Client responds slowly to questions and has reduced movement.
- **Mixed:** Hyperactive and hypoactive symptoms are evident.

Common Causes of Delirium

- Anemia
- Cardiovascular disorders
- Change of environment (e.g., from home to hospital)
- Chronic obstructive pulmonary disease
- Constipation
- Dehydration
- Dementia
- Diabetes mellitus
- Electrolyte imbalance
- Fever
- Head trauma
- Infections
- Medications
- Neurological conditions
- Pain
- Sleep deprivation
- Urinary retention

For health professionals, the primary goal of delirium treatment is to identify risk factors early, determine the underlying cause, and manage appropriately. Assessment begins by establishing rapport with the client and family members. Using an interdisciplinary approach, a comprehensive physical, psychosocial, neurological, and mental status examination is undertaken. An important component of the assessment is the history of the client's current medications (prescribed and over the counter) and any previous drug use.

Nurses and other health care providers are in a prime position to prevent, recognize, and manage delirium in hospitalized older adults if they know the best practice guidelines for delirium prevention and care. Such care focuses on early assessment and management that is person-centred and promotes positive clinical client outcomes. The Registered Nurses' Association of Ontario (RNAO) published best practice guidelines entitled *Delirium, Dementia, and Depression in Older*

Adults: Assessment and Care (2016) that support nurses and other members of the interprofessional health care team in working in partnership with persons and families who are experiencing a neurocognitive disorder.

Assessment

In assessing delirium, it is crucial that health care providers have the knowledge to recognize its presence and take steps to manage this acute clinical emergency to prevent negative client outcomes. A person with delirium may appear confused and distracted, and have difficulty with orientation (time, place, and person). For example, a woman with delirium may think it is 1998, that the hospital is home, and that the nurse is her son. Perceptual disturbances (hallucinations and delusions) may also be present. For example, the person may feel bugs crawling on or under their skin. This may cause the person to experience fear and anxiety and try to get away. If the person has intravenous lines or any type of tube or drain, they may pull on the tubes or try to get out of bed, which may lead to serious injury.

The Confusion Assessment Method (CAM) is a valid, reliable clinical instrument and is considered the gold standard for delirium recognition (Oh et al., 2017). The CAM used by clinicians focuses on the features of delirium:

- Acute onset and fluctuating course (change in mental status)
- Cognitive disorganization
- Inattention
- Alterations in consciousness

Another reliable and valid clinical instrument the nurse can use in assessment of delirium is the Mini Mental State Examination (MMSE) (Folstein et al., 1975). This tool is an 11-question measure, takes only 5–10 minutes to administer, and is used to assess mental status based on five areas of cognitive function:

- Orientation: "What is the (year) (season) (date) (day) (month)?"
- Registration: "Remember these three words: *cup*, *pen*, *airplane*." (Ask the client to say all three.)
- Attention and calculation
- Recall: "Please tell me the three words I gave you earlier."
- Language

The maximum score is 30, and a score of 23 or lower may indicate cognitive impairment. In the assessment process, it is critical that the nurse is aware if the client has special communication needs. For example, does the client use a hearing aid, eyeglasses, or have dentures? The nurse should also determine if the client has a vision or hearing impairment, or a speech or language disorder. These factors impact how the client will perform on the MMSE. To provide person-centred care, the nurse should be aware of the client's use of any aids and have knowledge of any communication disorders.

Some guidelines for MMSE assessment are as follows:

- Establish rapport (trust).
- Make sure the client has their hearing aid, dentures, or eyeglasses if used.
- Assess the client's need for comfort measures (due to pain, agitation, cold, tiredness).
- Assess for fluctuating levels of consciousness.
- Explain the purpose of the test.
- Administer the test in a quiet environment with no distractions.
- Ask one question at a time and allow time for response.
- Allow time for the client to ask questions.
- Provide reassurance throughout the assessment process.
- Document the findings.

It is also important that nurses caring for clients with delirium meet their physical, comfort, and safety needs. The physical environment should be free from hazards, the call bell within the client's reach, bed rails up as needed, and bed alarm in place to prevent potential falls and injury. Eyeglasses, hearing aids, and non-glare lighting contribute to the person's awareness of the environment, and objects such as clocks and large wall calendars can promote orientation to time. If the client is confused and experiencing perceptual disturbances, constant observation (one-on-one monitoring) may be necessary. The use of restraints is a controversial issue; best practice guidelines recommend using principles of least restraint, and if needed, only using restraints as a last resort (RNAO, 2016).

Case Example

A 55-year-old woman was admitted to the surgical floor following the repair of a ruptured spleen. On return to the floor, she was awake but drowsy, and her vital signs were normal. After 30 minutes she begins thrashing in the bed and yelling. The nurse enters the room and finds the client trying to climb over the bed rail. The client is anxious and unaware of her surroundings. Her speech is rapid but coherent. The nurse settles her back in bed and checks her vital signs, intravenous line, and abdominal dressing. The nurse calls the licensed practical nurse into the room to sit with client.

Exercise 9.1: Completion of MMSE

Purpose: To practise the use of the MMSE in the assessment of a client with delirium

Procedure

1. Work with a partner and complete the MMSE on each other. One student takes the role of client, and the other takes the role of nurse. See https://cgatoolkit.ca/Uploads/contentdocuments/mmse.pdf for the MMSE assessment tool.
2. Switch roles and complete the MMSE again.

Discussion

1. What was it like to be the nurse? The client?
2. Describe your feelings related to the questions asked and the score you achieved.
3. What factors must the nurse consider before administering the MMSE with a client?
4. What did you learn from doing this exercise?
5. How can the information gained in this exercise influence your future nursing practice?

DEMENTIA

Dementia is an umbrella term used to describe a decline in cognitive function that affects activities of daily living, caused by brain diseases and brain injuries (PHAC, 2017). According to the World Health Organization (2016), 47.5 million people worldwide live with dementia. Although dementia is not a normal part of aging, age is considered a risk factor, and with an aging Canadian population, the number of Canadians living with dementia is expected to increase dramatically. There are an estimated 564,000 Canadians living with dementia, and this number is expected to increase to 937,000 by 2031. Of the current number, two-thirds are women (Alzheimer Society of Canada, 2016b). Dementia has a major impact on the caregivers who are involved in staying home and providing care to their family members. Canadian singer and songwriter Jann Arden (2017) shared her experience of caring for her mother with Alzheimer's disease in the book entitled *Feed My Mother*. One in five Canadians have experience caring for someone living with dementia (Alzheimer Society of Canada, 2017). In June 2017, the Canadian government passed the National Strategy for Alzheimer's Disease and Other Dementias Act, which laid the foundation for the development of a dementia strategy for Canada (PHAC, 2019). Building upon this strategy, the federal government developed three national objectives to guide progress:

- Prevent dementia.
- Advance therapies and find a cure.
- Improve the quality of life of people living with dementia and caregivers.

A diagnosis of dementia is based upon a set of clinical features such as the 10 warning signs of dementia (Alzheimer Society of Canada, 2018):

1. Memory loss that affects day-to-day abilities
2. Difficulty performing familiar tasks
3. Problems with language such as forgetting or substituting words
4. Disorientation in time and space (not knowing how to get home)
5. Impaired judgment
6. Problems with abstract thinking
7. Misplacing things
8. Changes in mood and behaviour
9. Changes in personality
10. Loss of initiative

Some of the disorders most commonly associated with dementia are dementia of the Alzheimer's type, vascular dementia, Lewy body dementia, frontotemporal dementia (Pick's disease), Parkinson's disease, Huntington's disease, and Creutzfeldt-Jakob disease (Alzheimer Society of Canada, 2020). Alzheimer's disease is the most prevalent of the neurocognitive disorders. The cause is unknown, but it is believed to be multifactorial, and risk factors include age, genetics, family history, and head trauma. This disorder is characterized by a buildup of proteins in the brain called plaques (Lane et al., 2017). There is no known cure and symptoms are irreversible, but there are treatment options and lifestyle choices that may slow its progression.

Stages of Alzheimer's Disease

Alzheimer's disease is commonly divided into three stages (Alzheimer Society of Canada, 2016a):

- **Early stage**: Individual of any age who may have mild impairment. Symptoms include forgetfulness, communication difficulties, and changes in mood and behaviour. Person retains many of their abilities and requires little assistance.

- **Middle stage**: Decline in abilities but individual may have some awareness of their condition. Needs assistance with many tasks: shopping, finances, homemaking, dressing, bathing, and toileting. Persons in this stage have trouble with familiar surroundings—for example, may walk from home alone and be unable to find their way back.
- **Late stage**: Severe cognitive decline. Unable to communicate verbally or care for self. Twenty-four-hour-a-day care is necessary.

Case Example

Mrs. Jones is a 78-year-old woman who was admitted a week ago to the Psychogeriatric Assessment Unit for clinical evaluation. Mrs. Jones lives at home with her husband, Tom. He is finding it more difficult to manage things at home. He has reported that sometimes she doesn't know he is her husband. She is having difficulty with dressing and does not know what to do with her clothes. A week ago, she let the kettle on the stove go dry and started a small fire. He also noted that lately she has been following him from room to room in the home and crying out when he is not in sight. Mrs. Jones has dementia of the Alzheimer's type.

Assessment

It is important to determine the presence of Alzheimer's disease so appropriate interventions and treatment can be initiated. A complete history and a medical and physical examination, including a neurological assessment, are necessary. At this time, an interview with family members helps to complete the picture of what is happening with the client. Based upon the data obtained, further diagnostic tests may be ordered, such as laboratory tests (i.e., electrolytes, liver enzymes, glucose, folate, urinalysis) or radiology (e.g., computed tomography or magnetic resonance imaging scan). The MMSE is completed, and other screening instruments may be used to assess cognition and mental state, and track progression of the disease, including the clock drawing test and the Functional Dementia Scale.

Clock Drawing Test

This test is comparable with the MMSE. It is a reliable diagnostic tool that can be used easily in the clinical area (Shulman, 2000). The client is asked to draw a clock, put the numbers on it, and place the hands at 20 after 8, or 10 after 11. The test takes less than 10 minutes to administer, code, and score.

Functional Dementia Scale

This instrument is designed for use by health care providers in the assessment of degree of severity associated with dementia (Moore et al., 1983). It contains 20 items in three subscales: activities of daily living, orientation, and affect.

Upon assessment, some symptoms may be noted. Memory loss may be evident; most noticeable is impairment of short-term memory. As the disease progresses, the person may have issues with recent and remote memory. Other symptoms that may be observed are described as the four A's of Alzheimer's disease, which affect communication and the ability of the person to carry out activities of daily living:

- **Agnosia:** Impaired ability to recognize common objects, sounds, or persons
- **Apraxia:** Inability to carry out motor functions (e.g., loss of the ability to walk or dress)
- **Amnesia:** Impaired memory, inability to remember recent events
- **Aphasia**: loss of language, inability to express (expressive aphasia) or understand spoken words (receptive aphasia)

As the disease progresses, the person's ability to "be in the world" is greatly impacted. It is imperative that health care professionals provide person-centred care through the development of the therapeutic nurse-client relationship (Fazio et al., 2018). Through this relationship, the nurse provides evidence-informed interventions that promote client respect, autonomy, dignity, and safety. The focus of all health care team members is to support and maintain the person's optimum level of functioning and quality of life. Edvardsson et al. (2008) propose delivery of person-centred care for persons with Alzheimer's disease (AD) but acknowledge there is a risk that staff may focus only on the basic physical tasks and procedures and not on the development of a therapeutic relationship. These researchers advocate for the adoption of a person-centred care approach for persons with AD because of its value in contributing to respectful and ethical care practices in recognition of the person as an individual.

As a nurse working within the health care system, you may have the opportunity to provide care for persons in all stages of progression of Alzheimer's disease. These clients live in a variety of settings depending upon the level of care required. A person with a mild or moderate decrease in cognitive function may be living at home or in an assisted-living facility. Persons with a severe cognitive decline require assistance with all activities of daily living and constant supervision for mobility and safety concerns. They may live in a long-term care facility or at home, being cared for by family members.

To effectively communicate with persons with dementia, nurses and other health care providers need a good knowledge base of neurocognitive disorders, excellent communication skills, and an empathic, compassionate approach in providing person-centred care. The health care professionals need to practise with an approach that every client is unique and how the person engages in communication will depend upon the stage of their disease (Jootun & McGhee, 2011).

Communication Strategies for Use with Clients Experiencing Dementia

- Introduce yourself each time you meet—the client will not remember you.
- Approach the client from the front.
- Demonstrate respect.
- Take time to develop a therapeutic relationship (rapport).
- Ensure the environment is quiet, with no distractions (low stimulation).
- Make eye contact and call the person by name.
- Use a normal voice tone and be aware of your body language.
- Assess the client's verbal and nonverbal communication.
- When speaking, always face the client.
- Use short, simple sentences.
- Repeat sentences if necessary.
- Speak slowly and enunciate properly.
- Take time to listen.
- Allow the client time to respond—do not rush or finish their sentences.
- Introduce one topic/idea at a time. Use simple explanations.
- Avoid prolonged conversations. Brief interactions are best.
- Explain in simple terms what you are doing (activity/procedure, such as bathing).
- Do not use elderspeak (infantilization) communication.
- Assess the use of touch.
- Demonstrate empathy and show patience.
- Ask closed-ended questions, which require a yes/no response (e.g., "Are you thirsty?")
- Use memory aids, photographs, or familiar items as aids to communicate.
- Ensure aids the client needs are available and in place (e.g., eyeglasses, hearing aid, dentures).
- Avoid contradicting and arguing with the client.
- Avoid expressions of anger and frustration.
- Be aware of proxemics (not invading client's space).

Case Study 9.1

Mr. Stone is an 85-year-old man whose communication has progressively deteriorated due to the progression of his dementia. Over the past two weeks, while on the unit, he has experienced episodes of anger and disorientation. He has a history of a mood disorder that occurred when he lost his wife, Sara, after 45 years of marriage. She died suddenly when he was in his late seventies. The client and his wife operated a convenience store for many years, but they sold it when he retired at age 65. After his wife passed away, he was diagnosed with dementia. He was living at home by himself, but his son Peter has become concerned about his father, noticing lately that he is unable to care for himself and has become less communicative. He has been admitted to the hospital for assessment. You are a nursing student who has been assigned to Mr. Stone.

1. Describe how you would begin the orientation phase of the nurse-client therapeutic relationship.
2. Identify three nonverbal behaviours you could use to facilitate attentive listening.
3. What particular instruments would you use to assess Mr. Stone's cognitive function?
4. Identify particular strategies you would use to engage Mr. Stone in a nurse-client therapeutic relationship.

In person-centred care, nurses meet the individual client's needs through management of the environment to promote safety and security and provide an empathic presence and approach to meet physical and comfort needs (McCance et al., 2008). With progressive cognitive decline, the client will need interventions to promote or aid dressing, bathing, nutrition, bowel and bladder function, sleep hygiene, and social activities. Some clients may exhibit behavioural and psychological symptoms of dementia such as the following (Kales et al., 2015; Ooi et al., 2018):

- Agitation (e.g., pacing, crying out, inappropriate screaming)
- Anxiety
- Apathy
- Delusions
- Hallucinations
- Disinhibition (socially/sexually inappropriate behaviour)
- Wandering
- Rummaging
- Aggression (physical or verbal)

These behaviours may cause the nurse and other health care providers to disengage from the client and concentrate only on the physical tasks rather than coming to know the client through the development of an interpersonal relationship. However, it is critical that the nurse recognize and accept the person's reality and identify opportunities for meaningful engagement through relational practice (Fazio et al., 2018). How the nurse chooses to communicate and assess the client's ability to participate in care decisions must support the principles of a person-centred approach. The nurse uses assessment to gather information to determine the cause of the client's behaviour. They should consider what the client is trying to communicate through the behaviour: it may be related to an environmental trigger (e.g., noise, overcrowding); some unmet physical need, such as thirst, hunger, or the need to go to the bathroom; an underlying medical condition; or an adverse effect of prescribed medications (Kales et al., 2015). Several researchers have reported that aggressive behaviour may be related to pain, depression (Gerlach & Kales, 2017), or vision or hearing impairment (Vance et al., 2003). Others have reported that morning care, bathing, or toileting may trigger such behaviour (Brazil et al., 2013; Williams & Herman, 2011).

Research has shown that using a person-centred approach to care with a focus on social interaction with clients and staff promotes a culture for improvement in dementia care and appropriate behaviour management (Enmarker et al., 2010; Savundranayagam et al., 2016).

Research Highlight: An Education Intervention to Enhance Staff Self-Efficacy to Provide Dementia Care in an Acute Care Hospital in Canada: A Nonrandomized Controlled Study

Background

Dementia is on the rise globally as well as in Canada and will continue to increase as the population ages. Persons with neurocognitive disorders such as dementia will require care by staff in acute care. Acute care settings note an increase in the number of clients with dementia admitted for assessment, diagnosis, and treatment, and health care providers are often unprepared to care for those clients (Martin et al., 2016). Staff need to be knowledgeable about providing dementia care using a relational practice that is person-centred.

Purpose of the Study

- To identify the impact of a dementia education intervention, Gentle Persuasive Approaches (GPA), for health care providers
- To determine any change in the hospital staff's self-efficacy in interacting with clients with dementia

- To explore the lived experience of hospital staff who provide care to clients experiencing upset and stress during care interactions

Method

A nonrandomized, controlled research design was used to assess the impact of a GPA educational intervention (4 modules focused on person-centred care and dementia care) on staff from several clinical areas. The program was delivered to an intervention group (IG) (n = 468) of staff and a comparison wait-listed group (WLG) (n = 277). Data collection involved a focus group interview and the completion of the self-efficacy profile measurement tool at baseline and again eight weeks later.

Findings

The IG had significant improvement in self-efficacy scores from baseline to post-intervention at eight weeks (p < .001). No changes were reported for the WLG (p = .21). Qualitative data indicated that the IG gained insight into communicating with clients who exhibited acting out behaviours. This led to a change in their practice by applying a more person-centred approach to care. The WLG reported uncertainty and lack of skill in managing client behaviour. Their focus was on completing tasks and protecting client and staff safety.

Implications for Nursing Practice

The GPA program is effective in preparing staff to care for clients with dementia in acute care settings. The program provides an increase in staff knowledge and skill to manage and provide care for clients with dementia from a relational person-centred approach. Researchers suggest that the GPA program could benefit dementia education in Canada within health care settings.

Source: Martin, L. S., Gillies, L., Coker, E., Pizzacalla, A., Montemuro, M., Suva, G., & McLelland, V. (2016). An education intervention to enhance staff self-efficacy to provide dementia care in an acute care hospital in Canada: A nonrandomized controlled study. *American Journal of Alzheimer's Disease & Other Dementias, 31*(8), 664–677. https://doi .org/10.1177/15333/17516668574

Exercise 9.2: Therapeutic Environment

Nurses and other health care professionals working with persons with neurocognitive disorders will need to manage the environment. Making the environment conducive to the client's comfort and safety is essential in facilitating the development of the nurse-client relationship.

(Continued)

1. Identify some environmental factors that may contribute to confusion for clients living in a long-term care facility.
2. Identify some strategies that can be used to alleviate some of these issues and promote a dementia-friendly environment.

Treatment Options

There is no cure for Alzheimer's disease, but a variety of treatment options for persons with neurocognitive disorders that include a combination of nonpharmacological and pharmacological approaches are available. Nonpharmacological interventions are recommended as the first line of treatment in best practice guidelines for persons with dementia (RNAO, 2016). The treatment for delirium is early identification and management until the person's symptoms abate and they become stable. This section of the chapter presents an overview of the most common treatment approaches for dementia. As a health professional student, you may have an opportunity to observe and participate in some of these interventions during your clinical rotations.

Reminiscence Therapy

Reminiscence therapy is a psychosocial intervention that is used frequently with older adults in dementia care and treatment. It is consistent with a person-centred approach and is considered effective in helping to improve mood, cognition, communication, activities of daily living, and quality of life (Cuevas et al., 2020; Woods et al., 2018). This intervention involves the health care provider leading the discussion of past experiences or activities with the person or a small group of people. The facilitator encourages conversation among participants through a sharing of their experiences (Gonzalez et al., 2015). A variety of tools, such as photographs, books, movies, or music, can be used to prompt the person's memories or life history and aid well-being.

Validation Therapy

Another psychosocial intervention that fits with the approach of person-centred care is validation therapy. This therapy focuses on accepting the reality of the person living with dementia (Scales et al., 2018). In this intervention, the health care professional uses a number of communication techniques, such as eye contact, a gentle tone of voice, and touch, if appropriate, to validate the person's perceived emotional experience (e.g., anger, sadness). Validation therapy may enhance positive feelings and alleviate negative feelings.

Music Therapy

Research has shown that music therapy is appropriate for reducing behaviours such as anxiety, agitation, and depression (Moreno-Morales et al., 2020; van der Steen et al., 2018). This approach can include listening to music, playing instruments, or singing. These music-based interventions may also contribute to improvements in emotional well-being and quality of life.

Massage and Touch Therapy

Touch is an important means of communication for the practising nurse. It is powerful in promoting the development of a therapeutic nurse-client relationship as touch provides a means to express caring, reassurance, and understanding. Also, the nurse needs to be sensitive to all clients who may not be comfortable with touch and massage and assess their level of comfort. Touch therapy provides other benefits, such as decreasing anxiety, tension, fatigue, and depression. Wu et al. (2017), in a systematic review and meta-analysis of the effectiveness of massage and touch on behaviours of people with dementia, report that physical and verbal nonaggressive behaviours decrease significantly. In a similar study, Margenfeld et al. (2019) found that manual massage for individuals with dementia improves the behavioural and psychological symptoms of dementia. However, due to small sample size, both researchers recommend further research to determine the effectiveness of this intervention.

Pharmacological Interventions

Presently, there is no known cure for Alzheimer's disease and the other dementias. However, some drugs, classified as cholinesterase inhibitors, have been developed that have the potential to slow the progression of the disease. Alzheimer's disease has been linked to a deficiency of an enzyme called acetylcholine, so these drugs prevent acetylcholine (cholinesterase) from breaking down in the brain.

Case Study 9.2

You are a first-year nursing student on placement in a long-term care facility for older adults. Mrs. Pitcher, a 75-year-old woman, is a former elementary school teacher. She requires assistance with having a wash in the bathroom. She is able to ambulate, but her speech is impaired because of aphasia. She has some difficulty with hearing but does not use a hearing aid; she wears eyeglasses and has trouble speaking because of her dementia.

(Continued)

1. How would you approach Mrs. Pitcher?
2. In your interaction, identify two strategies you need to consider that support her inability to communicate.
3. Identify several aids that you could use to communicate with Mrs. Pitcher.

Caregiver Burden

Caregiver burden is a complex term that refers to the burden family caregivers experience as a result of caring for a family member with dementia. Caring for a person with dementia is an enormous task for family members. According to the Alzheimer Society of Canada (2020), one in five Canadians have experience caring for someone living with dementia. Caregivers spend, on average, about 26 hours per week supporting their family member. The literature reports that demands faced by caregivers of persons with dementia are greater than those experienced by the caregivers of seniors without dementia. Much of the burden experienced by families results from managing the behavioural and psychological symptoms of dementia and providing direct care.

According to the Canadian Institute for Health Information (2020), about four out of ten caregivers of seniors with dementia experience symptoms of caregiver distress. Many of these caregivers pay out-of-pocket expenses for a variety of services that are not fully covered by government funding or other programs. Some of these costs are attributed to medications, transportation, home modifications, or professional health care services. Nurses have an important role in supporting, advocating, and providing services and health teaching for clients and family caregivers. Nurses, when working with families experiencing dementia, need to consider the role they play in care. It is important to communicate with family members and assess their coping and available supports if they are the primary caregiver. In this capacity, nurses can provide information on respite care and facilitate referrals to other health care professionals or agencies to help meet family needs.

✚ Case Example

Elizabeth is a caregiver for her father, Daniel, who has dementia with Lewy bodies and is also being treated for Parkinson's disease. Daniel's dementia progressed quickly after his diagnosis in 2015. He experiences hallucinations and periods of paranoia at times. He now requires assistance with bathing, eating, dressing, and toileting.

Burden = responsibilities
Burnout = result of the responsibilities.

CHAPTER SUMMARY

The Canadian population is aging, and statistics indicate that seniors will make up 25 percent of the population by 2036. As a result, the number of persons living with neurocognitive disorders is expected to increase. The major neurocognitive disorders that are encountered in clinical practice are delirium and dementia. These disorders impact cognitive functioning, causing impairment in memory, confusion, agitation, restlessness, and perceptual disturbances. Delirium is a medical emergency, and immediate assessment and management are needed. Nurses and other health care providers need to know how to identify the difference between these disorders and use assessment skills so interventions can occur in a timely manner. Delirium is reversible; however, most types of dementia involve a progressive cognitive decline, which in most cases is not reversible. Some clients with dementia may exhibit changes in behaviour or lose the ability to speak or ambulate. Nursing care with these disorders is focused on communication, assessment, safety, and provision of a supportive environment using a person-centred approach. This approach supports the dignity of the person and provides the opportunity for client decision-making in care. There is no cure for dementia, but a combination of nonpharmacological and pharmacological therapies is available. Caregiver burden in families is common, and nurses can support these families by providing information, guidance, and support so they can participate in care and acquire knowledge to understand these disorders.

REVIEW QUESTIONS

Read the following three review questions and select the best option to answer each question. State your rationale for choosing your response. For the other four questions, identify your response.

1. On completing your admission assessment, you note that the client has a diagnosis of Alzheimer's disease and is experiencing aphasia. You understand this to mean that
   a. The client is no longer able to dress themselves
   b. The client is confused and unaware of surroundings
   c. The client is no longer able to speak
   d. The client is having difficulty forming words
2. Communication strategies for a client with dementia include all of the following *except*
   a. Sit by the client's side to provide support
   b. Introduce yourself each time you meet the client
   c. Assess the use of touch
   d. Use simple sentences when speaking

3. Which of the following are understood to cause delirium? Select all that apply.
   a. Anemia
   b. Dementia
   c. Constipation
   d. Dehydration
4. Differentiate between the terms *delirium* and *dementia*.
5. Identify the therapeutic communication strategies used by health care providers for clients with cognitive issues.
6. Identify the assessment strategies used by health care providers for clients with neurocognitive disorders.
7. Describe the guidelines for the MMSE assessment.

WEB RESOURCES

Alzheimer Society of Canada
https://www.alzheimer.ca/en
Canada Alzheimer's Association
https://www.alz.org/dementia-alzheimers-canada.asp
Parkinson Canada
https://www.parkinson.ca

REFERENCES

Alzheimer Society of Canada. (2016a). *Progression overview.* https://progression_overview.pdf

Alzheimer Society of Canada. (2016b). *Report summary: Prevalence and monetary costs of dementia in Canada (2016): A report by the Alzheimer Society of Canada.* https://www.canada.ca/content/dam/phac-aspc/migration/phac-aspc/publicat/hpcdp-pspmc/36-10/assets/pdf/ar04-eng.pdf

Alzheimer Society of Canada. (2017). *2017 awareness survey executive summary.* https://ilivewith dementia.ca/wp-content/uploads/2019/12/2017_awareness-survey_executive_summary.pdf

Alzheimer Society of Canada. (2018). *10 warning signs of dementia.* https://alzheimer.ca/en/about-dementia/do-i-have-dementia/10-warning-signs-dementia

Alzheimer Society of Canada. (2020). *I'm caring for a person living with dementia.* https://alzheimer.ca/en/help-support/im-caring-person-living-dementia

American Psychiatric Association. (2013). *Diagnostic and statistical manual of mental disorders* (5th ed.). https://doi.org/10.1176/appi.books.9780890425596

Arden, J. (2017). *Feed my mother.* Penguin Random House Canada.

Brazil, K., Maitland, J., Walker, M., & Curtis, A. (2013). The character of behavioural symptoms on admission to three Canadian long-term care homes. *Aging & Mental Health, 17*(8), 1059–1066. https://doi.org/10.1080/13607863.2013.807424

Canadian Institute for Health Information. (2020). *Dementia in Canada: Summary*. https:// www.cihi.ca/en/dementia-in-canada-summary

Cuevas, P. E. G., Davidson, P. M., Mejilla, L. J., & Rodney, T. W. (2020). Reminiscence therapy for older adults with Alzheimer's disease: A literature review. *International Journal of Mental Health Nursing, 29*(3), 364–371. https://doi.org/10.1111/inm.12692

Edvardsson, D., Winblad, B., & Sandman, P. O. (2008). Person-centred care of people with severe Alzheimer's disease: Current status and ways forward. *The Lancet Neurology, 7*(4), 362–367.

Enmarker, I., Olsen, R., & Hellzen, C. (2010). Management of person with dementia with aggressive and violent behaviour: A systematic literature review. *International Journal of Older People Nursing, 6*(2), 153–162. https://doi.org/10.1111/j.1748-3743.2010.00235.x

Fazio, S., Pace, D., Maslow, K., Zimmerman, S., & Kallmyer, B. (2018). Alzheimer's association dementia care practice recommendations. *The Gerontologist, 58*(1), s1–s9. https://doi.org/10.1093/geronto/gnx182

Folstein, M. F., Folstein, S. E., & McHugh, P. R. (1975). "Mini-mental state": A practical method for grading the cognitive state of patients for clinician. *Journal of Psychiatric Research, 12*(3), 189–198. https://doi.org/10.1016/0022-3956(75)90026-6

Gerlach, L. B., & Kales, H. C. (2017). Learning their language: The importance of detecting and managing pain in dementia. *American Journal of Psychiatry, 25*(2), 155–157. https://doi .org/10.1016/j.jagp.2016.11.012

Gonzalez, J., Mayordomo, T., Torres, M., Sales, A., & Meléndez, J. C. (2015). Reminiscence and dementia: A therapeutic intervention. *International Psychogeriatrics, 27*(10), 1731-1737. https://doi.10.1017/S1041610215000344

Harrison Dening, K. (2019). Differentiating between dementia, delirium, and depression. *Nursing Standard, 35*(1), 43–50. https://doi.org/10.7748/ns.2019.e11361

Inouye, S. K., Westendorp, R. G. J., & Saczynski, J. S. (2014). Delirium in elderly people. *Lancet, 383*(9920), 911–922. https //doi.org/10.1016/so140-6736(13)60688-1

Jootun, D., & McGhee, G. (2011). Effective communication with people who have dementia. *Nursing Standard, 25*(25), 40–46.

Kales, H. C., Gitlin, L. N., & Lyketsos, C. G. (2015). Assessment and management of behavioral and psychological symptoms of dementia. *BMJ, 350*, 1–33. https://doi .org/10.1136/bmj.h369

Lahariya, S., Grover, S., Bagga, S., & Sharma, A. (2016). Phenomenology of delirium among patients admitted to a coronary care unit. *Nordic Journal of Psychiatry, 70*(8), 626–632. https://doi.org/10.1080/08039488.2016.1194467

Lane, C. A., Hardy, J., & Schott, J. M. (2017). Alzheimer's disease. *European Journal of Neurology, 25*(1), 59–70. https://doi.org/10.1111/ene.13439

Margenfield, F., Klocke, C., & Joos, S. (2019). Manual massage for persons living with dementia: A systematic review and meta-analysis. *International Journal of Nursing Studies, 96*, 132–142. https://doi.org/10 1016/j.ijnurstu.2018.12.012

Martin, L. S., Gillies, L., Coker, E., Pizzacalla, A., Montemuro, M., Suva, G., & McLelland, V. (2016). An education intervention to enhance staff self-efficacy to provide dementia care in an acute care hospital in Canada: A nonrandomized controlled study. *American Journal of Alzheimer's Disease & Other Dementias, 31*(8), 664–677. https://doi.org/10.1177/15333/ 17516668574

McCance, T., Slater, P., & McCormack, B. (2008). Using the caring dimensions inventory as an indicator of person-centred nursing. *Journal of Clinical Nursing, 18*(3), 409–417. https:// doi.org/10.1111/j.1365-2702.2008.02466.x

Moore, J. T., Bobula, J. A., Short, T. B., & Mischel, M. (1983). A functional dementia scale. *The Journal of Family Practice, 16*(3), 499–503.

Moreno-Morales, C., Calero, R., Moreno-Morales, P., & Pintado, C. (2020). Music therapy in the treatment of dementia: A systematic review and meta-analysis. *Frontiers in Medicine, 7*(160), 1–11. https://doi.org/10.3389/fmed.2020.00160

Mossello, E., Tesi, F., Di Santo, S. G., & Italian Study Group on Delirium. (2018). Recognition of delirium features in clinical practice: Data from the "Delirium Day 2015" national survey. *Journal of the American Geriatric Society, 66*, 302–308. https://doi .org/10.1111/jgs.15211

Oh, E. S., Fong, T. G., Hshieh, T. T., & Inouye, S. K. (2017). Delirium in older persons. *JAMA, 318*(12), 1161–1174. https://doi.org/10.1001/jama.2017.12067

Ooi, C. H., Yoon, P. S., How, H. C., & Poon, N. Y. (2018). Managing challenging behaviours in dementia. *Singapore Medical Journal, 59*(10), 514–518. https://doi.org/10.11622/ smedj.2018125

Pryor, C., & Clarke, A. (2017). Nursing care for people with delirium superimposed on dementia. *Nursing Older People, 29*(3), 18–21. https://doi.org/10.7748/nop.2017.e887

Public Health Agency of Canada. (2017). *Dementia in Canada, including Alzheimer's disease: highlights from the Canadian chronic disease surveillance system.* https://dementia-highlights-canadian-chronic-disease-surveillance.pdf

Public Health Agency of Canada. (2019). *A dementia strategy for Canada: Together we aspire.* https://www.canada.ca/en/public-health/services/publications/diseases-conditions/ dementia-strategy.html

Registered Nurses' Association of Ontario. (2016). *Clinical best practice guidelines: Delirium, dementia, and depression in older adults: Assessment and care.* https://rnao.ca/bpg./guidelines

Savundranayagam, M. Y., Sibalija, J., & Scotchmer, E. (2016). Resident reactions to person-centered communication by long-term care staff. *American Journal of Alzheimer's Disease & Other Dementias, 31*(6), 530–537. https://doi.org/10.1177/153331751562291

Scales, K., Zimmerman, S., & Miller, S. J. (2018). Evidence-based nonpharmacological practices to address behavioral and psychological symptoms of dementia. *The Gerontologist, 58*(1), S88–S102. https://doi.org/10.1093/geront/gnx167

Seeganna, C., & Antai-Otong, D. (2016). Managing the care of the older patient with delirium and dementia. *Nursing Clinics of North America, 51*(2), 261–273. https://doi.org/10.1016/ j.cnur.2016.01.009

Shulman, K. I. (2000). Clock-drawing: Is it the ideal cognitive screening test? *International Journal of Geriatric Psychiatry, 15*(6), 548–561. https://doi.org/10.1002/1099-1166(200006)15:6<548::AID-GPS242>3.0.CO;2-U

Vance, D. E., Burgio, L. D., Roth, D. L., Stevens, A. B., Kaci Fairchild, J., & Yurick, A. (2003). Predictors of agitation in nursing home residents. *The Journal of Gerontology, 58*(2), 129–137. https://doi.org/10.1093/geronb/58.2p129

van der Steen, J. T., Smaling, H. J., van der Wouden, J. C., Bruinsma, M. S., Scholten, R. J., & Vink, A. C. (2018). Music-based therapeutic interventions for people with dementia. *Cochrane Database System Review, 7*(7), https://doi.org/10.1002/14651858.CDOO3477.pub.4

Weldingh, N. M., Mellingsaeter, M. R., Hegna, B. W., Benth, J. S., Einvik, G., Thommessen, B., & Kirkevold, M. (2022). Impact of a dementia-friendly program on detection and management of patients with cognitive impairment and delirium in acute-care hospital units: A controlled clinical trial design. *BMC Geriatrics, 22*(266), https://doi.org/10.1186/s12877-022-02949-0

Williams, K. N., & Herman, R. E. (2011). Linking resident behavior to dementia care communication: Effects of emotional tone. *Behavior Therapy, 42*(1), 42–46. https://doi.org/10.1016/j.beth.2010.03.003

Woods, B., O'Philbin, L., Farrell, E. M., Spector, A. E., & Orrell, M. (2018). Reminiscence therapy for dementia. *Cochrane Database System Review, 3*(3), https://doi.org/10.1002/14651858.CD001120.pub3

World Health Organization. (2016). *World Alzheimer report 2016: Improving healthcare for people living with dementia.* https://www.alz.co.uk/research/worldalzheimerreport2016.pdf

Wu, J., Wang, Y., & Wang, Z. (2017). The effectiveness of massage and touch on behavioural and psychological symptoms of dementia: A quantitative systematic review and meta-analysis. *Journal of Advanced Nursing, 73*(10), 2283–2294. https://doi.org/10.1111/jan.13311

CHAPTER 10

Communication with Clients Experiencing Loss, Grief, Dying, and Death

LEARNING OBJECTIVES

After reading this chapter, you will be able to

1. Define the terms *loss*, *grief*, and *bereavement*
2. Identify types of loss that people experience
3. Discuss communication practices in end-of-life care
4. Identify end-of-life care nursing interventions for clients and family members
5. Indicate the purpose of an advance directive
6. Define the term *medical assistance in dying* (MAiD)
7. Discuss self-care strategies used by nurses who provide end-of-life care

KEY TERMS

Acute grief

Advance directive

Anticipatory grief

Bereavement

Chronic sorrow

Cultural safety

Disenfranchised grief

MAiD

Palliative care

INTRODUCTION

This chapter introduces the concept of loss and the associated concepts of grief and bereavement. The theories and models related to grief, loss, and grieving applicable to clinical practice are introduced. In addition, aspects of person-centred care by nurses for clients in hospice palliative care and their families are discussed. Also addressed are nurses' attitudes toward end-of-life care for clients who are dying and the communication challenges in working with clients and families experiencing loss. Resources nurses use for self-care, due to numerous stress factors they experience in providing end-of-life care, are described.

LOSS, GRIEF, AND BEREAVEMENT

Loss is a common phenomenon that is experienced by everyone at some point in their lives. Loss, as defined by Townsend (2015), is the "experience of separation from something of personal importance" (p. 831). There are many kinds of loss that can occur throughout life, including the loss of a person or pet, a possession such as a home or family photographs, or a job, or loss through illness or situation (e.g., "empty nest"), divorce, or death. Whatever the loss, the significance of the object for the person triggers emotions and behaviours associated with the grieving process (Townsend, 2015). Grief is the person's emotional response to the loss, which is shaped by the loss's value, cultural influences, and societal norms (Slade & Hoh, 2020). Bereavement refers to the period after loss during which the person may experience a variety of feelings and behaviours such as insomnia, anxiety, helplessness, or hyperactivity. The experience of bereavement in coping with grief following the death of a significant other is very individual. Nurses, as well as other health care providers, have an important role in providing bereavement care to clients and families during end-of-life care (Buglass, 2010; Raymond et al., 2016). Nurse assessment of the needs of families receiving bereavement care should begin prior to the client's death, ideally at the time of admission to a health facility and throughout the illness journey. How well grief resolves itself following a death depends upon the grieving process of and support available to survivors. Some family members may require professional support following the death of a loved one.

Case Example

A 70-year-old man had been in declining health for about three years after a myocardial infarction. These 36 months were marked by numerous visits to the hospital, progressive angina, and worsening congestive heart failure. The client, however, was able to spend some time at home with his family until his last admission, when he died quietly with his wife and sons at his hospital bedside.

DEATH: LIFE'S FINAL JOURNEY

Death and dying is an event and a process that is universal and is a regular occurrence in many health care settings (Zheng et al., 2017). Irrespective of the cause of death or whether it is unexpected, sudden, or prolonged, the death of a loved one results in an irreversible loss and is considered one of the most stressful life events. Families who experience a significant loss because of death display a combination of emotional, behavioural, cognitive, and physical responses. Nurses need to be attuned to these behaviours to provide bereavement care for families. Without appropriate support, grief and bereavement may affect personal health.

Health professionals, regardless of the clinical setting, encounter death as part of their daily work (Nyatanga, 2016). Nurses view the loss of a client as one of the most challenging and demanding clinical practice issues (Zheng et al., 2017). Health professionals working in hospice palliative care or other clinical settings provide support for clients and families who are coping with a terminal illness. In this work, they are witness to the phenomenon of death but may suppress their feelings as they provide care, presence, and support to clients and families. This approach leads to stress, anxiety, decreased job satisfaction, and compassion fatigue (Andersson et al., 2016; Harder et al., 2020; Melvin, 2015), which can impact care provision and nurses' well-being. Nurses and other health care professionals need to practise and prioritize self-care to offset the stressors in their profession (Scruth & Allen, 2022). Health care professional students may not have experience with death or dying, and during their clinical rotations, emotions may surface related to their fear of caring for clients with death or dying (Petrongolo & Toothaker, 2021). Due to the complexity of providing end-of-life care in health care settings, it is recommended that nurses and nursing students receive more support and education than they currently receive on caring for clients who are dying (Andersson et al., 2016; Berndtsson et al., 2019; Henoch et al., 2017).

GRIEF AND BEREAVEMENT THEORIES AND MODELS

There are several theories of grief and dying that have guided health care professionals' understanding, assessment, and clinical interventions for clients and families during the grieving process. Several theorists considered pioneers in this area—Lindemann, Engel, and Kübler-Ross—describe an individual's grief process as occurring in phases or stages. Despite their importance, these theories have been challenged and criticized over the years and are seldom used in practice for grief and bereavement support/counselling (Corr, 2021; Corr & Corr, 2020; Davies, 2004, Silverman et al., 2021).

Loss, grief, and bereavement are considered unique components of the grieving process. Health professionals need to consider, accept, and recognize the process of personal grieving for each individual and provide support (Corr & Corr, 2020). Grief is considered a diverse experience shaped by social, cultural, and political factors (Silverman et al., 2021). Corr and Corr contend that the key to becoming effective in care provision is to listen actively to those who are dying and others coping with grief. Through relationships, health care providers come to understand the psychosocial and spiritual needs of the client. They need to work with family members to understand their process of grief. The new models of grief support the importance of family holding on to or forming new relationships with the person who is no longer present (Davies, 2004).

Exercise 10.1: Experiences of Loss

Purpose: Reflecting on an experience of loss helps us to think on our own mortality as a person. This helps us, as health care providers, bridge our understanding of others who have experienced a loss and are grieving.

Procedure
Complete each statement and reflect on your answers.

The first experience with loss that I can remember was _____
I was _____ years of age at the time
My feelings at the time were _____
The thing that puzzled me the most about the experience was _____
When I think about the loss now, I remember _____
I coped with the loss by _____

_____

My sources of support during this period of loss were _____
Reflecting on this experience, what was most helpful was

_____

This experience may help me in my clinical work to support others who have also experienced loss because _____

Source: Adapted from Mallon, B. (2008). *Dying, death and grief: Working with adult bereavement* (p. 16). Sage. https://doi.org/10.4135/9781446214510

Grief and Patterns of Grieving

Nurses and other health professionals will be working with clients and families who experience grief because of a loss. Nurses work very closely with clients who are dying and their families, so it is important that they have a good understanding of the reactions and responses to grief. This knowledge enhances nurses' ability to support clients and families through the grieving process. Several patterns of grieving have been identified:

Acute Grief

Acute grief is defined as a normal reaction to a stressful situation (e.g., loss of a loved one). Exactly how people respond to loss varies, so it is necessary for the health care professional to have awareness that an individual's response to a loss is influenced by their culture, history of previous loss, coping skills, and support resources (Meichsner et al., 2020). Some emotions expressed by individuals experiencing acute grief may include anxiety, anger, or guilt (Meichsner et al., 2020).

Anticipatory Grief

Anticipatory grief is a process in which individuals confronted with the expectation that they will experience a significant loss in the future begin the grieving process. This usually occurs at the time of diagnosis, so it may provide some benefit by giving time to the client to prepare for the loss of their health (e.g., cognitive ability, body part), and in case of death, to plan their funeral, complete unsettled business, and prepare family members to take on some new responsibilities. Unfortunately, this process does not lessen the loss experienced by the spouse/partner, family members, friends, and caregivers who may grieve for the client's loss as well as their own (Coelho & Barbosa, 2017).

Disenfranchised Grief

Disenfranchised grief occurs when a person experiences a loss but it "cannot be openly acknowledged, publicly mourned, or socially supported" (Tsui et al., 2019, p. 285). The term is used to refer to grief experienced by health care workers, including nurses, after client death. It is suggested that nurses may form closer relationships with clients than those formed by other health care providers and experience a greater sense of loss when clients die (Anderson & Gaugler, 2007).

Chronic Sorrow

Chronic sorrow is a concept that was derived from research on parents of children who had a physical, emotional, or chronic illness. The impact on the parents' psychological and physical health from caring for a child with chronic health issues created a sense of sadness and chronic sorrow. Health care professionals should understand that chronic sorrow is a normal consequence of having a child with a chronic illness. All support and health care interventions should be guided by a family-centred approach (Coughlin & Sethares, 2017).

Maladaptive Responses to Loss

Everyone will experience grief resulting from the loss of a loved one, but no two people will experience grief the same. Some individuals may have a delay in the grief response and experience a complicated grief due to their inability to cope with a profound loss (Townsend, 2015). Complicated grief is seen in individuals who experience a sudden or traumatic loss, multiple losses, and those not having any support resources (Slade & Hoh, 2020). Persons with complicated grief report symptoms of loss of interest in daily life, emotional numbing, and negative memories of the deceased. Professional help provided by a grief therapist or counsellor is recommended (LeBlanc et al., 2016).

END-OF-LIFE CARE

Although Canadians are living longer, some struggle with poor health caused by chronic conditions, degenerative diseases, or cancer. Many Canadians with these conditions are admitted to acute care hospitals seeking treatment but are designated as palliative clients after a change in their health status. Most clients who are palliative prefer to die at home, but few Canadians receive formal palliative care outside of hospitals. Of all deaths in Canada, about 60 to 70 percent occur in hospitals, and only a small number of Canadians die in specialized palliative care units (Canadian Institute for Health Information, 2020). Access to palliative care is not equitable across all provinces and territories. The Government of Canada (2018a) released a document entitled *Framework on Palliative Care in Canada* that laid out a five-year plan to improve and enhance access to palliative care for all Canadians.

Palliative care is offered to clients who have a life-threatening condition or a serious illness and focuses on helping them to live as actively as possible by doing the following:

- Improving quality of life
- Reducing or relieving physical and psychological symptoms
- Contributing to a more peaceful and dignified death
- Supporting the client and their family while dying and afterward

Clients in palliative care are managed by an interdisciplinary team that uses a person-centred treatment plan with a focus on the following:

- Pain management
- Symptom management (e.g., nausea, anxiety, depression)
- Social, psychological, spiritual, and emotional support
- Caregiver support

Although each team member brings a particular expertise to palliative care, nurses provide around-the-clock care and have the most contact with the client and family members.

Additional assistance to meet the comfort needs of dying persons and their families is offered through hospice palliative care in some provinces and territories in Canada. Various models of hospice exist in Canada, including home care programs and hospice palliative care provided by institutions that exist in the community. For example, British Columbia provides palliative care in homes, hospices, and hospitals through its regional health networks.

Another option for end-of-life care that is now available to Canadians who have an incurable illness, disease or disability, or state of decline is medical assistance in dying (MAiD). In 2016 the Government of Canada passed Bill C-14, an act to amend the Criminal Code prohibiting physician-assisted suicide. The act stipulates that physicians and nurse practitioners (NPs) may offer MAiD to persons who are facing foreseeable death. Persons (aged 18 or older) who meet the eligibility criteria can make a written request and pursue an assisted death. Two forms of MAiD are available (Beuthin et al., 2018; Government of Canada, 2018b):

- **Clinician-assisted MAiD**: Provider (physician or NP) directly administers medication that causes death.
- **Self-administered MAiD**: A physician or NP provides a prescribed medication, which is taken by the client with the intent of causing death.

The Canadian Hospice Palliative Care Association, established in 1991, serves as a national voice advocating for quality end-of-life hospice palliative care, public policy, and public education and awareness. This agency is a good resource for clients and families, health professionals, and the public, who can access online information on advance care planning for end-of life.

Nurses' Role in End-of-Life Care

Nurses working in the health care setting can encounter clients anywhere who require end-of-life care. In some health care facilities, specialized units or beds have been allocated to provide care to clients with life-threatening illnesses. The Canadian Palliative Care Nursing Association (2021) has standards of practice that are relevant to nurses who work with people with end-of-life care needs and their families. These standards can be used to guide practice, practice environment supports, and policy development. The Canadian Nurses Association (2022) recognizes nurses who work in this speciality area of palliative care practice. They offer a certification program in palliative care; nurses who write the national examination and are successful obtain the credential Certified in Hospice Palliative Care Nursing Canada, or CHPCN(C). This certification demonstrates to clients, employers, the public, and professional licensing bodies that the nurse is qualified and competent in a nursing speciality (CNA, 2022). The use of effective and compassionate communication is a critical attribute for nurses working with clients who are dying and their families. Nurses in these settings need competency in clinical assessment, "attention to physical symptoms and psychosocial concerns, responses to suffering, listening to expressions of loss and grief, and recognition of ethical or spiritual concerns" (Malloy et al., 2010, p. 167). These qualities are paramount in facilitating a therapeutic relationship, as described by a nurse who works in the speciality of palliative care practice:

> I would say within palliative care there is a strong focus on interpersonal skills and a sensitivity and a perceptiveness of how to interact with other people, and particularly patients and families, for their best outcome … managing, manoeuvring … negotiating your way through an interaction [keeping] in mind their best outcome at the end of it. (Canning et al., 2007, p. 226)

To develop a therapeutic relationship, nurses need to be competent in clinical and interpersonal skills. As discussed in chapter 2, nurses should use the core skills of communication: active listening, open-ended questioning, reflection of feeling, and empathy building. When meeting the client and family for the first time, it is important to have an awareness of what the client and family have been told about the diagnosis. The nurse can ask some open-ended questions to facilitate the process:

- "What have you been told about your illness so far?"
- "What is your understanding of the reasons you were admitted to this unit?"
- "What do you understand palliative care to mean?"
- "Do you have any questions about what the doctor has told you?"

Having this information helps to promote nurses' ability to talk about the end of life before the end of life, with the client and family. As health professionals, we need to be sensitive to the client's and family's need to talk about dying and end-of-life care. Most clients know when their time is getting short but may not bring it up for fear of upsetting their spouse, partner, or family members. Some may not be ready, so nurses must be attuned to the client's readiness to talk and acquire information. Clients and families may want to discuss information around disease progression, the dying process, and pain management. It is best to provide information without overloading the client or family. Information should be presented in a clear, simple, and jargon-free manner, allowing time for questions. Repeat information during the progression of care and supplement with written material, as stress may hinder their ability to remember what has been discussed.

In working with clients with serious illness and providing holistic end-of-life care, nurses get to the know the client and family through their "therapeutic use of self." Clients who are at the end of life need caring, empathic, and supportive nurses who are engaged in authentic humanistic caring practices. Through their verbal and nonverbal communication, nurses are instrumental in supporting the client's decisions about their treatment and care. They work with the family in providing support and keeping them informed about the client's status during this difficult time. Family members may have anxiety about the dying process and one of them may wish to stay with the client while they are receiving care. This request should be accommodated and, ideally, the family should name a family contact who will act as a liaison between the client and health care providers. This nurse narrative demonstrates how nurse presence and actions (therapeutic use of self), a form of nonverbal communication, is expressed to the client and their family through caring behaviours:

It was not the conversation that made a difference in one patient that I took care of; it was how I spoke to family and involved them in bedside care. The child was a drown victim and was brain dead. I spoke to the child and bathed him and held him as if he was asleep. My action spoke louder than words. I treated him as if he were still alive, and the parents were truly touched. (Malloy et al., 2010, p. 169)

Following the plan of care and using an interdisciplinary palliative care team approach, nurses can coordinate the services of other clinicians (e.g., physicians, social workers, dietitians, and clergy) to meet client and family needs. Knowing and discussing all aspects of end-of-life care provides the client and family the opportunity to express their fears and concerns and receive appropriate support. The goal of the nurse and the interdisciplinary team is to provide an environment to support a good death (Krikorian et al., 2020).

Nurses have an important role in guiding and comforting clients and families experiencing the dying process. Nursing *presence* consists of not only the physical presence but also the relationship that is developed through connection with the client and family. Nurses have the privilege to be sharing the journey with clients and families coping with life-threatening illnesses. Being present involves the use of self, meaning being attentive, sensitive, accountable, and open, and actively listening (Schaffer & Norlander, 2009). The nurse, while "being," is totally focused on the client and meeting their needs of symptom management and issues specific to the living-dying experience. One of the priorities for nurses working with clients in end-of-life care is informing the family that death is approaching. If the family is not present at the time, the nurse needs to contact the designated family member and communicate in a sensitive way that there has been a change in the status of their loved one.

Guidelines for Communicating with Clients in Hospice Palliative Care

- Listen actively (a critical care component).
- Use honest, direct language (avoid medical jargon).
- Avoid stereotypical responses and false reassurances.
- Use pacing and staging when presenting/providing information.
- Assess their understanding of information.
- Use open-ended questioning.
- Use nursing presence—silence and touch (keeping in mind cultural implications).
- Provide a quiet, private environment.
- Display and demonstrate empathy through verbal and nonverbal behaviours.
- Maintain professional boundaries.
- Ask about their values and goals.
- Use the communication skills of reflection, paraphrasing, and summarizing.
- Be sensitive to the client's readiness to talk. Take time to listen and do not rush.
- Be cognizant of the use of nonverbal body language and voice.
- Be self-aware of your own values, beliefs, fears, and needs.
- Use alternative methods of communication as needed (e.g., ASL).

In client-centred care, nurses play an important role in providing end-of-life care by meeting the comfort needs of clients who are dying. Nurses spend the most time with clients, so they help provide comfort care: personal hygiene, nutrition, mouth care, pain and symptom management, and emotional, spiritual, and psychological support. This can be described as the "being" and the "doing" in nursing that aid the development of trust in therapeutic relationships. They also contribute to overall client comfort, quality of life, and peaceful death.

INVOLVEMENT OF CLIENT IN END-OF-LIFE DECISIONS

When clients enter a facility to receive end-of-life care, nurses have an ethical obligation to assess clients' and families' responsibility and understanding around end-of-life decisions. Some clients may have already made advance care planning decisions prior to being admitted to a health facility.

Advance Directives

In Canada, every province and territory has legislation that adult clients must be given information about advance health directives. *Advance directives* is a term that refers to advance care planning, a process in which individuals make decisions ahead of time about their preferred type of medical care in case they are incapacitated and unable to speak for themselves. Families whose loved one has completed an advance directive are obligated to inform health care providers who are involved in the person's care. The two main elements in an advance directive are a living will and a durable power of attorney.

- **Living will**: A living will is a written document that informs health care providers how a person wishes to be treated when dying, unconscious, and unable to make decisions about care.
- **Durable power of attorney**: A durable power of attorney for health care is a legal document naming a health care proxy (surrogate or representative) who should be familiar with the person's values and wishes. This person is responsible to make decisions about treatment.

When a person completes an advance directive, they can choose to create other documents that speak to specific medical issues that might arise at the end of life. These may include allow natural death (AND) orders: an allow natural death order informs health care providers that the person does not want their heart returned to a normal rhythm if it stops. They should receive no cardiopulmonary resuscitation (CPR) or other life-support. Some hospitals still use the obsolete term DNR (do not resuscitate) or DNAR (do not attempt resuscitation), although the recommended name in most settings is AND (allow natural death) as the meaning is clear (Piryani & Piryani, 2018). As a health professional student, you may become aware of these terms throughout your specific clinical rotations.

When clients are receiving end-of-life care and are competent but have not made an advance directive, the nurse can provide information about the process. It is best to begin the advance care planning discussions at an early stage of the life-threatening illness so that clients can be involved in the decision-making around their treatment and illness management (Head et al., 2018). However, in some cases, clients may lack the capacity (competency) to be involved in advance care decisions and the substitute decision-maker would decide on end-of-life treatment decisions.

Exercise 10.2: End-of-Life Care—the Nurse's Role

Purpose: To consider what constitutes a "good death"

Procedure
Pair up with a partner. Individually, write some brief notes on what you think would be considered having a "good death" or "dying well."

Questions
1. In today's chaotic health care system, is this possible?
2. How can a "good death" or "dying well" be facilitated by health care providers?

Discussion
1. Discuss your ideas/comments with your partner.
2. How similar/different were your ideas/comments?
3. As a class, share responses and discuss.

Communication with and Preparation of the Client

Nurses throughout the complete journey of end-of-life care communicate caring to clients through their verbal and nonverbal behaviours. In interactions with the client, it is important to assess their readiness to talk about death and dying. Sometimes clients are aware that they have little time left and feel relieved when they are asked about it by their care providers. Some questions to guide discussion could be "How do you imagine spending your last days? Is there anything special you would like to do?" or "Have you had any thoughts about where you would like to spend your last days?"

Communication with the client's relatives is an important component of end-of-life care. Poor communication from health care professionals is a common concern of the families of clients approaching the end of life. During this time, you should provide information on the client's health status and deterioration and involve the family in decision-making (Anderson et al., 2019). In the later stages of dying, when the client is unconscious or unable to speak, the nurse's presence and use of silence can be comforting for the client and family. The nurse may be checking in and asking the family, "How are you doing?" "This must be difficult or hard for you," or "Do you have any questions?"

Nurses, in a natural approach, can consider the use of touch as appropriate. The offer of a simple cup of tea or coffee may provide comfort to family members. Encouraging family to take some time away from the bedside allows them some quiet respite. These behaviours demonstrate the nurse's caring, understanding, and involvement in sharing the family's experience with loss and grief.

The final stage in the client's journey in receiving end-of-life care is death. This is a highly sensitive and emotional time for the nurse and the family. At this time, when care of the body is undertaken by the health care providers, it should reflect the client's and family's wishes and their cultural, ethnic, and spiritual beliefs. In the assessment and preparation of the body, nurses should be aware of the hospital or agency policy related to care of the body. In addition, they should have knowledge of any social, cultural, and/or religious considerations that should be observed during the procedure. It is impossible for nurses to be aware of all religions in Canada, so having knowledge of the client's and family's wishes is important and should take precedence. For example, in Islam, it is believed that death is in Allah's (God's) plan. The client should not be touched for 30 minutes after death. When providing care, nursing staff should adhere to specific religious duties (e.g., facing the client's body head-first and pointing toward Mecca) (Pattison, 2008).

Preparing the Client (Post-Mortem Care)

Following the death of a client, be sensitive to the family's wish to spend time with their loved one. It is important to inform the family of the process that will be undertaken; simple and brief information is best. Determine the client's previous wishes for washing; this may be noted in the nursing Kardex, or if not, check with the family. Maintain cultural safety in recognizing and having awareness of certain cultural and religious rituals for end-of-life care. For example, when caring for a client who is Islamic, the washing of the body is performed by family members who are of the same sex as the deceased (Gatrad & Sheikh, 2002). If clients have religious artifacts or objects (e.g., bracelets, feathers, amulets), they should be left with the body, and the family should be asked if there are any special procedures regarding their placement.

In most settings, it is usually the nurse who will prepare the client for the family to view. As before death, the body should be treated with dignity and respect. Health care providers should follow guidelines as outlined by the organization's policy and procedure. There may be religious or cultural implications for washing that must be followed, and in some cases, the family may wish to be involved, as already discussed. Other aspects of care that demonstrate a peaceful environment include the cleaning/combing of the client's hair, inserting clean dentures (if worn), dressing them in their own clothes (at the client or family's request) or hospital gown, covering them with sheets or blankets, and ensuring that the room is tidy. Provide privacy for the client and family, and if they request to speak to clergy or a representative from pastoral care, that should be accommodated. During this time, the silence and presence of the health care provider demonstrate respect for the family and the deceased. The nurse can also use other communication techniques, such as the use of touch or a simple response such as "I'm sorry for your loss." The most therapeutic approach is to be genuine, sensitive, and natural in all interactions with the family.

Assessment of Spiritual Needs and Cultural Safety

In providing end-of-life care using a person-centred approach, health care professionals can focus on supporting and facilitating the client's spiritual and cultural ways of being.

Spiritual Care

Spiritual care is recognized as a critical component of palliative care, which is facilitated through the nurse's understanding of their own spirituality and manifested through their caring actions in providing client care (Ricci-Allegra, 2018). *Spirituality* has many definitions and sometimes people confuse the term with *religion*, but the two are different. Spirituality can be defined as the beliefs and values that give meaning to a person's life and existence, "whether or not they believe in a higher being or are affiliated to a religion" (Quinn, 2020, p. 61). Religion can be defined as a component of spirituality in which the person follows specific practices and beliefs associated with an organized group (Kruse et al., 2007). For example, if a client is Catholic, the nurse can inquire if a visit from the priest would provide comfort. Spirituality is a resource for clients who are dealing with a life-threatening illness as it can assist them in coping and help them find purpose in their illness (Speck, 2016).

When caring for clients with a terminal illness, nurses should do an assessment of their spiritual needs. According to Bash (2004), spirituality is "what each person says it is, and the task of nurses is to identify and respect that person's expression of their spiritual experience and to offer them appropriate support" (p. 14). The assessment can be done formally or informally by using a qualified spiritual assessment tool or simply asking the question "Do you have a faith or spirituality that helps you cope (or that is important to you)?" or "Do you have a religious or spiritual support to help you during difficult times?" Some clients may state that they do not or may not disclose, as they wish to keep that information private. An evaluation tool for spiritual assessment that nurses can use is the FICA (Borneman et al., 2010):

- **Faith, belief, and meaning**: What is their faith, if they have one?
- **Importance**: How important is it to them?
- **Community**: What links, if any, do they have with a faith community?
- **Address in care**: How can their religious needs be addressed in their care?

This is a very simple standardized tool comprising a set of questions that nurses can use to ensure they have the information to provide holistic care and best practice in end-of-life care.

In addressing the client's spirituality, a caring presence is a crucial attribute for the nurse to bring to the clinical situation in providing end-of-life care. This caring presence is demonstrated by using a person-centred approach in developing the nurse-client relationship (Quinn, 2020). Ramezani et al. (2014), in their concept analysis of spiritual care in nursing, identified seven specific attributes to support best practice and competency for nurses' provision of spiritual care:

- Healing presence
- Therapeutic use of self
- Intuitive sense
- Exploration of the spiritual perspective (assessment of client's spiritual needs)
- Client-centredness
- Meaning-centred therapeutic intervention
- Creation of a spiritually nurturing environment (aids comfort and contributes to a peaceful death)

Nurses who understand the art of a caring presence will facilitate quality of life for clients who are receiving end-of-life care (Schaffer & Norlander, 2009).

Cultural Safety

Culture is "concerned with the language, knowledge, beliefs, assumptions and values that shape how we see the world and our place in it" (Speck, 2016, p. 341).

Health care professionals providing end-of-life care will encounter clients from diverse cultural backgrounds. It is impossible to be an expert in all cultures, so nurses need to understand and respect cultural diversity. Nurses bring their own values, beliefs, and judgments, which may be different from those of their clients, into their clinical practice. They need to have an awareness of their own cultural and personal influences and not impose them on the clients and families at the end of life.

Cultural safety is a concept that stresses the delivery of quality care through changes in thinking about power relationships and clients' rights, with an emphasis on recognizing and respecting the difference among individuals. Cultural safety encompasses cultural awareness, sensitivity, and cultural competency (e.g., skills to build and maintain trusting relationships), and health professionals are responsible for providing cultural safety (Tremblay et al., 2020). Cultural safety implementation within health care in Canada has the potential to improve the health inequities between Indigenous and non-Indigenous Canadians (Brooks-Cleator et al., 2018).

Nurses working in community, hospital, and palliative care settings demonstrate an understanding of cultural safety by providing comfort to the dying person and asking them about their own values and issues, respecting the client's and family's religious and spiritual beliefs, using a person-centred approach, inquiring about and creating a space for cultural expression, and involving the client in health decisions. Once the nurse understands the client's cultural and spiritual needs, they can be assured that they will receive high-quality end-of-life care (Cain et al., 2018).

SELF-CARE FOR NURSES IN PROVIDING END-OF-LIFE CARE

All health care professionals face the dying and death of clients, so it is a source of occupational stress. Hospice and palliative care professionals spend more time in direct contact with clients who are dying from life-threatening illness than nurses in other clinical settings (Melvin, 2015). Nurses may have a close connection with clients and families in these situations and experience grief when clients die. As a result, these nurses are at risk of developing emotional and physical distress, which can impact their well-being, client care and outcomes, job satisfaction, and work-life balance (Sinclair et al., 2017). In the following narrative, the nurse demonstrates this connection and verbalizes how they were impacted by the death of a client:

> I felt that I really shared in their painful experience. I felt really close to the family because I had been there since the moment he (client) was admitted to the moment he died. I'd been there through it all and really felt as though I was going through it with them. (Bloomer et al., 2022, p. 14)

Nurses can experience *compassion fatigue*, which is a state of complete physical, emotional, and spiritual exhaustion related to repeated exposure to others' suffering, impacting their caregiver role (Peters, 2018). Without recovery, nurses may decide to leave the profession, suffer burnout, or provide suboptimal client care (Linton & Koonmen, 2020). Self-care interventions completed by nurses may offset compassion fatigue. Nurses can reduce their stress and maintain their overall well-being if they adopt self-care practices (Linton & Koonmen, 2020). Simple strategies for self-care, including mindfulness, meditation, yoga, exercise, journaling, or prayer, can help achieve work-life balance. Some work-related strategies include self-reflection, debriefing, and talking to colleagues and managers about feelings that stem from caring for clients and their families in end-of-life care. Students entering nursing programs are educated about the importance of self-care and the use of reflection to help develop critical thinking and professional competency.

Case Study 10.1

Mr. Asikinach is a 65-year-old Indigenous man of the Anishinabek Nation who is admitted to the hospital from the emergency department with a diagnosis of terminal lung cancer. For the past three weeks he has not been feeling well, with complaints of stomach pain, nausea and vomiting, and shortness of breath. On admission to the unit, he is accompanied by his wife and two members of his family. When he gets up from the wheelchair, you notice that he is short of breath. As you settle him in bed, he asks, "Am I going to die?"

1. What would be your response to Mr. Asikinach?
2. His wife and two members of his family ask if they can have a pipe ceremony for Mr. Asikinach at the bedside. (For information on the pipe ceremony see Longboat, D. M. [2002]. *Indigenous perspectives on death and dying.* https://www.cpd.utoronto.ca) What would be your response to the family?
3. What steps can you take to accommodate this request? Think about what you, as the nurse, can facilitate within your facility. For example, perhaps you can turn off the smoke detectors in the client area or find an area with an exhaust fan. Another option, if the client is able, is to inquire if the ceremony can take place outside on facility grounds.

CHAPTER SUMMARY

This chapter describes the process of loss, grief, and bereavement. Loss is a part of life, and grief is the normal response to loss. Loss includes loss of health, object, person, security, or lifestyle. Everyone may demonstrate different behaviours and experience loss, grief, and bereavement in an individual way. Health care profession-als' role is to explore those grief experiences with clients and their families. Culture plays a large part in determining a person's response to death, and denial and fear of death are common in Canadian culture. People who have a life-threatening illness obtain care from nurses in hospital or hospice palliative care settings. Nurses play a critical role in helping clients and families during times of loss. Nurses provide sup-port, guidance, and information through authentic, compassionate communication, presence, and caring to help ease reactions to death and dying.

In providing end-of-life care, nurses use "self" therapeutically in the develop-ment of the nurse-client relationship to understand the client's and family's physical, psychological, cultural, and spiritual needs in response to the client's terminal ill-ness. Nurses must facilitate and support the death rituals and grief responses of cli-ents and families, which help to contribute to a "good death." Nurses have an ethical responsibility to assess client understanding of and provide information on advance directives. This removes the burden from families in making decisions for loved ones at a difficult time. Death is a challenging situation for nurses in end-of-life care and practising self-care helps to strike a work-life balance. If nurses do not manage the stressors in their work of end-of-life care, compassion fatigue (burnout) or leaving the profession may result.

REVIEW QUESTIONS

Read the following three review questions and select the best option to answer each question. State your rationale for choosing your response. For the other four questions, identify your response.

1. When asked by a client's family member about what an advance directive is, the nurse should respond that it states
    a. The health care professional's role in care provision at the end of life
    b. What treatment should be provided or omitted if a person becomes incapacitated
    c. The clinicians who are involved in the client's "circle of care"
    d. The competency framework necessary in the provision of end-of-life care
2. One of the factors that influence the relationship between health care professionals and relatives of clients at the end of life is
    a. Health care providers' lack of knowledge on how to provide end-of-life care
    b. Health care providers' lack of knowledge on disenfranchised grief
    c. Poor communication from health care professionals
    d. Health care professionals' inability to use grief theory in practice

3. Anticipatory grief
   a. Occurs due to the loss of a significant other/partner in a major motor vehicle accident
   b. Occurs due to the loss of those whose death occurs unexpectedly
   c. Occurs when individuals grieve prior to the actual loss
   d. Occurs from the sudden loss of a family pet
4. A nurse has worked for over 20 years in a busy critical care unit. They were just recently diagnosed as having compassion fatigue. Define the term and identify several activities that the nurse can use to promote self-care.
5. Identify several communication practices for use in end-of-life care.
6. Define the terms loss, grief, and bereavement.
7. Discuss the reasons why nurses must have knowledge of cultural safety when providing care to clients with a terminal illness.

WEB RESOURCES

Canadian Hospice Palliative Care Association
www.chpca.ca/resource-group/patients/
Indigenous Voices: Honouring Our Loss and Grief
https://livingmyculture.ca

REFERENCES

Anderson, K. A., & Gaugler, J. E. (2007). The grief experiences of certified nursing assistants: Personal growth and complicated grief. *OMEGA—The Journal of Death and Dying, 54*(4). https://doi.org/10.2190/T14N-W223-7612-0224

Anderson, R. J., Bloch, S., Armstrong, M., Stone, P. C., & Low, J. S. (2019). Communication between healthcare professionals and relatives of patients approaching the end-of-life: A systematic review of qualitative evidence. *Palliative Medicine, 33*(8), 926–941. https://doi.org/10.1177/0269216319852007

Andersson, E., Salickiene, Z., & Rosengren, K. (2016). To be involved—a qualitative study of nurses' experiences of caring for dying patients. *Nurse Education Today, 38*, 144–149. https://doi.org/10.1016/j.nedt.2015.11.026

Bash, A. (2004). Spirituality: The emperor's new clothes? *Journal of Clinical Nursing, 13*(1), 11–16. https://doi.org/10.1046/j.1365-2702.2003.00838.x

Berndtsson, I. E. K., Karlsson, M. G., & Renjo, A. C. U. (2019). Nursing students' attitudes toward care of dying patients: A pre- and post-palliative course study. *Heliyon, 5*(10). https://doi.org/10.1016/j.heliyon.2019.e02578

Beuthin, R., Bruce, A., & Scaia, M. (2018). Medical assistance in dying (MAiD): Canadian nurses' experiences. *Nursing Forum, 53*(4), 511–520. https://doi.org/10.1111/nuf.12280

Bloomer, M. J., Ranse, K., Adams, L., Brooks, L., & Coventry, A. (2022). "Time and life is fragile": An integrative review of nurses' experiences after patient death in adult critical care. *Australian Critical Care*. https://doi.org/10.1016/j.aucc.2022.09.008

Borneman, T., Ferrell, B., & Puchalski, C. M. (2010). Evaluation of the FICA tool for spiritual assessment. *Journal of Pain and Symptom Management*, 40(2), 163–173. https://doi.org/10.1016/j.jpainsymman.2009.12.019

Brooks-Cleator, L., Phillipps, B., & Giles, A. (2018). Culturally safe health initiatives for Indigenous peoples in Canada: A scoping review. *Canadian Journal of Nursing Research*, 50(4), 202–213. https://doi.org/10.1177/0844562118770334

Buglass, E. (2010). Grief and bereavement theories. *Nursing Standard*, 24(41), 44–47. https://doi.org/10.7748/ns2010.06.24.41.44.c7834

Cain, C. L., Surbone, A., Elk, R., & Kagawa-Singer, M. (2018). Culture and palliative care: Preferences, communication, meaning, and mutual decision making. *Journal of Pain and Symptom Management*, 55(5), 1408–1419. https://doi.org/10.1016/j.jpainsymman.2018.01.007

Canadian Institute for Health Information. (2020). *Your health system: Hospital deaths.* https://yourhealthsystem.cihi.ca/hsp/inbrief?lang=en#/indicators/005/hospital-deaths-hsmr/;mapC1:map1.eve12:/

Canadian Nurses Association. (2022). *Certification.* https://www.cna-aiic.ca/en/certification

Canadian Palliative Care Nursing Association. (2021). *Canadian palliative care nursing standards of practice.* https://www.cpcna.ca/-files/ugdb8al_7cd2666999d34/96ace7807a221da76f.pdf

Canning, D., Rosenberg, J. P., & Yates, P. (2007). Therapeutic relationships in specialist palliative care nursing practice. *Journal of Palliative Nursing*, 13(5), 222–229. https://doi.org/10.12968/ijpn.2007.13.5.23492

Coelho, A., & Barbosa, A. (2017). Family anticipatory grief: An integrative literature review. *American Journal of Hospice & Palliative Medicine*, 34(8), 774–785. https://doi.org/10.1177/1049909116647960

Corr, C. A. (2021). Should we incorporate the work of Elisabeth Kübler-Ross in our current teaching and practice and, if so, how? *OMEGA-Journal of Death and Dying*, 83(4), 706–728. https://doi.org/10.1177/0030222819865397

Corr, M. D., & Corr, C. A. (2020). Elisabeth Kübler-Ross and the 5 stages model in a sampling of recent North American nursing textbooks. *Journal of Hospice & Palliative Nursing*, 22(1), 61–67. https://doi.org/10.1097/NJH.0000000000000615

Coughlin, M. B., & Sethares, K. A. (2017). Chronic sorrow in parents of children with a chronic illness or disability: An integrative literature review. *Journal of Pediatric Nursing*, 37, 108–116. https://doi.org/10.1016/j.pedn.2017.06.011

Davies, R. (2004). New understandings of parental grief: Literature review. *Journal of Advanced Nursing*, 46(5), 506–513. https://doi.org/10.1111/j.1365-2648.2004.03024.x

Gatrad, R., & Sheikh, A. (2002). Palliative care for Muslims and issues after death. *International Journal of Palliative Nursing*, 8(12), 594–597. https://doi.org/10.12968/ijpn.2002.8.12.10977

Government of Canada (2018a). *Framework on palliative care in Canada.* https://www.canada
.ca/en/health-canada/services/health-care-system/reports-publications/palliative-care/
framework-palliative-care-canada.html

Government of Canada. (2018b). *Legislative summary: Library of Parliament: Bill C-14: An act to
amend the criminal code and to make related amendments to other acts (medical assistance in
dying).* https://lop.parl.ca

Harder, N., Lemoine, J., & Harwood, R. (2020). Psychological outcomes of debriefing
healthcare providers who experience expected and unexpected patient death in clinical or
simulation experiences: A scoping review. *Journal of Clinical Nursing, 29*(3–4), 330–346.
https://doi.org/10.1111/jocn.15085

Head, B. A., Song, M., Wiencek, C., Nevidjon, B., Fraser, D., & Mazanec, P. (2018). Nurses
leading change and transforming care: The nurse's role in communication and advance care
planning. *Journal of Hospice & Palliative Nursing, 20*(1), 23–29. https://doi.org/10.1097/
NJH.0000000000000406

Henoch, I., Melin-Johansson, C., Bergh, I., Strang, S., Ek, K., Hammarlund, K.,
Hagelin, C. L., Westin, L., Osterlind, J., & Browall, M. (2017). Undergraduate nursing
students' attitudes and preparedness toward caring for dying persons — A longitudinal
study. *Nurse Education in Practice, 26*, 12–20. https://doi.org/10.1016/j.nepr.2017.06.007

Krikorian, A., Maldonado, C., & Pastrana, T. (2020). Patient's perspectives on the notion of a
good death: A systematic review of the literature. *Journal of Pain and Symptom
Management, 59*(1), 152–164. https://doi.org/10.1016/j.jpainsymman.2019.07.033

Kruse, B. G., Ruder, S., & Martin, L. (2007). Spirituality and coping at the end of life. *Journal
of Hospice and Palliative Nursing, 9*(6). https://doi.org/10.1097/01.NJH.0000299317

LeBlanc, N. J., Unger, L. D., & McNally, R. J. (2016). Emotional and physiological reactivity
in complicated grief. *Journal of Affective Disorders, 194*, 98–104. https://doi.org/10.1016/
j.ad.2016.01.024

Linton, M., & Koonmen, J. (2020). Self-care as an ethical obligation for nurses. *Nursing Ethics,
27*(8), 1694–1702. https://doi.org/10.1177/0969733020940371

Longboat, D. M. (2002). *Indigenous perspectives on death and dying.* https://www.cpd.utoronto.ca

Mallon, B. (2008). *Dying, death and grief: Working with adult bereavement.* Sage. https://doi
.org/10.4135/9781446214510

Malloy, P., Virani, R., Kelly, K., & Munevar, C. (2010). Beyond bad news: Communication
skills of nurses in palliative care. *Journal of Hospice and Palliative Nursing, 12*(3), 166–174.
https://doi.org/10.1097/NJH.0b013e3181d99fee

Meichsner, F., O'Connor, M., Skritskaya, N., & Shear, K. (2020). Grief before and after
bereavement in the elderly: An approach to care. *The American Journal of Geriatric
Psychiatry, 28*(5), 560–569. https://doi.org/10.1016/j.jagp.2019.12.010

Melvin, C. S. (2015). Historical review in understanding burnout, professional compassion
fatigue, and secondary traumatic stress disorder from a hospice and palliative nursing
perspective. *Journal of Hospice & Palliative Nursing, 17*(1), 66–72. https://doi.org/10.1097/
NJH.0000000000000126

Nyatanga, B. (2016). Challenges of loss and grief in palliative care nursing. *British Journal of Community Nursing, 21*(2). https://doi.org/10.12968/bjcn.2016.21.2.106

Pattison, N. (2008). Care of patients who have died. *Nursing Standard, 22*(28), 42–48. https://doi.org/10.7748/ns2008.03.22.28.42.c6434

Peters, E. (2018). Compassion fatigue in nursing: A concept analysis. *Nursing Forum, 53*(4), 466–480. https://doi.org/10.1111/nuf.12274

Petrongolo, M., & Toothaker, R. (2021). Nursing students perceptions of death and dying: A descriptive quantitative study. *Nursing Education Today, 104*, 1–4. https://doi.org/10.1016/j.nedt.2021.104993

Piryani, R. M., & Piryani, S. (2018). Do-not-resuscitate (DNR). *Journal of Kathmandu Medical College, 7*(4), 187–190. https://doi.org/10.3126/jkmc.v7i4.23327

Quinn, B. G. (2020). Responding to people who are experiencing spiritual pain. *Nursing Standard, 35*(4), 59–65. https://doi.org/10.7748/ns.2020.e11523

Ramezani, M., Ahmadi, F., Mohammadi, E., & Kazemnejad, A. (2014). Spiritual care in nursing: A concept analysis. *International Nursing Review, 61*(2), 211–219. https://doi.org/10.1111/inr.12099

Raymond, A., Lee, S. F., & Bloomer, M. J. (2016). Understanding the bereavement care roles of nurses within acute care: A systematic review. *Journal of Clinical Nursing, 26*(13–14), 1787–1800. https://doi.org/10.1111/jocn.13503

Ricci-Allegra, P. (2018). Spiritual perspective, mindfulness, and spiritual care practice of hospice and palliative nurses. *Journal of Hospice & Palliative Nursing, 20*(2), https://doi.org/10.1097/NJH.0000000000000426

Schaffer, M., & Norlander, L. (2009). *Being present: A nurse's resource for end-of-life communication.* Edward Brothers.

Scruth, E. A., & Allen, A. (2022). Self-care: The ethical imperative for nurses and other healthcare professionals. *Clinical Nurse Specialist, 36*(4), 181–182. https://doi.org/10.1097/NUR.0000000000000683

Sinclair, S., Raffin-Bouchal, S., Venturato, L., Mijovic-Kondejewski, J., & Smith-MacDonald, L. (2017). Compassion fatigue: A meta-narrative review of the healthcare literature. *International Journal of Nursing Studies, 69*, 9–24, https://doi.org/10.1016/j.ijnurstu.2017.01.003

Silverman, G. S., Baroiller, A., & Hemer, S. R. (2021). Culture and grief: Ethnographic perspectives on ritual, relationships and remembering. *Death Studies, 45*(1), 1–8. https://doi.org/10.1080/07481187.2020.1851885

Slade, J. D., & Hoh, N. Z. (2020). Employing Watson's theory of human caring with people experiencing loss and grief. *International Journal for Human Caring, 24*(1), 4–11. https://doi.org/10.20467/1091-5710.241.4

Speck, P. (2016). Culture and spirituality: Essential components of palliative care. *Postgraduate Medical Journal, 92*, 341–345 https://doi.org/10.1136/postgradmedj-2015-133369

Townsend, M. C. (2015). The bereaved individual. In M. C. Townsend (Ed.), *Psychiatric mental health nursing: Concepts of care in evidence-based practice* (8th ed., pp. 830–850). F. A. Davis.

Tremblay, M., Graham, J., Porgo, T. V., Paquette, J.-S., Careau, E., & Witteman, H. O. (2020). Improving cultural safety of diabetes care in Indigenous populations of Canada, Australia, New Zealand, and the United States: A systematic rapid review. *Canadian Journal of Diabetes*, *44*(7), 670–678. https://doi.org/10.1016/j.jcjd.2019.11.006

Tsui, E. K., Franzosa, E., Cribbs, K. A., & Baron, S. (2019). Home care workers' experiences of client death and disenfranchised grief. *Qualitative Health Research*, *29*(3), 382–392. https://doi.org/10.1177/1049732318800461

Zheng, R., Lee, S. F., & Bloomer, M. J. (2017). How nurses cope with patient death: A systematic review and qualitative meta-synthesis. *Journal of Clinical Nursing*, *27*(1–2). https://doi.org/10.1111/jocn.13975

CHAPTER 11

Communication with Health Care Teams and Other Health Care Professionals

LEARNING OBJECTIVES

After reading this chapter, you will be able to

1. Identify the difference between a team and a group
2. Describe the characteristics of effective teams
3. Discuss the benefits of interprofessional teams
4. Identify the challenges of being a member of a health care team
5. Describe strategies for effective team communication
6. Define *conflict* and *incivility*
7. Discuss the concept of conflict in health care organizations
8. Describe effective techniques for conflict competency
9. Identify principles of communication for working in teams

KEY TERMS

Collaboration	Incivility
Conflict	Interprofessional collaboration
Groups	Intra-professional collaboration

INTRODUCTION

This chapter introduces the topic of teams and their importance within the health care system. One of the key factors necessary for working in health care is the ability to work in teams. Presently the emphasis in health care is on collaboration among health professionals for delivery of effective and safe client care. Attributes necessary for the development of effective teams are discussed. Successful teams within health care contribute to effective communication, client safety, collaboration, work satisfaction, personal well-being, and quality client outcomes. However, team performance and cohesiveness are impacted by poor communication and conflict. Conflict is everywhere and is unavoidable for those working in health care, so it is best to have knowledge of strategies for conflict management within these settings

(Kfouri & Lee, 2019; McKibben, 2017). Different conflict management styles used by health care providers are identified, and effective strategies to help constructively manage conflict are described.

TEAMS AND GROUPS

As students, you may be familiar with the terms *teams* and *groups* as most of you have participated in one or both of those throughout your lives. Some of you may have been a member of a specific sports team or a school, church, or university/college group. A team is defined as a group of people that come together to work on a particular task, and teamwork is what transpires among its members to complete the task (Rydenfalt & Odenrick, 2017). Teams in health care can take many forms, be large or small, and comprise members with a variety of expertise. Some teams may be nursing-specific, for example, registered nurses, licensed practical nurses, registered practical nurses, and personal care attendants who have similar backgrounds and work together on a given client care unit or setting. Other teams may be comprised of physicians, pharmacists, dietitians, registered nurses, and nurse practitioners who have different skill sets but work with an interdisciplinary approach for the provision of quality client care.

An interdisciplinary team is composed of members who have clinical expertise from a variety of disciplines and who meet on a regular basis to discuss and collaborate on treatment goals and plans of care for clients. A multidisciplinary team is represented by a variety of disciplines, but the physician is at the top of the line of authority, and all other professionals provide input to them on client treatment plans. The physician communicates with each team member, and little or no communication occurs among the team members (Korner, 2010). An interprofessional (IP) health care team is composed of team members from two or more different professions (e.g., physicians, nurses, pharmacists) who collaborate on a client's plan of care. These IP teams enhance the quality of safe care and promote best client health outcomes (Wranik et al., 2019).

As a student, you have probably interacted with a variety of groups beginning at a young age. As you reflect on your time in school, and now in university/college, how many group projects have you worked on with fellow classmates? One group with which you are familiar is family; it is considered a specialized type of group. A group is defined as "two or more people together functioning interdependently" (Tusaie, 2017, p. 138), established for a common purpose or goal. In health care there are therapeutic groups, psychoeducation groups, stress management groups, and support groups (e.g., for bereavement). In the community there are also self-help groups, which may be led by professionals or nonprofessionals, that provide support and education for individuals with health issues (e.g., Alcoholics Anonymous).

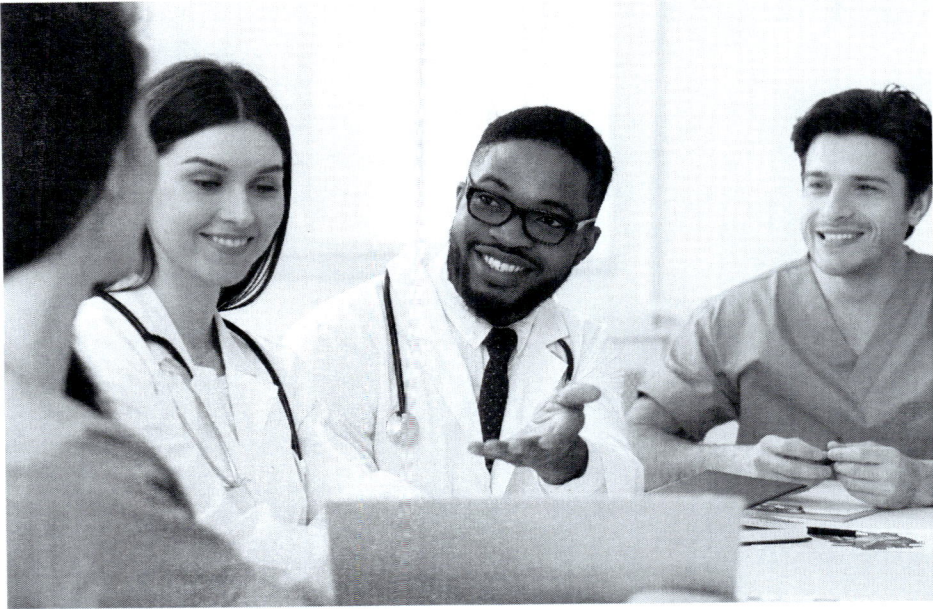

Figure 11.1: Health care team communicating

Source: Adobe Stock/Prostock-studio

QUALITIES NECESSARY FOR EFFECTIVE TEAMS

In health care there are many teams that provide care for clients in a variety of settings. Communication among team members is identified as a significant attribute for effective team functioning (Cutler et al., 2019), along with these other attributes that contribute to team effectiveness (Gluyas, 2015; Stoller, 2021):

- **Open communication:** Information is shared and communication is clear. Appropriate terminology and objective language are used. Clear roles and responsibilities are evident. Communication is acknowledged and checked for correct interpretation. All members are engaged and not afraid to provide an opinion.
- **Listening:** Active listening, with use of effective listening techniques (e.g., questioning, validation, summarizing), is practised.
- **Mutual support:** There is mutual trust, and members are comfortable and feel safe. Decisions are made via consensus. Conflict is acknowledged, and members collaborate for management of issues.
- **Shared leadership:** Members demonstrate effective leadership behaviour. Everyone is aware of roles, responsibilities, and plan. Workload is shared. Members' diverse skills are recognized and appreciated.

- **Self-assessment:** Team self-assesses performance in meeting plan/goals on an ongoing basis. Members evaluate, adapt, adjust, and reassign responsibilities and tasks as necessary.

Effective teamwork in health care requires interprofessional collaboration to ensure the best client care and safety. A positive workplace culture (e.g., cohesive, supportive, collaborative, and inclusive) is associated with best client outcomes, while a negative culture is associated with mortality, impaired physician-nurse relationships, medication errors, and other adverse events (Braithwaite et al., 2017). Within interprofessional teams, communication, respect, and collaboration among members contribute to a quality practice environment that values the well-being and safety of clients and health care providers (Canadian Nurses Association [CNA], 2019).

BARRIERS TO EFFECTIVE TEAM COMMUNICATION

Various barriers that hinder communication are classified as behavioural, cognitive, linguistic, environmental, or technological (Guttman et al., 2021).

- **Behavioural:** There is a lack of communication. Health care providers are afraid to use "speak up" behaviour, meaning they are reluctant to ask questions, ask for further information, or voice concerns.
- **Cognitive:** Cognition becomes a barrier to communication when information exchange is interrupted, contains insufficient information, lacks context, or includes extraneous information.
- **Linguistic:** An individual's style, tone, syntax, or use of language contributes to communication breakdown. For the receiver of messages, using explicit and closed-loop communication (feedback) is recommended to ensure message and information are accurate and precise.
- **Environmental:** In health care settings, environmental noise is common (e.g., staff-related noise, equipment, alarms, and machinery), as well as physical environmental barriers such as drapes and masks, which impact the line of vision of speaker and listener.
- **Technological:** Health care providers are spending increased time in documentation. Use of the electronic medical record and involvement in other duties leave less time to spend with clients. Staff are caught up with technological functions and spend less time in care activities (Schenk et al., 2018). These factors impede development of the nurse-client relationship.

STRATEGIES FOR ENHANCED COMMUNICATION WITHIN TEAMS

To offset communication failures in health care, several team-building strategies and communication tool components of the TeamSTEPPS program are currently used: CUS, TeamSTEPPS, and SBAR.

CUS is a standardized communication tool that can be used in health care for conflict resolution or advocacy to discuss an issue that is identified as a safety concern:

- **C:** I am concerned (about …).
- **U:** I am uncomfortable (because …).
- **S:** This is a safety issue (because …).

Case Example

Mr. Learner is a 45-year-old male who was admitted to the acute care unit with a diagnosis of chronic schizophrenia. He has been on the unit for about a week and was prescribed quetiapine (Seroquel) 300 mg BID (twice a day). Following a morning round, you find Mr. Learner lying on his bed, sweating and drooling. You take his vital signs and note he is hypertensive and tachycardiac, and has hyperpyrexia.

C: "I am concerned about possible neuroleptic malignant syndrome."

U: "I am uncomfortable that he may lose consciousness and have other complications."

S: "This is a safety issue because it can be life-threatening."

TeamSTEPPS

TeamSTEPPS is an acronym that refers to Team Strategies and Tools to Enhance Performance and Patient Safety, a program developed by the Joint Commission and Agency for Healthcare Research and Quality (AHRQ) and the Department of Defense in the United States to integrate teamwork in practice and improve communication, quality, and safety in health care (Coolen et al., 2020; Plonien & Williams, 2015). The TeamSTEPPS program is also offered to health care providers in Canada through the agency Healthcare Excellence Canada. The evidence-based toolbox includes a standardized framework for health care team members to use when communicating about a client's condition. The tools most often used are the following (Weller et al., 2014):

- SBAR
- Call out (step back)
- Closed-loop communication
- Structured handover

SBAR

SBAR is a mnemonic for Situation, Background, Assessment, and Recommendation (Muller et al., 2018; see table 11.1 on the following page for a case example). This structured tool demonstrates collaboration between physicians and nurses using effective communication when providing information about a client's change in status and an intervention that is needed. It is recognized as an effective technique for promotion of client safety and best practice in critical clinical situations.

Call Out (Step Back)

This communication technique involves taking a step back from the environment and situation. The health care provider who is the lead for the team calls the attention of the team, provides a situation update and the plan, and seeks suggestions for management of the situation.

Closed-Loop Communication

This communication strategy uses a three-step approach: (1) a team member sends a message to a recipient (calling them by name); (2) the receiver checks that they understood the message; and (3) the sender confirms that the receiver's understanding is correct. This technique is used in acute care settings and during codes (e.g., cardiac arrest). For example, the client has arrested; the team arrives and directs the scene. The physician (team lead) takes charge and, as the sender, states, (1) "Okay, let's administer epinephrine 1 mg IVP" (intravenous push). The nurse preps the medication and, as the receiver, states, (2) "Yes, epinephrine 1 mg IVP given." The team lead says, (3) "Okay, thanks. (1) Can we get a set of vital signs, please?" The nurse (receiver) states, (2) "Yes, taking now. Vital signs are …" The team lead states, (3) "Thanks. (1) What's showing on the monitor?"

Structured Handover

This communication tool is recognized as an important element in clinical handover for nurses and other health care providers in health care settings.

Table 11.1: SBAR Case Example

SBAR	Question	Description	Example
Situation	What is going on with the client?	Speaker presents client information, and briefly describes the problem.	"Dr. Greene, I am calling about Mrs. Forest, who has fallen out of bed."
Background	What is the background/context of the client?	Provides background: diagnosis, reason for admission, medical status/history. Client's chart is reviewed.	"She is 78 years of age, admitted with a bowel obstruction three days ago. She had a bowel resection yesterday morning. No past medical history."
Assessment	What is the problem?	Provides specific information, vital signs, lab data, and any information related to the client's current condition.	"She climbed over the bed rails. Pupils are PERRLA. Vital signs: BP: 128/78, p: 120 bpm, R: 28, rapid and shallow breathing. T: 37.5ºC. Has an IV of RL running at 125 cc/hr. She has a large black bruise with some slight swelling on her right (R) hip. She is talking and complains of pain in R hip.
Recommendation	What's the next step(s) in the management of the client?	Specific continued care of the client is suggested by speaker in a clear manner.	"I need you to see her right away. I think she may have a broken hip. She may need some X-rays."

Source: Muller et al. (2018). Impact of the communication and patient hand-off tool SBAR on patient safety: A systematic review. *BMJ Open*. https://doi.org/10.1136/bmjopen-2018-022202.

There are a variety of templates available that provide a combination of verbal and written information on clients' needs and clinical status during huddles, handover, or debriefs. One structured handover tool that is widely used in a hospital setting is the iSoBAR (Beament et al., 2018).

- **Identify**: Introduce self and the client.
- **Situation**: Why are you calling? Briefly state the problem.
- **Observation**: Observe recent vital signs and clinical assessment data.
- **Background**: Review pertinent information related to client and medical history.
- **Agreed plan**: What needs to happen? Assess the situation.
- **Read back**: Clarify and check for understanding. Who is responsible for what and what is the time frame?

This tool promotes continuity of care and reduces risk of miscommunication. It supports "closed-loop communication" by acknowledging communication and checking for correct interpretation.

Quality Practice Environments

Nurses are considered the "backbone" of the health care system in Canada and work around the clock to provide direct client care despite the physical and mental demands of their role. These health professionals are faced with many challenges such as heavy workloads, clients with complex health needs, incivility (lateral violence), bullying, conflict, lack of resources, and disrespectful communication. Positive practice environments for health care professionals are influenced by supportive management, autonomy in clinical practice, collegial professional relationships, and appropriate staffing (Erickson et al., 2017).

The Canadian Nurses Association (CNA, 2019) and the Canadian Federation of Nurses Unions issued a joint position statement that advocates for a quality practice environment for nurses. Nurses who work in a quality practice environment experience respect and are involved in decision-making. These organizations identify the following attributes of a quality practice environment:

- Communication and collaboration (considered the foundation of nursing)
- Responsibility and accountability
- Safe and realistic workload
- Leadership
- Support for information and knowledge management (technologies to support nurses' work and provision of safe, effective care)

- Professional development opportunities (e.g., continuing education supports, workshops/seminars)
- Workplace culture (values the well-being of clients and employees)

Quality practice environments contribute to nurse empowerment, client safety, best client outcomes, effective teamwork, and nurse satisfaction (Braithwaite et al., 2017; Prentice et al., 2020).

COLLABORATION

The World Health Organization (2010) defines collaborative practice in health care as occurring "when multiple health workers from different professional backgrounds provide comprehensive services by working with patients, their families, carers and communities to deliver the highest quality of care across settings" (p. 13). In Canada, professional associations and nurses propose that *intra-professional collaboration* (collaboration among team members from the same profession) is essential for ensuring optimal quality client care and relational practice for all regulated nurses. The Canadian Nurses Association (2020) issued a position statement on intra-professional collaboration to highlight its importance in improving nurses' professional practice and safe health care outcomes for clients.

Interprofessional collaboration is a process where health care professionals from different professions, such as physicians and nurses, work together to maximize client outcomes (Schot et al., 2020). In the context of health care delivery, the process of collaboration maintains an emphasis on person-centred care influenced by the relationship between team members, understanding and knowledge of each other's roles, mutual respect, and effective communication. For over a decade, an organization called the Canadian Interprofessional Health Collaborative (CIHC) has advocated for health professionals' collaborative practice because of its benefits for clients and the health care system. The CIHC's framework (CIHC, 2022) comprises six competency domains necessary for collaborative practice:

- **Role clarification:** Practitioners/learners understand their role as well as the roles of other health professionals. This knowledge helps to establish and meet client/family and community goals.
- **Team functioning:** Practitioners/learners have knowledge of team dynamics and group processes to enable effective interprofessional collaborative practice.
- **Interprofessional communication:** Practitioners/learners from a variety of professions learn to communicate collaboratively and respectfully.

- **Client/family/community-centred care**: Practitioners/learners seek input from client/family/community in designing and implementing care/services to meet client health care needs.
- **Interprofessional conflict resolution:** Practitioners/learners engage client/family to deal effectively with interprofessional conflict.
- **Collaborative leadership:** Practitioners/learners work collaboratively with all participants to design, implement, and evaluate care/services to promote best client outcomes.

The competency domains of the CIHC framework have been integrated into courses within health professional programs across Canada to prepare students for interprofessional and collaborative practice in health care organizations.

Incivility in Clinical Environments

Despite the call for a healthy work environment, it is well documented that health care settings where nurses work are difficult. On a day-to-day basis, nurses work under very stressful situations that include heavy workloads, limited resources, disrespectful behaviour, conflict, and incivility. This impacts their work and leads to dissatisfaction with work, negative mental and physical health, impaired team performance, interpersonal conflict, and poor client outcomes (Anusiewicz et al., 2020; Keller et al., 2020). Negative relationships among nurses are common in the workplace and across all care settings (Bambi et al., 2018; Crawford et al., 2019). The incidence of workplace nurse-to-nurse incivility has challenged the work of nurses, leading to negative consequences on client care (Armstrong, 2018; Logan, 2016; Taskaya & Aksoy, 2021). *Incivility* has been defined as the use of negative verbal behaviours such as threats, insults, name-calling, gossip, yelling, putdowns, and non-verbal behaviour such as rolling eyes (Keller et al., 2020; Layne et al., 2019). Some other labels used to describe these behaviours include verbal abuse, lateral violence, horizontal violence, harassment, and bullying. Incivility in the workplace directed at nurses may come from other nurses, clients, families, or other health professionals (Taskaya & Aksoy, 2021). These practices hinder communication and development of the nurse-client relationship and lead to interpersonal or intra-professional conflict, disrespect, and toxic work environments (Anusiewicz et al., 2020; Boateng & Adams, 2016; Clark, 2019). Incivility also affects the organization through an increase in employee absenteeism and through some nurses leaving to seek employment elsewhere (Solis, 2019).

The following are some common examples of uncivil behaviours observed in the workplace (Pattani et al., 2018; Sanner-Stiehr & Ward-Smith, 2017; Solis, 2019):

- Gossiping about co-workers

- Refusing to offer help or provide information
- Eye-rolling or sighing in front of a co-worker
- Yelling at a co-worker (e.g., calling them stupid because they are not familiar with a particular procedure)

Case Example

Nurse Gerry asks Nurse Madison to show them how to flush a subclavian line on the client in Room 225. Madison, sighing and rolling eyes, states, "I'll guess I'll have to!" Nurse Gerry responds, "I sense there may be something you want to say to me. It's okay, you can tell me."

Some interventions that organizations can make to address incivility in nursing include (but are not limited to) the following (Kroning, 2019; Sanner-Stiehr & Ward-Smith, 2017):

- Commit to creating and supporting a culture of safety (using evidence-based strategies).
- Model respectful, effective communication, and adhere to professional codes (conduct) (CNA, 2017, 2019).
- Ensure all employees are aware of their own behaviour and are able to receive and accept feedback from others to promote change.
- Implement mandatory education on zero-tolerance policy.
- Put process in place for reporting of behaviours and following up.
- Put supports in place for individuals who require services.
- Collaborate with academics to develop curricula on cultures of civility.
- Educate health care staff to identify incivility and respond appropriately.

Bullying of nurses is a well-documented phenomenon in health care workplaces in Canada. Although nurses suffer negative health outcomes when bullied, nursing students are also vulnerable. While undertaking their clinical placements, 70 percent of nursing students in Eastern Canada report experiencing incivility from registered and licensed practical nurses (MacDonald et al., 2022). More than thirty-five years ago, Meissner (1986) asked, "are we eating our young?" to generate dialogue among nurses about their treatment of other current nurses and future nurses entering the profession, and this is still relevant to how nurses treat other practising and future nurses today. Nurses need to support the profession and use respectful communication and collaboration in the workplace for the benefit of clients, colleagues, and the organization. The Canadian Nurses Association (2017) states in its Code of Ethics that nurses should "treat each other, colleagues, students and other health-care providers in a respectful manner, and work with others to honour dignity and resolve differences in a constructive way" (p. 41).

CONFLICT

Conflict is a common phenomenon, evident in the various daily news reports from around the world. Health care environments are high-pressure areas, so conflict is common and is sometimes an unavoidable issue within clinical settings. Miscommunication is a critical factor in conflict. Communication scholars Miller and Steinberg (1975) classified conflict as having three distinct forms:

- *Pseudoconflict* entails a basic lack of understanding; a person misunderstands the meaning in a message.
- *Simple conflict* relates to differences in perceptions, ideas, or goals.
- *Ego conflict* occurs when conflict gets personal and individuals attack each other's self-esteem.

Health care work environments are often a contributing factor to the development of conflict. Nursing professionals try to balance multiple demands with limited resources, more acutely ill clients, increased workloads, and less staff. These consistent pressures weaken work and team performance, foster interpersonal and intra-professional conflict, and result in practitioner burnout and poor client outcomes (Almost et al., 2016; Boateng & Adams, 2016). Conflict is perceived as either constructive (positive) or destructive (negative), depending on how it is managed. According to Kim et al. (2015), constructive outcomes entail improved decision-making, synergized solutions to problems, individual and group performance growth, and the search for innovative approaches to conflict resolution. Destructive outcomes lead to occupational stress, dissatisfaction, impaired communication between individuals and groups, decreased work performance, distrust, and burnout. All health care providers need to have knowledge and awareness of conflict and use effective collaborative interventions to manage and mitigate its effects (Almost et al., 2016).

Conflict Management Styles

Five styles or approaches of conflict management are identified in the literature (Labrague et al., 2018):

- **Avoiding** is a common response to conflict and is used to prevent an escalation of the actual conflict. Sometimes the experience is so uncomfortable that the nurse avoids the other person or the situation to prevent escalation of conflict. In many health care situations, the decision to use this style may be appropriate when the other person is more powerful. This strategy results in an *I lose, you lose* situation and is seen as an unassertive, uncooperative approach.
- **Accommodating** is another common response. This is an unassertive approach that employs cooperation to satisfy the concerns of others. It is used when the issue is more important to the other person. One person is accommodating the other to preserve or maintain harmony. This is an *I lose, you win* situation. This is the second-most frequently used strategy by nurses.
- **Collaborating** (also known as integrating) is a solution-focused approach where everyone works cooperatively to meet the needs/goals and confront the issues of the situation. Open-loop communication is used to gain understanding and insight into the issue, leading to a mutually agreeable solution. This is an *I win, you win* situation. This is the most frequently used conflict management style among nurses.
- **Competing** is an assertive approach but is uncooperative and more power controlled. A person has high concern for self and meeting their needs regardless of the concerns of others. This approach is used when quick decisions are needed within organizations. This is an *I win, you lose* situation. This approach can lead to more conflict. This is the least employed approach in conflict resolution.
- **Compromising** is seen as a "quick fix" approach for managing conflict situations temporarily. One person gives up something to satisfy the goals/needs of others. In this situation there is some cooperation to reach a solution, but neither party is completely satisfied. It becomes an *I lose, you lose* situation. This style is still sometimes employed by nurses in conflict management.

The nursing literature suggests that individuals experience less conflict using an accommodating or collaborating style approach, whereas those using the other forms of conflict management experience more conflict (Almost et al., 2016; Labrague et al., 2018; Nicotera, 2021). Similarly, in an integrative review on conflict management styles among nursing students, Labrague & McEnroe-Petitte (2017) found that students utilized a collaborating approach to resolve conflict.

Communication Approaches for Conflict Management

Think about what happens when you face a conflict situation. In most cases, a feeling of fear, anger, and anxiety takes over, which clouds your ability to think, make decisions, and respond to the conflict experience. These strategies may help:

- Select a mutually acceptable time and place to discuss a conflict. This provides time for you to think about the situation. When you are angry and upset, it is best to take time to think; this helps prevent the risk of an emotionally charged confrontation. Do not take things personally. This interaction should take place in private, not on an open nursing unit.
- Plan your message. If you plan to meet, take time to prepare your response. Identify your goals and the outcome of the situation. Rehearse with a friend or family member what you plan to say before having the actual interaction.
- Monitor verbal and nonverbal messages. Have awareness of your own and others' body language. Use respectful communication, speak calmly using a moderate pitch and tone, use direct eye contact, and maintain a relaxed body posture.
- Use active listening skills.
- Avoid personal attacks, name calling (becoming defensive), emotionally charged statements, or use of profanity.
- Don't blame the person (e.g., client, colleague, physician): "You made me mad" or "You called me a terrible name." Use "I" language instead of "you" language to create a supportive climate. "I" statements are considered more assertive: "I feel hurt when my work ethic is discussed in the unit hallway because someone might overhear personal information."
- Check your understanding of what others say and do. Assess information and ask questions. Summarize and rephrase what has been said to clarify understanding. Maintain an open dialogue.

TEAMSTEPPS COMMUNICATION STRATEGY

The TeamSTEPPS curriculum that was previously discussed has a tool that can be used by nurses and teams to manage and resolve conflict: DESC.

- **D**: Describe specific situation or behaviour (source of conflict) and provide concrete data.
- **E**: Express how the situation makes your feel or what your concerns are.

- **S:** Suggest alternatives and seek agreement (solutions).
- **C:** Consequences should be stated in terms of impact on established team goals. Strive for consensus—this results in an improved relationship.

When using the DESC tool, the goal is to resolve the interpersonal conflict and obtain a win-win outcome for all involved.

Using the DESC Tool: An Example

- **D:** "I do not appreciate you shouting at me in the client's presence. I ask that you please leave the room. I need to finish hanging this unit of blood."
- **E:** "Dr. White, I feel that you undermined my competency in front of the client. Could you and I meet in private to discuss this further?" Doctor: "Sure, not a problem. I have some time now before going to the OR."
- **S:** "Dr. White, I felt put on the spot in Mr. Bellow's room. Let's discuss the situation." Doctor: "I had some written orders for Mrs. White, but they were not followed correctly."
- **C:** "I see the order was not clearly written; I understand how the order was misinterpreted. I would suggest in the future, to promote clarity for nursing staff, that you write clearly to prevent errors in transcription. In addition, I would expect to be treated respectfully. I wish that you would apologize." Doctor: "I really was disrespectful to you. I am very sorry."

NURSE-PHYSICIAN COMMUNICATION

Although nurses and physicians are the largest group of health care providers who work in close contact with each other, effective communication in health care is a challenge due to workplace cultures and practices, institutions' hierarchical structure, and workflow patterns (Manojlovich et al., 2020; Tan et al., 2017). Poor communication between nurses and physicians impacts team performance and client safety, leading to adverse events such as unexpected client deaths and medication errors (Kang et al., 2020; Tsz-Sum Lee & Doran, 2017). Healthy work environments are critical for effective nurse-physician communication and client safety. Interprofessional teamwork and collaboration are recognized as important in facilitating effective nurse-physician communication (Jones et al., 2019; Tan et al., 2017; Vatn & Dahl, 2021). Some of the communication strategies described in this chapter are useful for improving collaboration and interprofessional teamwork among health professionals.

Summary of Principles for Effective Communication and Collaboration in Health Care

- Use respectful and professional communication (avoid gossip).
- Listen actively.
- Respect each person's skill set.
- Know your own communication style.
- Have awareness of your own body language (e.g., eye contact, body position).
- Avoid using stereotypes or relying on biases and move beyond them.
- Do not take things personally.
- Make clear statements.
- Acknowledge communication and check for correct interpretation.
- Avoid "why" or "you" statements (e.g., "Why did you say that? It was hurtful." or "You don't know what you're doing. Let me do that.").
- Use "I" statements (e.g., "I feel disrespected when my opinion is not considered in care provision for ...").
- Describe the conflict, taking into account all information.
- Be assertive, not aggressive.
- Use a collaborative approach for consensus building.
- Use a calm, normal vocal tone.
- Take accountability for your feelings and behaviours. If at fault, offer an apology.

Exercise 11.1: Sources of Workplace Conflict

Purpose: To understand the sources of behaviours in workplace settings that contribute to conflict. This exercise will help you become aware of the behaviours in the workplace that lead to conflict and take the necessary steps to determine a strategy for intervention.

Procedure

This exercise can be completed during class time or as a reflection or an online activity.

1. Write down behaviours that can be considered sources of conflict within the workplace.
2. Recommend a strategy that would be effective in managing each behaviour.
3. In your small group, share and discuss your answers. Have one student act as the recorder and present your findings to the whole class.

Discussion

1. In a group of three to four students, discuss the similarities and differences in your responses.
2. Describe effective ways nurses can deal with nurse-to-nurse conflict situations.
3. What are some organizational strategies for conflict prevention and resolution?

Exercise 11.2: Role Play Scenario—Response to Conflict

Purpose: To understand the process of being assertive in response to conflict situations

Procedure

This exercise can be completed during class time. Work with a partner. Each of you will role-play the specific scenario assigned by your instructor. With your partner, describe how you can communicate assertively in the role play and arrive at a win-win solution.

Role Play A

Student 1: You are Student 2's supervisor. You feel frustrated and angry because Student 2 is always late returning from coffee and lunch breaks while on the unit. As the supervisor, you have received complaints from nursing staff about Student 2's behaviour. You are also aware that work is left undone, and the night staff are left to pick up the workload.

Role Play B

Student 1: You are a new graduate who has recently been hired to work on a 28-bed surgical unit. While you are still getting used to the routine on the floor, you ask the staff questions about policies and treatments on most of your shifts. Student 2 (a nurse colleague) confronts you in a client room and tells you, while rolling their eyes, "I am tired of your questions. You should know that stuff by now. What did they teach you in that university program?" and abruptly leaves the room.

Role Play C

Student 1: You are the doctor who has been on the unit, and you call out for the nurse in charge of a client. Mrs. Winters. She is a 45-year-old woman with a broken

(Continued)

right radius. She is scheduled for surgery in the afternoon for an open reduction and insertion of a metal plate. The doctor on the unit yesterday had ordered a specific bone prep for the client, but it was not completed. Student 2 is the nurse, who enters the room and asks, "How can I help you?" You shout at the nurse, "This client's bone prep is not completed as ordered, and she is going to the OR in a couple of hours. I can't depend on you nurses to follow a simple order! Now I will have to cancel her surgical procedure. I'll talk to your manager about this incompetence!"

CONFLICT PREVENTION AND RESOLUTION STRATEGIES

A healthy workplace is important in conflict prevention and resolution. The Canadian Nurses Association (2019), in collaboration with the Canadian Federation of Nurses Unions, advocates for healthy practice environments that support the health, safety, and well-being of clients and nurses. At the organizational level, many health care facilities in Canada have policies that promote civility and respect in the workplace. For example, Eastern Health (2022) regional health authority in Newfoundland and Labrador has adopted the concepts outlined in the book *Trust Your Canary: Every Leader's Guide to Taming Workplace Incivility* by Bar-David (2015) to guide the enhancement of respect and civility throughout the organization.

Leadership within teams and organizations is critical for implementation of policies on fostering a culture of civility and respect in health care facilities. Specific strategies from the literature include a management and organizational commitment to a zero-tolerance policy to foster a safe and healthy workplace environment; adoption of employee policies that detail how bullying should be reported and addressed in clinical practice environments; and implementation of ongoing policy education and information sharing for employees, nurses, physicians, and students on conflict awareness and resolution (Smith et al., 2020). Resources to encourage nurses and other employees to seek employee assistance if health support is needed should be available, and educational programs for managers and nurses on management of workplace incivility, lateral violence, and bullying are recommended (Armstrong, 2018). Educational sessions on incivility and effective communication should be provided to students who plan to work in health care settings. These programs will help students gain knowledge and practise the management of disruptive behaviours in the workplace (Bambi et al., 2018). In addition, team building exercises can help health care providers be effective team members through promotion of interdisciplinary communication and collaboration (Logan, 2016). TeamSTEPPS is an evidence-based method that has been used to enhance clinical communication within teams and improve client safety. Several structured tools used to enhance communication among health care teams (e.g., SBAR) have been described in this chapter.

CHAPTER SUMMARY

It is important that health care professionals have the knowledge to develop skill in conflict prevention and resolution. Incivility is common in the nursing workforce and throughout health care settings. Such behaviour contributes to adverse outcomes for health professionals, clients, and organizations. Communication and collaboration of health professionals is critical for the provision of safe client care. Interpersonal conflicts between health care providers have negative effects on health care teams. A collaborative work environment contributes to employee satisfaction, respectful communication, and effective team behaviours. The use of structured communication tools and educational training on workplace incivility management and resolution helps to build open communication, which is necessary for effective interprofessional health care teams. Clinical practitioners with communication and collaborative skills are fundamental for the creation of a healthy work environment.

REVIEW QUESTIONS

1. Describe the difference between a team and a group.
2. Identify characteristics of effective teams.
3. Describe barriers to effective team communication.
4. Define *conflict* and *incivility*.
5. Identify several strategies to enhance communication within teams.
6. Describe communication approaches for conflict management.

WEB RESOURCES

Healthcare Excellence Canada
https://www.healthcareexcellence.ca
Psychological Health and Safety in the Workplace
Mental Health Commission of Canada National Standard
https://www.mentalhealthcommission.ca/national-standard/

REFERENCES

Almost, J., Wolff, A. C., Stewart-Pyne, A., McCormick, L. G., Strachan, D., & D'Souza, C. (2016). Managing and mitigating conflict in healthcare teams: An integrative review. *Journal of Advanced Nursing, 72*(7), 1490–1505. https://doi.org/10.1111/jan.12903

Anusiewicz, C. V., Ivankova, N. V., Swiger, P. A., Gillespie, G. L., Li, P., & Patrician, P. A. (2020). How does workplace bullying influence nurses' abilities to provide patient care? A nurse perspective. *Journal of Clinical Nursing, 29*(21–22), 4148–4160. https://doi.org/10.1111/jocn.15443

Armstrong, N. (2018). Management of nursing workplace incivility in the health care settings. *Workplace Health & Safety, 66*(8), 403–410. https://doi.org/10.1177/2165079918771106

Bambi, S., Foa, C., De Felippis, C., Lucchini, A., Guazzini, A., & Rasero, L. (2018). Workplace incivility, lateral violence and bullying among nurses. A review about their prevalence and related factors. *Acta Biomedica, 89*(6-S), 51–79. https://doi.org/10.23750/abm.v89i6-S.7461

Bar-David, S. (2015). *Trust your canary: Every leader's guide to taming workplace incivility.* Fairleigh Press.

Beament, T., Ewens, B., Wilcox, S., & Reid, G. (2018). A collaborative approach to the implementation of a structured clinical handover tool (iSoBAR), within a hospital setting in metropolitan Western Australian: A mixed methods study. *Nurse Education in Practice, 33*, 107–113. https://doi.org/10.1016/j.nepr.2018.08.019

Boateng, G. O., & Adams, T. L. (2016). "Drop dead … I need your job": An exploratory study of intra-professional conflict amongst nurses in two Ontario cities. *Social Science & Medicine, 155*, 35–42. https://doi.org/10.1016/j.socscimed.2016.02.045

Braithwaite, J., Herkes, J., Ludlow, K., Testa, L., & Lamprell, G. (2017). Association between organisational and workplace cultures, and patient outcomes: Systematic review. *BMJ Open, 7*(11). https://doi.org/10.1136/bmjopen-2017-017708

Canadian Interprofessional Health Collaborative. (2022). *CIHC framework.* https://www.mcgill.ca/ipeoffice/ipe-curriculum/cihc-framework

Canadian Nurses Association. (2017). *Code of ethics for registered nurses.* https://cna-aiic-ca/en/nursing/regulated-nursing-in-Canada/nursing-ethics

Canadian Nurses Association. (2019). *Joint position statement: Practice environment: Maximizing outcomes for clients, nurses, and organizations.* https://www.nursesunions.ca

Canadian Nurses Association. (2020). *Position statement: Interprofessional collaboration.* https://hl-prod-ca-oc-download.s3-ca-central-1.amazonaws.com/CNA/2f975e7e-4a40-45ca-863c-5ebf0a138d5e/UploadedImages/documents/Interproffessional_Collaboration_position_statement.pdf

Clark, C. M. (2019). Fostering a culture of civility and respect in nursing. *Journal of Nursing Regulation, 10*(1), 44–52. https://doi.org/10.1016/S2155-8256(19)30082-1

Coolen, E., Engbers, R., Draaisma, J., Heinen, M., & Fluit, C. (2020). The use of SBAR as a structured communication tool in the pediatric non-acute care setting: Bridge or barrier for interprofessional collaboration? *Journal of Interprofessional Care.* https://doi.org/10.1080/13561820.2020.1816936

Crawford, C. L., Chu, F., Judson, L. H., Cuenca, E., Jadalia, A. A., Kawar, L. N., Runnels, C., & Garvida, R. (2019). An integrative review of nurse-to-nurse incivility, hostility, and workplace violence: A GPS for nurse leaders. *Nursing Administration Quarterly, 43*(2), 138–156. https://doi.org/10.197/NAQ.0000000000000338

Cutler, S., Morecroft, C., Carey, P., & Kennedy, T. (2019). Are interprofessional healthcare teams meeting patient expectations? An exploration of the perceptions of patients and informal caregivers. *Journal of Interprofessional Care, 33*(1), 66–75. https://doi.org/10.1080/13561820.2018.1514373

Eastern Health. (2022). *Healthy workplace—Eastern Health Regional Health Authority, Newfoundland & Labrador.* https://www.easternhealth.ca/employees-and-physicians/healthy-workplace/

Erickson, J. I., Duffy, M. E., Ditomassi, M., & Jones, D. (2017). Development and psychometric evaluation of the professional practice work environment inventory. *The Journal of Nursing Administration, 47*(5), 259–265. https://doi.org/10.1097/NNA.0000000000000476

Gluyas, H. (2015). Effective communication and teamwork promotes patient safety. *Nursing Standard, 29*(49), 50–57. https://doi.org/10.7748/ns.29.49.50.e10042

Guttman, O. T., Lazzaru, E. H., Keebler, J. R., Webster, K. L., Gisick, L. M., & Baker, A. L. (2021). Dissecting communication barriers in healthcare: A path to enhancing communication resiliency, reliability, and patient safety. *Journal of Patient Safety, 17*(8), e1465–e1471. https://doi.org/10.1097/PTS.0000000000000541

Jones, L., Cline, G. J., Battick, K., Burger, K. J., & Amankwah, E. K. (2019). Communication under pressure. *Journal for Nurses in Professional Development, 35*(5), 248–254. https://doi.org/10.1097/NND.0000000000000573

Kang, X. L., Brom, H. M., Lasater, K. B., & McHugh, M. D. (2020). The association of nurse-physician teamwork and mortality in surgical patients. *Western Journal of Nursing Research, 42*(4), 245–253. https://doi.org/10.1177/0193945919856338

Keller, S., Yule, S., Zagarese, V., & Parker, S. H. (2020). Predictors and triggers of incivility within healthcare teams: A systematic review of the literature. *BMJ Open, 10*(6). https://doi.org/10.1136/bmjopen-2019-035471

Kfouri, J., & Lee, P. E. (2019). Conflict among colleagues: Health care providers feel undertrained and unprepared to manage inevitable workplace conflict. *JOGC, 41*(1), 15–20. https://doi.org/10.1016/j.joc.2018.03.132

Kim, W., Nicotera, A. M., & McNulty, J. (2015). Nurses' perceptions of conflict as constructive or destructive. *Journal of Advanced Nursing, 71*(9), 2073–2083. https://doi.org/10.1111/jan.12672

Korner, M. (2010). Interprofessional teamwork in medical rehabilitation: A comparison of multidisciplinary and interdisciplinary team approach. *Clinical Rehabilitation, 24*(8), 745–756. https://doi.org/10.1177/0269215510367538

Kroning, M. (2019). Be civil: Committing to zero tolerance for workplace incivility. *Nursing Management, 50*(10), 52–54. https://doi.org/10.1097/01.NUMA.0000580628.91369.50

Labrague, L. J., Hamdan, Z. A., & McEnroe-Petitte, D. M. (2018). An integrative review on conflict management styles among nursing professionals: Implications for nursing management. *Journal of Nursing Management, 26*(8), 902–917. https://doi.org/10.1111/jonm.12626

Labrague, L. J., & McEnroe-Petitte, D. M. (2017). An integrative review on conflict management styles among nursing students: Implications for nurse education. *Nurse Education Today, 59.* https://doi.org/10.1016/j.nedt.2017.09.001

Layne, D. M., Anderson, E., & Henderson, S. (2019). Examining the presence and sources of incivility within nursing. *Journal of Nursing Management, 27*(7), 1505–1511. https://doi.org/10.1111/jonm.12836

Logan, T. R. (2016). Influence of teamwork behaviors on workplace incivility as it applies to nurses. *Creighton Journal of Interdisciplinary Leadership*, *2*(1), 47–53. https://doi .org/10.17062/CJIL.v2i1.28

MacDonald, C. M., Hancock, P. D., Kennedy, D. M., MacDonald, S. M., Watkins, K. E., & Baldwin, D. D. (2022). Incivility in practice—incidence and experiences of nursing students in eastern Canada: A descriptive quantitative study. *Nurse Education Today*, *110*. https://doi.org/10.1016/j.nedt.2021.105263

Manojlovich, M., Harrod, M., Hofer, T. P., Lafferty, M., McBratnie, M., & Krein, S. L. (2020). Using qualitative methods to explore communication practices in the context of patient care rounds on general care units. *Journal of General Internal Medicine*, *35*, 839–845. https://doi.org/10.1007/s11606-019-05580-9

McKibben, L. (2017). Conflict management: Importance and implications. *British Journal of Nursing*, *26*(2), 100–103. https://doi.org/10.12968/bjon.2017.26.2.100

Meissner, J. E. (1986). Nurses: Are we eating our young? *Nursing*, *16*(3), 51–53. https://journals .lww.com/nursing/citation/1986/03000/nurses_are_we_eating_our_young_.14.aspx

Miller, G. R., & Steinberg, M. (1975). *Between people: A new analysis of interpersonal communication*. Science Research Associates.

Muller, M., Jurgens, J., Rendaelli, M., Klingberg, K., Hautz, W., & Stock, S. (2018). Impact of the communication and patient hand-off tool SBAR on patient safety: A systematic review. *BMJ Open*. https://doi.org/10.1136/bmjopen-2018-022202

Nicotera, A. M. (2021). Nursing and conflict communication: A review. *Nursing Communication*, *1*(1). https://repository.usfca.edu/nursingcommunication/vol1/iss1/6

Pattani, R., Ginsberg, S., Johnson, A. M., Moore, J. E., Jassemi, S., & Straus, S. E. (2018). Organizational factors contributing to incivility at an academic medical center and systems-based solutions: A qualitative study. *Academic Medicine*, *93*(10), 1569–1575. https://doi.org/10.1097/ACM.0000000000002310

Plonien, C., & Williams, M. (2015). Stepping up teamwork via TeamSTEPPS. *AORN Journal*, *101*(4), 465–470. https://doi.org/10.1016/j.aorn.2015.01.006

Prentice, D., Moore, J., Crawford, J., Lankshear, S., & Limoges, J. (2020). Collaboration among registered nurses and licensed practical nurses: A scoping review of practice guidelines. *Nursing Research and Practice*. https://doi.org/10.1155/2020/5057084

Rydenfalt, C., & Odenrick, P. (2017). Organizing for teamwork in healthcare: An alternative to team training? *Journal of Health Organization and Management*, *31*(3), 347–362. https://doi .org/10.1108/JHOM.12.2016.0233

Sanner-Stiehr, E., & Ward-Smith, P. (2017). Lateral violence in nursing: Implications and strategies for nurse educators. *Journal of Professional Nursing*, *33*(2), 113–118. https://doi .org/10.1016/j.profnurs.2016.08.007

Schenk, E., Schleyer, R., Jones, C. R., Fincham, S., Daratha, K. B., & Monsen, K. A. (2018). Impact of adoption of a comprehensive electronic health record on nursing work and caring efficacy. *CIN: Computers, Informatics, Nursing*, *36*(7), 331–339. https://doi.org /10.1097/CIN.0000000000000441

Schot, E., Tummers, L., & Noordegraaf. M. (2020). Working on working together: A systematic review on how healthcare professionals contribute to interprofessional collaboration. *Journal of Interprofessional Care, 34*(3), 332–342. https://doi.org/10.1080/135 61820.2019.1636007

Smith, C. R., Palazzo, S. J., Grubb, P. L., & Gillespie, G. L. (2020). Standing up against workplace bullying behavior: Recommendations from newly licensed nurses. *Journal of Nursing Education and Practice, 10*(7). https://doi.org/10.5430/jnep.v10n7p35

Solis, S. (2019). A lesson on incivility: Application of an ethical decision-making model. *The Journal of Nurse Practitioners, 15*(8), 592–594. https://doi.org/10.1016/j.nurpra.2019.05.014

Stoller, J. K. (2021). Building team in health care. *Chest, 159*(6), 2392–2398. https://doi .org/10.1016/j.chest.2020.09.092

Tan, T., Zhou, H., & Kelly, M. (2017). Nurse-physician communication—an integrated review. *Journal of Clinical Nursing, 26*, 3974–3989. https://doi.org/10.1111/jocn.13832

Taskaya, S., & Aksoy, A. (2021). A bibliometric analysis of workplace incivility in nursing. *Journal of Nursing Management, 29*(3), 518–525. https://doi.org/10.1111/jonm.13161

Tsz-Sum Lee, C. & Doran, D. M. (2017). The role of interpersonal relations in healthcare team communication and patient safety: A proposed model of interpersonal process in teamwork. *Canadian Journal of Nursing Research, 49*(2), 75–93. https://doi .org/10.1177/0844562117699349

Tusaie, K. R. (2017). Systems concepts and working in groups. In J. S. Jones, J. J. Fitzpatrick, & V. L. Rogers (Eds.), *Psychiatric mental health nursing: An interpersonal approach* (2nd ed., pp. 135–155). Springer.

Vatn, L., & Dahl, B. M. (2021). Interprofessional collaboration between nurses and doctors for treating patients in surgical wards. *Journal of Interprofessional Care.* https://doi.org/10.1080/ 13561820.2021.1890703

Weller, J. Boyd, M., & Cumin, D. (2014). Teams, tribes and patient safety: Overcoming barriers to effective teamwork in healthcare. *BMJ Post graduate Medical Journal, 90*(1061), 149–154. https://doi.org/10.1136/postgradmedj-2012-131168

World Health Organization. (2010). *Framework for action on interprofessional education & collaborative practice.* https://www.who.int/publications/i/item/framework-for-action-on-interprofessional-education-collaborative-practice

Wranik, W. D., Price, S., Haydt, S. M., Edwards, J., Hatfield, K., Weir, J., & Doria, N. (2019). Implications of interprofessional primary care team characteristics for health services and patient health outcomes: A systematic review with narrative synthesis. *Health Policy, 123*, 550–563. https://doi.org/10.1016/j.healthpol.2019.03.015

CHAPTER 12

Communication with Children and Adolescents

INTRODUCTION

Health care professionals are integral to the care of children and their families. Nurses' competency in the provision of family-centred care is dependent upon their knowledge of the child or young person's cognitive and psychosocial development to enact appropriate communication. Family-centred care is defined as placing the family and client at the centre of care. In this approach, family members are partners in collaboration with health care providers to plan, provide, and meet their health care needs (Kokorelias et al., 2019). Effective communication with children and their families allows facilitation of the nurse-client relationship, and the communication skills presented in previous chapters are fundamental for communicating with children at different age levels. This chapter will provide an overview of the theoretical stages of development for infants, children, and adolescents, as well as the communication skills used by nurses and the role of play in communicating with children. The impact of the child's or young person's illness on families is presented, and nurses' interventions are described.

The World Health Organization's (2018) child and adolescent framework standards focus on improving the quality of care for children and their families in health facilities. These standards highlight children's rights to health care and suggest that their needs are different from those of adults. Two standards within the framework specifically focus on the communication approach with children and their families:

> **Standard 4.** "Communication with children and their families is effective, with meaningful participation, and responds to their needs and preferences" (p. 4).
>
> **Standard 7.** "For every child, competent, motivated, empathic staff are consistently available to provide routine care and management of common childhood illnesses" (p. 6).

Are we meeting these standards? Nurses and other health care professionals work with children and their families in the clinical speciality of pediatrics or provide care to children and adolescents in an outpatient area. To communicate effectively and appropriately with infants and young people requires health care professionals to adapt their interpersonal skills. Effective communication enhances family-centred care and supports relationships between the family and health care providers (Dryden & Greenshields, 2020).

DEVELOPMENTAL THEORIES

Health care providers need knowledge of the theories of cognitive and psychosocial development in children to assess, understand, and determine young people's perceptions of hospitalization and ability to engage in communication. Jean Piaget's theory of cognitive development provides a description of the child's cognitive ability over time as they mature and negotiate their environment. Table 12.1 presents a summary of Piaget's four stages of cognitive development (Piaget, 1997). These stages are influenced by the child's experiences, culture, and environment.

Erik Erikson (1963) was a psychoanalyst with an interest in human development from a humanistic and phenomenological perspective (Maree, 2021). He described development as comprising eight life stages, beginning at birth and continuing into late adulthood. The completion of specific stages is dependent upon dealing with a conflict (psychosocial crisis) before progressing to the next stage. These stages are influenced by the person's specific circumstances, environment, culture, and education (Maree, 2021). Table 12.2 provides an overview of these developmental stages.

Table 12.1: Piaget's Stages of Cognitive Development

Stage	Age Range	Description
Sensorimotor	Birth–2 years	Infants and toddlers understand the world through the senses (e.g., sucking) and motor actions (e.g., shaking a rattle). They develop an awareness that people and things continue to exist even when out of sight (object permanence).
Preoperational	2–7 years	Child development is characterized by egocentric and concrete thinking and thinking in absolutes (good/bad). Language is developing. Children may benefit from play sessions.
Concrete Operational	7–11 years	Reasoning skills become more logical. Children can view a situation from more than one point of view. They have improved language and neuro-muscular skills. Peers start to gain importance. Children have an increased awareness of internal body parts.
Formal Operational	11 years and older	Abstract thinking begins. Independence from parents begins; body image and peer groups are important. Children are able to problem solve.

Source: Based on Piaget, J. (1997). *The child's conception of the world.* Routledge.

COMMUNICATING WITH CHILDREN IN A CLINICAL/OUTPATIENT SETTING

When nurses and other health care providers communicate with an infant, child, or young person, to be effective, they need to have knowledge of speech and language milestones. This information will influence the communication approach used by the nurse as well as in the provision of health information (Dryden & Greenshields, 2020). Table 12.3 presents a summary of speech development in the first five years of life.

COMMUNICATING WITH PARENTS AND THE CHILD OR YOUNG PERSON IN A HEALTH CARE SETTING

A hospital is a strange place to a child or young person who is admitted because of illness or injury. The child feels vulnerable because of their fear and anxiety around strangers, medical equipment, separation from family and pets, limited understanding of treatments, and the unfamiliar environment. The nurse has a critical role in

Table 12.2: Erikson's Stages of Development

Stage and Age	Developmental Task	Resolution
Trust vs. Mistrust, Infancy, 1–2 years	Early attachment figure—mother or caregiver—lays foundation for trust development in others.	If needs are met, sound basis for relating and trusting others. If not met, infant may be anxious or fearful of others and learn to mistrust others.
Autonomy vs. Shame and Doubt, Early childhood, 2–4 years	Learning to achieve a sense of self. Trying to become a little independent, exploring their environment and toilet training.	Becoming independent and developing their own will: "I can do this."
Initiative vs. Guilt, Preschool age, 4–5 years	Trying to do things on their own, complete certain tasks.	Gaining a sense of determination to achieve and accomplish tasks.
Industry vs. Inferiority, School age, 5–12 years	Gaining a sense of confidence to complete activities. Developing social and school skills.	Sense of proficiency increased. Belief in their ability to accomplish tasks.
Identity vs. Role Confusion, Adolescence, 13–19 years	Support from others helps achieve a sense of self. Learning to become more independent, with guidance and support.	Aware of who they are as a person. Successful in completing complex tasks.
Intimacy vs. Isolation, Early and middle adulthood, 20–40 years	Making transition from adolescence. Establishing relationships with others, love, and intimate bonds.	Developing relationships with others they can trust. Becoming aware of their vulnerabilities.
Generativity vs. Stagnation, Adulthood, 40–65 years	Fulfilling life's goals. Caring about others, not only themselves.	Experiencing a sense of meaning and purpose in life.
Ego Integrity vs. Despair, 65+ years	Reflecting on life. Sense of fulfillment, sense of wisdom.	Willing to face death. Seeing their life as successful.

Source: Based on Erikson, E. H. (1963). *Childhood and society* (2nd ed.). W. W. Norton; and Maree, J. G. (2021). The psychosocial development theory of Erik Erikson: Critical overview. *Early Child Development and Care, 191*(7–8). https://doi.org/10.1080/03004430.2020.1845163

Table 12.3: Summary of Speech Development

Age	Language Comprehension Skills	Expressive Speech and Language Skills
Birth–3 months	Startles to loud sounds Quiets or smiles to familiar voice	Cries to communicate needs Coos to indicate pleasure
4–8 months	Localizes to sound Reacts to changes in tone of voice	Babbles (e.g., bababa) Makes vowel sounds and uses voice to communicate excitement and displeasure
7–14 months	Listens to speech and localizes to sound Recognizes words for common items (e.g., *daddy* or *juice*)	Babbles with short sentences Uses one or two words (e.g., *bye-bye* or *mama*) Uses speech or non-crying sounds to get and keep attention
1–2 years	Follows simple commands Points to familiar pictures in a book	Uses at least 10 words by 18 months Begins to combine words into two-word phrases and questions
2–3 years	Follows two-part commands (e.g., "Get your shoe and bring it here.") Consistently identifies body parts	Speech is understood by caregivers most of the time Uses speech to request or get attention
3–4 years	Learns vocabulary and sentence structure from adult conversation and being read to	Uses longer sentences of four or more words. Listeners can understand most of child's speech
4–5 years	Attends to and understands short stories Can answer questions about a story	Voice sounds clear Communicates easily and clearly Says most sounds correctly

Source: Based on Dryden, P., & Greenshields, S. (2020). Communicating with children and young people. *British Journal of Nursing, 29*(20). https://doi.org/10.12968/bjon.2020.29.20.1164

helping the child and the family adjust to the new environment. This process begins at the initial meeting, with the health care professional and the communication approach used with the child and the parents or caregivers. The nurse's communication is dependent upon the stages of development and comprehension of the client.

Davison and her colleagues (2021) suggest that health care professionals use child-centred communication in building trusting relationships with children and young people. This approach involves a series of four steps as illustrated in figure 12.1. The centre circle represents the child (infant, adolescent), who is the focus for the nurse. The four small circles represent the strategies for communicating and engaging with children who are visiting a health care facility. The health care provider uses a friendly, nonjudgmental approach to greet the child. This includes being sensitive to the child's fears and perspectives as they enter a strange environment.

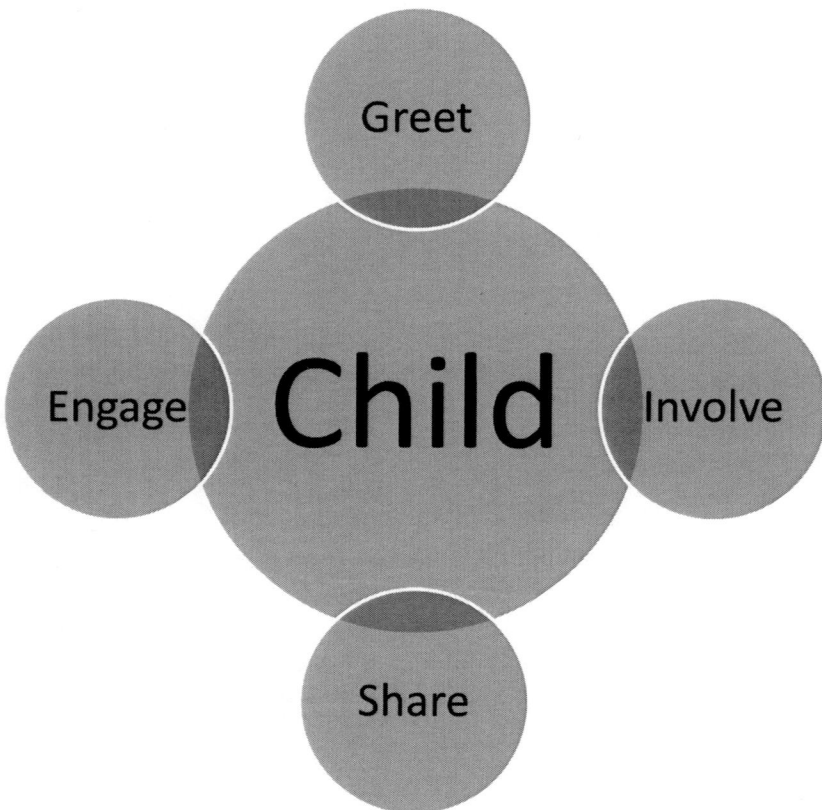

Figure 12.1: Steps for Child-Centred Communication

Source: Adapted from Davison, G., Conn, R., Kelly, M. A., Thompson, A., & Dornan, T. (2021). Fifteen-minute consultation: Guide to communicating with children and young people. *Archives of Disease in Childhood-Education and Practice*, 1–5. https://doi.org/10.1136/ archdischild-2021-323302

As a part of the greeting, verbal and nonverbal behaviours lay the foundation for child-centred communication. The nonverbal attending behaviours identified by the acronym SOLER or SURETY, as discussed in chapter 2, serve as an effective guide for the nurse in rapport building with the child and family. Some strategies are recommended during these steps:

Step I: Greet children (Davison et al., 2021)

- Greet the child as a person, even though they are accompanied by an adult. Communication and language should be tailored to the child or young person's age and developmental level.
- Maintain good eye contact. For children, it is best to sit or kneel when speaking. This position puts the health care provider at their eye level. This position is less threatening for the child and provides an opportunity to observe facial expressions (Stock et al., 2012). Attentively listen, and demonstrate interest and respect.
- Smile. Introduce yourself with your name and title, for example, "Call me Nurse Tom." Children remember first names best, and using your first name also narrows the power gap between health care provider and client. Check that you are pronouncing the child's name correctly; for older children, check which pronouns they prefer.
- Use welcome hand gestures (wave) and touch if appropriate (seek permission). Have awareness of proxemics during interaction.

Step II: Engage children (Davison et al., 2021)

- Build some rapport with the child and help them become less anxious and more relaxed before asking questions. Talk person-to-person, including some small talk. Focus questions, and ask about clothes, pets, hobbies, games, school, and outside interests. For toddlers or infants, use of toys such as bubbles, play dough, or colouring books may help to engage the child. These activities also help to build trust, which is important for children (Sheehan & Fealy, 2020).

Step III: Involve children (Davison et al., 2021)

- Although the caregiver or parent is present, it is important not to leave the child out of the conversation. Depending upon the child's developmental level, they should be involved in clinical conversations by asking, for example, "May I ask you a few questions about why you came to the hospital (clinic / emergency department) today?" Give them ample time to respond and do not rush them. You show respect by involving them in dialogue and seeking their input into care decisions.

- Start with some open-ended questions: "What has brought you here today?" or "Tell me about how you have been feeling." Depending upon their response, ask more focused or closed-ended questions.
- Speak slowly in a child-friendly manner and avoid the use of medical terms. Allow time for them to ask questions. Explain all tests, procedures, or treatments in language they can understand. The use of pictures, books, drawings, or other visual aids appropriate to the child's developmental level and age helps with communication and understanding.
- Ask the child for permission to question their parent or caregiver about their illness or condition, but advise the child that they can interrupt. The child may add to the information or validate the parent's information. It is important to share decision-making with parents by facilitating discussions with children. Thank children for their involvement in providing information and tell them that if at any time they have any concerns or questions, they can ask their health care provider.

STRATEGIES FOR COMMUNICATING WITH CHILDREN AND ADOLESCENTS

Infants

Infants from birth to 12 months communicate through their senses of touch, sight, and hearing. Crying is their main form of communication to indicate needs such as hunger, discomfort, or pain. After attending to the child's needs, the nurse can provide comfort by holding and singing softly to the infant. Speech vocalizations and eye gaze are infants' preferred ways to communicate with adults. Vocalization may occur if the infant is alone or when engaged in interactions with adults. When health professionals talk to infants, a soothing and calm tone of voice, smile, and touch provide a sense of comfort. Communicating through play can be effective for infants; the nurse can play peek-a-boo or make silly faces or noises. Toys like rattlers, music toys, and mobiles are also effective in fostering play for infants. Playing with a familiar item or toy helps infants to feel secure, so nurses can suggest bringing a favourite toy or blanket from home.

Toddlers and Preschoolers

Toddlers (ages 1–2) and preschoolers (ages 3–5) have some language acquisition as they build on their word vocabularies. Toddlers are wary of strangers, so the health care provider needs to take time to build rapport. If an examination is necessary, the parent can hold the child while the nurse completes the assessment, maintaining a calm, gentle, easygoing approach. If asking questions, the nurse should use simple child-appropriate language and allow time for response. To engage the toddler, the nurse can use a variety of toys, such as dolls and books, to capture the child's interest. During the toddler years, as the sense of self is being developed, the child is striving for independence and a sense of control and tends to be possessive. The nurse should promote independence by allowing them to complete tasks and offering choices (Lambert et al., 2012).

Preschoolers may ask many questions; the nurse should provide a simple response. Children at this developmental level have fears about hospitalizations, so the health care provider needs to provide reassurance and support to help them feel safe. As these children have a short attention span, limit-setting is needed, and information provided should be simple and appropriate. Preschool children can be engaged in communication through drawing, colouring, storytelling, or puppetry (Lambert et al., 2012; Tilbrook et al., 2017).

School-Age Children

School-age children (ages 6–12) have greater cognitive ability and can problem solve and comprehend information. They have a better understanding of their body as well as the physical and emotional impact of hospital procedures (Seibold, 2014). The nurse providing information and answering questions needs to be sensitive to the child's ability to express their feelings. In providing information and explanations, they should use simple, common words. For therapeutic communication, drawing, painting, writing, and mutual storytelling are helpful for children to express feelings and concerns regarding hospitalization or undergoing a medical procedure. Altay et al. (2017) found that school-aged children receiving inpatient cancer treatment experienced a reduction in their anxiety through drawing, writing, and mutual storytelling.

Adolescents

Adolescence (ages 13–18) is considered a period of transition where the young person is experiencing puberty, establishing self-identity, separating from parents, and placing more importance on peers and peer groups. When admitted to a health facility, adolescents have fears of being judged by health care providers and are concerned about their privacy and the sharing of information (Kim & White, 2018). When meeting the adolescent, the nurse should try to make a person-to-person connection with the client and family; this creates a foundation for a positive and trusting environment. After introductions, the nurse needs to explain the concept of confidentiality and the limits on how information is shared. Although they are accompanied by a parent, the young person should be the focus of the communication and involved in decision-making with respect to their health care (Smith et al., 2020).

During the admission process, the nurse collects information on the reason for hospitalization. A psychosocial history is obtained during the interview, along with a physical examination. The health care professional should conduct the interview and assessment with the adolescent in private. Parents, if present, may limit the sensitive information that the adolescent will provide. The HEEADSSS framework is a validated tool that is frequently used by clinicians to complete a thorough psychosocial assessment for young people (Klein et al., 2014; Smith & McGuinness, 2017). HEEADSSS is an acronym for home, education and employment, eating, activities (peer- / family- / social media–related), drugs, sexuality, suicide (depression), and safety. The following are some sample questions from the domains of the instrument (Klein et al., 2014):

- **Home**: "How are things at home? Anything stressful recently? Where do you live, and who lives with you?"
- **Education and employment**: "Are you still in school? Which school/college? Tell me more about school."
- **Eating**: "Have there been any recent changes in your weight?"
- **Activities**: "What do you do for fun? How many hours do you spend on any given day in front of a screen, such as a computer, TV, or phone?"
- **Drugs**: "Do any of your friends or family members use tobacco? Alcohol? Other drugs? Do you use tobacco or electronic cigarettes?"
- **Sexuality**: "Have you ever been in a romantic relationship?"
- **Suicide/depression:** "Do you feel 'stressed' or anxious more than usual or more than you prefer to feel? Have you thought about hurting yourself or someone else?"
- **Safety**: "Have you ever been seriously injured? How?"

Using HEEADSSS, the health care professional can begin from any domain to interview the adolescent. It is best to start the interview with nonthreatening questions to foster rapport and trust, facilitating disclosure. The nurse can explore topics with the adolescent based upon the information disclosed. In starting the interview, as noted above, the concept and limitations of confidentiality are discussed as part of the initial conversation (Klein et al., 2014).

Exercise 12.1: Communication with Children in a Clinical Setting

You are completing a clinical placement in a pediatric setting. Your clinical teacher assigns you to administer an immunization to a toddler.

1. How will you communicate?
2. How would this change for a preschooler, a school-aged child, and an adolescent?

In formulation of your responses, keep in mind that for communication to be effective, it must be appropriate to one's age, understanding, and communication abilities.

THE IMPORTANCE OF PLAY DURING HOSPITALIZATION OF CHILDREN

Hospitalization causes a major disruption in the lives of children and young people and can produce feelings of fear, anxiety, and loneliness (Koukourikos et al., 2015). The nurse needs to work collaboratively with the family as the child's hospitalization causes concern for all members. One of the strategies to help young children who are hospitalized is to make use of the therapeutic benefits of play. Play is an important component in children's lives from infancy through adolescence. Play is a key factor contributing to children's healthy physical, social, emotional, and cognitive development (Nijhof et al., 2018). Through play, young children can learn to cope with their fears and concerns about being in a health care setting.

Health care professionals can use play as a treatment and care strategy to help children to express their feelings when facing illness and hospitalization, or an invasive procedure. Jones (2018) identified three forms of play interventions that health care professionals can use in their work with children:

Normalizing Play

Play is a normal part of being a child and is fun, but being a client in hospital interrupts normal play activities. Familiar objects and family are absent, so encouraging parents to bring in decorations, blankets, pictures, and toys from home can help to make the environment more comforting. The nurse can use toys, storytelling, or any other age-appropriate toy or activity to communicate and engage with children. Today technology is influencing the ways in which young people play. More children and young people are using technology (e.g., smartphones, tablets, or other digital devices) as a component of play, which is evident within health care settings (Slutsky & DeShetler, 2017).

Preparation Play and Distraction

When coming into the hospital, children are exposed to medical equipment such as stethoscopes, masks, gloves, and different types of treatments involving needles or other instruments, which are unfamiliar and frightening. Medical or focused play can be used in preoperative preparation, invasive procedures, and treatments by gradually introducing the child or young person to the equipment (Koukourikos et al., 2015). This enables children to explore, ask questions, and become familiar with the supplies and equipment used in the hospital (Burns-Nader & Hernandez-Reif, 2016). The child can use a doll, puppet, or teddy bear to carry out the procedure and play out their emotions related to the situation.

Play is recommended as a distraction technique for children undergoing a medical procedure in a health care setting (Drape & Greenshields, 2020). Toys, picture books, bubbles, and videos have been used as distractions during procedures. In a Canadian study, Ballard et al. (2017) used distraction kits (containing toys such as a flute, stickers, finger puppets, and a windmill) developed for infants, toddlers, and preschool children visiting the emergency department and requiring a needle-related procedure. The distraction kits were effective as a nonpharmacological intervention that provided nurses with a technique to distract children and improve their hospital experience.

Expressive Arts Play

This technique provides an opportunity for children to use play as a form of expression of their feelings and fears through drawing, colouring, writing, or mutual storytelling (Altay et al., 2017). These play activities allow children to express themselves in a creative way and develop an understanding of their feelings, thoughts, and experiences during hospitalization. Such emotional expression for children can also include role-playing, arts and crafts, poetry, and painting (Delamerced et al., 2021; Jepsen et al., 2019).

PLAY THERAPY

Play is an effective tool for enabling children to express themselves and alleviate the impact of stress (Jones, 2018). Health care professionals can incorporate play activities to enhance development in young children and promote a trusting and caring experience during illness and hospitalization. Play therapy is a formalized psychological intervention in which "therapists use the therapeutic power of play to help children prevent or resolve psychosocial difficulties and achieve optimal growth" (Koukourikos et al., 2021, p. 293). It was initially developed as a treatment approach for children who had experienced emotional abuse or for those who had developmental delays, but it is used today for children with post-traumatic stress disorder, chronic illness, and a variety of disorders and health conditions (Porter et al., 2009; Thomas et al., 2021). Play therapy as an intervention for children was developed by Virginia Axline (1947), who, in her classic text *Play Therapy*, identified eight basic principles of nondirective play therapy, which are still used by clinicians in practice:

- Establish rapport and a warm, friendly relationship with the child. This provides a climate for the child to express their feelings in a caring environment.
- Accept the child and follow their lead in conversation.
- Maintain a consistent approach and set limits as necessary to promote safety and security.
- Recognize the child's feelings and reflect them back so that the child can gain insight into their behaviour.
- Show respect for the child's ability to solve personal problems.

COMMUNICATING WITH CHILDREN AND THEIR FAMILIES AT THE CHILD'S END OF LIFE

A child being diagnosed with a life-threatening illness and admitted to hospital has a devastating effect on the parents and the family unit. Health care professionals face the challenge of how to communicate with the parent and the child on admission to the clinical area. Despite this challenge, nurses play an important role in providing comfort and support to the child and family facing this difficult situation.

The death of a child is one of the most life-altering events in a parent's life and one of the most stressful for nurses and other health care providers (Butler et al., 2018; Yadegari et al., 2019). Nurses who are caring for the child and the family need knowledge of the grieving process and therapeutic communication skills to provide appropriate nursing interventions. They also need to have awareness of the cognitive, emotional, and psychological development of children. See chapter 10, which provides an overview of the concepts of grief and loss, and death and dying. When meeting the child and the family for the first time, the nurse needs to establish rapport to facilitate development of the therapeutic nurse-client relationship. This begins with greeting the family and child in a respectful way, making a professional introduction, and conducting a formal child assessment as part of the admission process. The nurse's communication approach is influenced by the knowledge and awareness children have related to their illness, diagnosis, and prognosis. The child's age, developmental level, and cultural and religious beliefs of the child and family influence disclosure of such information (Stein et al., 2019). Table 12.4 presents information on a child's developmental understanding of the concept of death (Bates & Kearney, 2015; Stein et al., 2019).

Table 12.4: Child's Developmental Understanding of Death

Age	Concept of Death	Recommended Communication Approaches with the Child
Birth–2 years	No concept of death	Maintain normal routines. Has awareness of object permanence.
2–5 years	Death seen as departure but not seen as permanent. May be confused with sleeping. Magical thinking—believe their illness attributed to their thoughts, wishes, and behaviour.	Be honest with child in explanation; use simple, clear language. Use the terms *dying*, *death*, or *dead*. Do not use euphemisms. If you say, "When you die, you will go to sleep," the child may be afraid if they go to sleep, they might not wake up. Use play or drawing to express feelings.
6–9 years	Death seen as possible but not for them. Child may feel responsible for death.	Explore family's spiritual and cultural beliefs about death and afterlife. Provide reassurance and support. Discuss fears of death. Can use books to explain concept of death and dying, for example, *The Invisible String* by Patrice Karst.
10–12 years	Understands that death is final. Understands causality and universality of death.	Provide reassurance to child that their feelings/fears are normal. Use open, honest communication. Explore their concerns and fears.
12 years+	Understands concept of death and its implications.	Have an open conversation about death and its impact on the family unit. Discuss religious and cultural rituals of funeral.

Sources: Based on Bates, A. T., & Kearney, J. A. (2015). Understanding death with limited experience in life: Dying children's and adolescents' understanding of their own terminal illness and death. *Current Opinion in Supportive and Palliative Care, 9*(1). https://doi.org/10.1097/SPC.0000000000000118; and Stein et al., (2019). Communication with children and adolescents about diagnosis of their own life-threatening condition. *The Lancet, 393*(10176). https://doi.org/10.1016/s0140-6736(18)33201-x

If health professionals have an awareness of what children and young people with a terminal illness understand about death and dying, this creates an opening for end-of-life care discussions. As it is an emotionally difficult time for the child or young person, parents may be reluctant to talk about the prospect of death and dying. Bates and Kearney (2015) suggest that if young clients are not informed about their prognosis, they are prevented from authentically discussing their fears and concerns or seeking comfort from family and friends. Nurses, in collaboration with the health care team and parents, need to address the situation and plan how the information can be shared in a sensitive way with the child or young person. Once the information is shared, the nurse has a major role in providing emotional support and information and facilitating the coping process for parents and the child. Using a family-centred approach, nurses are at the bedside, with the child and parent engaged in every aspect of end-of-life care. The focus is the child and the family unit, "addressing needs during life, through the dying phase, and into the bereavement period" (Larkin, 2012, p. 93).

Self-Awareness

Caring for the child and the family at end of life may bring up nurses' and other health care providers' own anxieties about death and dying. This is challenging work for nurses, so self-care is critical. Awareness, which is essential for practising self-care, involves being "consciously aware of one's physical, mental, and emotional reactions in different situations" (Crane & Ward, 2016, p. 389). Self-inventory (checking in) is a strategy for nurses in the moment of stressful or unique situations to centre themselves and mentally review their reactions, thoughts, and emotions. Other techniques recommended for self-care include the following:

- Relaxation techniques (e.g., guided imagery)
- Mindfulness
- Exercise
- Nutrition
- Body awareness (body scanning)
- Yoga

COMMUNICATING WITH CHILDREN WHO HAVE A NEURODEVELOPMENTAL DISORDER

Neurodevelopmental disorders (NDDs) are a group of conditions that cause abnormal functioning of the brain and central nervous system. Children with these disorders demonstrate issues with language, speech, memory, learning, and motor functioning (American Psychiatric Association [APA], 2013). Autism spectrum disorder (ASD) and attention-deficit/hyperactivity disorder (ADHD), which are some of the most common NDDs (Francés et al., 2022), are discussed in this section of the chapter. Children who have an NDD such as ASD will have deficits in social communication and social interaction that cause significant impairment in social, occupational, and other areas of functioning (APA, 2013). A report by the Public Health Agency of Canada (2018) reports that ASD in children is on the increase in Canada, with approximately 1 in 66 children and youth diagnosed with the disorder.

ASD is on a spectrum, so the severity of the symptoms experienced by children will vary; some may have severe impairment, while others only minimal. Common symptoms associated with ASD are presented in table 12.5 (APA, 2013).

Nurses who work in a clinical setting may have the opportunity to provide care for a child or young person with ASD. Hospitalization for this population can be overwhelming, so nurse interventions are focused on the needs of the child,

Table 12.5: Common Symptoms Associated with ASD

Type	Symptoms
Behavioural	Routines or rituals involving taste, smell, or touch
	Repetitive movements (e.g., hand flapping, finger flicking, rocking)
	Constant movement
	Self-injurious behaviours (e.g., head banging)
	Disruptive, challenging behaviours
	Fixated interest with unusual objects
	Heightened sensation
	Inflexibility
Communication	Delayed speech, no speech
	Loss of language or words
	Echolalia (repeating what has been said, e.g., Nurse: "Do you want a cookie?" Child: "Do you want a cookie?" [Child doesn't provide an answer])
	Lack of facial expression
	Difficulty initiating or sustaining conversations
	Difficulty sending and receiving messages
Social	Little or no eye contact
	No interest in developing peer relationships
	No sharing of emotions
	Preference for solitary play

Source: Based on American Psychiatric Association. (2013). *Diagnostic and statistical manual of mental disorders* (5th ed.). https://doi.org/10.1176.appi.books.9780890425596

provision of quality care, and reduction of stress for the client and family (Brown & Elder, 2014; Jolly, 2015). When the child is admitted, the health care provider, in partnership with the parent, will conduct a complete assessment to facilitate an appropriate interdisciplinary plan of care Some relevant initial assessment questions include the following (Scarpinato et al., 2010):

- How does your child communicate? Verbally/nonverbally?
- Does (name) prefer to use picture cards, writing, drawing, or electronic devices to communicate?
- Is (name) comfortable with eye contact?
- Is (name) able to understand emotional cues?
- How does your child report or show pain?
- How does your child tolerate new faces?
- How does (name) react to other children their age? To adults?
- Is (name) sensitive to touch, taste, noise, or sight?
- What is (name)'s comfort with personal space?
- What is the best way to approach (name)?
- If (name) becomes agitated or overstimulated, what are the interventions that work best?
- What is (name)'s schedule at home?
- What are (name)'s strengths?

This information helps to promote a safe and low-sensory environment and determine the best communication approach during the child's inpatient stay. For children who struggle with new faces, it is best to pre-assign primary staff to provide consistency. The nurse can encourage the family to bring in favourite objects or food from home to provide comfort and regular routine. The nurse can advocate for the family, who know the child best, to be involved in their care (Brown & Elder, 2014; Jolly, 2015; Scarpinato et al., 2010).

The following is a summary of recommended guidelines for health care professionals when caring for a child with ASD (Brown & Elder, 2014; Jolly, 2015):

- Conduct admission interview with family member present.
- Provide continuity of health care provider.
- Encourage family to stay.
- Use different modes to communicate (e.g., visuals, pictures, digital devices).
- Use low vocal tone and pitch when speaking.
- Avoid closed nonverbal body language.
- Use short, succinct commands. Avoid using the command "no."

- If child is nonverbal, label room items/objects with words or pictures; child may point to desired object as needed.
- Decrease environmental stimulation (e.g., noise, lights, smells). Assign private room if possible.
- Avoid restraining an agitated child. Intervene if there is a risk of harm to client or others.
- Provide a reward system for positive behaviour.
- Use the r-FLACC (an observational pain scale used by nurses to assess pain in children who are nonverbal) or other pain tool to identify discomfort in child with ASD.

ATTENTION-DEFICIT/HYPERACTIVITY DISORDER

This disorder affects both children and adults. Individuals demonstrate an inability to sustain attention, difficulty organizing tasks and activities, hyperactivity, and impulsivity (APA, 2013). Nurses have an important role in working with these children and their families through the provision of education about disorder management at home and school. Management may consist of a combination of medication and behavioural interventions (e.g., cognitive behavioural therapy, social skills training) (Leahy, 2018). The Canadian ADHD Resource Alliance (2020) has practice guidelines available online for health professionals. Their site also has information on disorder management available for clients and families.

Case Study 12.1

Bobby is a four-year-old toddler who is going to have a lumbar puncture. This is an uncomfortable procedure where a thin needle is inserted into the spinal canal to collect cerebrospinal fluid. Answer the following questions:

1. Write out the narrative script of the conversation you have with Bobby to prepare him for the procedure.
2. How can you use play to provide Bobby with information about the procedure?
3. How will you address any concerns that Bobby may have about the procedure?

Case Study 12.2

Jamie is a 10-year-old schoolchild who is admitted to hospital with a diagnosis of an intestinal obstruction. Following assessment by the physician, an order for intravenous fluids of normal saline at 100 cc/hour and insertion of a nasogastric tube (insertion of a tube through the nose and into the stomach) is ordered. Answer the following questions:

1. Write out the narrative script of the conversation you have with Jamie to prepare them for the procedures.
2. How can you use play to provide Jamie with information about the procedures?
3. How will you address any concerns Jamie may have about the procedures?

Case Study 12.3

John is a 14-year-old adolescent who has autism spectrum disorder, which was diagnosed at age five. He is being admitted to the medical unit for investigation of type 1 diabetes mellitus. He is accompanied to the unit by his mother, Mrs. Hill. You are assigned to complete the admission interview with John. Answer the following questions:

1. Identify how you will approach John and his mother. What will you include in your introduction?
2. What questions will you want to ask John and his mother?
3. From the assessment interview, you find out from Mrs. Hill that John is nonverbal. How will you communicate with John?
4. Identify strategies you will implement to promote a safe and low-sensory environment for John.
5. What will be important in John's nursing plan of care?

CHAPTER SUMMARY

Communicating with children and young people is an essential role for health care professionals. Being ill and having to be hospitalized is a stressful experience for children and their families. Nurses need knowledge of child development theories and communication skills to work with children and families during these challenging times. Developmentally appropriate communication is recommended for children and young people, and this chapter highlights various strategies for communicating with children and young people. When a child is hospitalized, nurses are responsible for supporting the child and their families through family-centred care. This entails assessing coping, providing medical information, providing direct care, and being a resource for the child and family. Finally, play is an important coping strategy for ill children, and suggested strategies for health care professionals to incorporate play in health care situations for children of all ages are effective in child-centred care.

REVIEW QUESTIONS

1. Describe how play is used as a tool to enhance communication with a preschool child.
2. Identify communication interventions for a child with ASD.
3. Define *family-centred care.*
4. Identify the interpersonal skills health care professionals need in order to communicate with parents of children who are dying.
5. Describe several distraction techniques a nurse may use for a toddler who is undergoing a blood test.

WEB RESOURCES

Canadian ADHD Resource Alliance
https://www.caddra.ca

REFERENCES

Altay, N., Kilicarslan-Toruner, E., & Sari, C. (2017). The effect of drawing and writing technique on the anxiety level of children undergoing cancer treatment. *European Journal of Oncology Nursing, 28,* 1–6. https://doi.org/10.1016/j.ejon.2017.02.007

American Psychiatric Association. (2013). *Diagnostic and statistical manual of mental disorders* (5th ed.). https://doi.org/10.1176.appi.books.9780890425596

Axline, V. (1947). *Play therapy.* Houghton Mifflin.

Ballard, A., Le May, S., Khadra, C., Fiola, J. L., Charrette, S., Charest, M.-C., Gagnon, H., Bailey, B., Villeneuve, E., & Tsimicalis, A. (2017). Distraction kits for pain management of children undergoing painful procedures in the emergency department: A pilot study. *Pain Management Nursing, 18*(6), 418–426. https://doi.org/10.1016/j.pmn.2017.08.001

Bates, A. T., & Kearney, J. A. (2015). Understanding death with limited experience in life: Dying children's and adolescents' understanding of their own terminal illness and death. *Current Opinion in Supportive and Palliative Care, 9*(1), 40–45. https://doi.org/10.1097/SPC.0000000000000118

Brown, A. B., & Elder, J. H. (2014). Communication in autism spectrum disorder: A guide for pediatric nurses. *Pediatric Nursing, 40*(5), 219–225. https://pubmed.ncbi.nlm.nih.gov/25929112/

Burns-Nader, S., & Hernandez-Reif, M. (2016). Facilitating play for hospitalized children through life services. *Children's Health Care, 45*(1), 1–21. https://doi.org/10.1080/02739615.2014.948161

Butler, A. E., Hall, H., & Copnell, B. (2018). Becoming a team: The nature of the parent-healthcare provider relationship when a child is dying in the pediatric intensive care unit. *Journal of Pediatric Nursing, 40*, e25–e32. https://doi.org/10.1016/j.pedn.2018.02.002

Canadian ADHD Resource Alliance. (2020). *Canadian ADHD practice guidelines* (4.1 ed.). https://www.caddra.ca/

Crane, P. J., & Ward, S. F. (2016). Self-healing and self-care for nurses. *AORN Journal, 104*, 386–400. https://doi.org/10.1016/j.aorn.2016.09.007

Davison, G., Conn, R., Kelly, M. A., Thompson, A., & Dornan, T. (2021). Fifteen-minute consultation: Guide to communicating with children and young people. *Archives of Disease in Childhood-Education and Practice*, 1–5. https://doi.org/10.1136/archdischild-2021-323302

Delamerced, A., Panicker, C., Monteiro, K., & Chung, E. Y. (2021). Effects of a poetry intervention on emotional wellbeing in hospitalized pediatric patients. *Hospital Pediatrics, 11*(3). https://doi.org/10.1542/hpeds.2020-002535

Drape, K., & Greenshields, S. (2020). Using play as a distraction technique for children undergoing medical procedures. *British Journal of Nursing, 29*(3), 142–143. https://doi.org/10.12968/bjon.2020.29.3.142

Dryden, P., & Greenshields, S. (2020). Communicating with children and young people. *British Journal of Nursing, 29*(20), 1164–1166. https://doi.org/10.12968/bjon.2020.29.20.1164

Erikson, E. H. (1963). *Childhood and society* (2nd ed.). W. W. Norton.

Francés, L., Quintero, J., Fernández, A., Ruiz, A., Caules, J., Fillon, G., Hervás, A., & Soler, C. V. (2022). Current state of knowledge on the prevalence of neurodevelopmental disorders in childhood according to the DSM-5: A systematic review in accordance with the PRISMA criteria. *Child and Adolescent Psychiatry and Mental Health, 16*(1), https://doi.org/10.1186/s13034-022-00462-1

Jepsen, S. L., Haahr, A., Eg, M., & Jorgensen, L. B. (2019). Coping with the unfamiliar: How do children cope with hospitalization in relation to acute and/or critical illness? *Journal of Child Health Care, 23*(4), 534–550. https://doi.org/10.1177/1367493518804097

Jolly, A. A. (2015). Handel with care: Top ten tips a nurse should know before caring for a hospitalized child with autism spectrum disorder. *Pediatric Nursing, 41*(1), 11–22.

Jones, M. (2018). The necessity of play for children in health care. *Pediatric Nursing, 44*(6), 303–305.

Kim, B., & White, K. (2018). How can health professionals enhance interpersonal communication with adolescents and young adults to improve health care outcomes? Systematic literature review. *International Journal of Adolescence and Youth, 23*(2), 198–218. https://doi.org/10.1080/02673843.2017.1330696

Klein, D. A., Goldenring, J. M., & Adelman, W. P. (2014). Probing for scars: How to ask the essential questions. *Contemporary Pediatrics, 31*(1), 16–28. https://www.researchgate.net/publication/279767065_Probing_scars_for_how_to_ask_the_essential_questions

Kokorelias, K. M., Gignac, M. A., Naglie, G., & Cameron, J. I. (2019). Towards a universal model of family centered care: A scoping review. *BMC Health Services Research, 19*(564). https://doi.org/10.1186/s12913-019-4394-5

Koukourikos, K., Tsaloglidou, A., Tzeha, L., Iliadis, C., Frantzana, A., Katsimbeli, A., & Kourkouta, L. (2021). An overview of play therapy. *Materia Socio-Medica, 33*(4), 293–297. https://doi.org/10.5455/msm.2021.33.293-297

Koukourikos, K., Tzeha, L., Pantelidou, P., & Tsaloglidou, A. (2015). The importance of play during hospitalization of children. *Materia Socico-Medica, 27*(6), 438–441. https://doi .org/10.5455/msm.2015.27.438-441

Lambert, V., Long, T., & Kelleher, D. (2012). *Communication skills for children's nurses.* Open University Press.

Larkin, P. (2012). Communicating with children and their families during sensitive and challenging times. In V. Lambert, T. Long, & D. Kelleher (Eds.), *Communication skills for children's nurses* (pp. 90–104). Open University Press.

Leahy, L. G. (2018). Diagnosis and treatment of ADHD in children vs adults: What nurses should know. *Archives of Psychiatric Nursing, 32*(6), 890–895. https://doi.org/10.1016/j.apnu.2018.06.013

Maree, J. G. (2021). The psychosocial development theory of Erik Erikson: Critical overview. *Early Child Development and Care, 191*(7–8), 1107–1121. https://doi.org/10.1080/03004430 .2020.1845163

Nijhof, S. L., Vinkers, C. H., van Geelen, S. M., Dujiff, S. N., Achterberg, E. J. M., van der Net, J., Veltkamp, R. C., Grootenhuis, M. A., van de Putte, E. M., Hillegers, M. H. J., van der Brug, A. W., Wierenga, C. J., Benders, M. J. N. L., Engels, R. C. M. E., van der Ent, C. K., Vanderschuren, L. J. M. J., & Lesscher, H. M. B. (2018). Healthy play, better coping: The importance of play for the development of children in health and disease. *Neuroscience and Biobehavioral Reviews, 95*, 421–429. https://doi.org/10.1016/j.neubiorev.2018.09.024

Piaget, J. (1997). *The child's conception of the world.* Routledge.

Porter, M. L., Hernandez-Reif, M., & Jessee, P. (2009). Play therapy: A review. *Early Child Development and Care, 179*(8), 1025–1040. https://doi.org/10.1080/03004430701731613

Public Health Agency of Canada. (2018). *Autism spectrum disorder among children and youth in Canada.* https://www.canada.ca/en/public-health/services/publications/diseases-conditions/autism-spectrum-disorder-children-youth.canada-2018.html

Scarpinato, N., Bradley, J., Kurbjun, K., Bateman, X., Holtzer, B., & Ely, B. (2010). Caring for the child with an autism spectrum disorder in the acute care setting. *Pediatric Nursing, 15*(3), 244–254. https://doi.org/10.1111/j.1744-6155.2010.00244.x

Seibold, E. (2014). Talking with children: Working with families. In L. Kennedy Sheldon & J. B. Foust (Eds.), *Communication for nurses: Talking with patients* (3rd ed., pp. 143–150).

Sheehan, R., & Fealy, G. (2020). Trust in the nurse: Findings from a survey of hospitalised children. *Journal of Clinical Nursing 29*(21–22), 4289–4299. https://doi.org/10.1111/jocn.15466

Slutsky, R., & DeShetler, L. M. (2017). How technology is transforming the ways in which children play. *Early Child Development and Care, 187*(7), 1138–1146. https://doi.org/10.1080/03004430.2016.1157790

Smith, G. L., & McGuinness, T. M. (2017). Adolescent psychosocial assessment: The HEEADSSS. *Journal of Psychosocial Nursing and Mental Health Services, 55*(5), 24–27. https://doi.org/10.3928/02793695-2017420-03

Smith, L. A. M., Critoph, D. J., & Hatcher, H. M. (2020). How can health care professionals communicate effectively with adolescent and young adults who have completed cancer treatment? A systematic review. *Journal of Adolescent and Young Adult Oncology, 9*(3), 328–340. https://doi.org/10.1089/jayao.2019.0133

Stein, A., Dalton, L., Rapa, E., Bluebond-Langer, M., Hanington, L., Stein, K. F., Ziebland, S., Rochat, T., Harrop, E., Kelly, B., Bland, R., & Communication Expert Group. (2019). Communication with children and adolescents about diagnosis of their own life-threatening condition. *The Lancet, 393*(10176), 1150–1163. https://doi.org/10.1016/so140-6736(18)33201-x

Stock, A., Hill, A., & Babl, F. E. (2012). Practical communication guide for paediatric procedures. *Emergency Medicine Australasia, 24*, 641–646. https://doi.org/10.1111/j.1742-6723.2012.01611.x

Thomas, S., White, V., Ryan, N., & Byrne, L. (2021). Effectiveness of play therapy in enhancing outcomes in children with chronic illness: A systematic review. *Journal of Pediatric Nursing, 63*. E72–E81. https://doi.org/10.1016/j.pedn.2021.10.009

Tilbrook, A., Dwyer, T., Reid-Searl, K., & Parson, J. A. (2017). A review of the literature — The use of interactive puppet simulation in nursing education and children's healthcare. *Nurse Education in Practice, 22*, 73–79. https://doi.org/10.1016/j.nepr.2016.12.001

World Health Organization. (2018). *Standards for improving the quality of care for children and young adolescents in health facilities.* https://cdn.who.int/media/docs/default-source/mca-documents/child/standards-for-improving-the-quality-of-care-for-children-and-young-adolescents-in-health-facilities—policy-brief.pdf?sfvrsn=1e568644_1

Yadegari, M., Rankin, J., & Johnson, J. M. (2019). Nurses' communication with dying children and their families in pediatric oncology: A literature review. *Journal of Nursing Education and Practice, 9*(2), 37–41. https://doi.org/10.5430.jnep.v9n2p37

Index

Page numbers in italics denote figures, tables, and boxes.